Foreword From Migraineurs Who Read the 1st Edition

The usual practice of publishing a book is to start with blurbs of recommendation written by well-known experts. The experts whose blurbs start this book are migraineurs who have read the 1st edition of this book and who have joined the Facebook migraine group. They are the real experts and these are their selected testimonials. You can find the originals on Facebook at "Migraine Sufferers Who Want to be Cured".

A complete manual for migraine free living as well as healthy eating! Dr. Angela Stanton is a revolutionary in this field and thanks to her research and book I can now live without being dependent on triptan drugs!
-- Paula S.

After going to every Headache/Neurology specialist in our area I was so overwhelmed with the growing number of medications they always wanted to prescribe. The day I stumbled across Fighting The Migraine

Epidemic and Angela Stanton was one of the best days of my life! It wasn't easy for the first few weeks. I feel so much better now, I have my life back! I thank God for Angela often.
-- Sue Bidwell

After two years on the Stanton Migraine Protocol, I continue to be migraine free. My overall health is better; instead of two different medications to control my hypertension, I no longer take any meds, my BP has remained consistently normal. Best of all, no migraines- no ER's- no migraine meds. Thank you, Angela Stanton for changing my life
-- Michaelyn (Miki) Denny

I suffered daily migraines for 17 years until I stumbled across Angela Stanton and her book online. It has been completely life changing. I feel like I'm back in the world again and not a few steps behind in a mask of pain. One of my biggest worries was my young daughters' memories of me would always be mummy had a headache. The protocol has changed everything.
-- Tracey Cawdrey

The Stanton Protocol has changed my life from barely coping with chronic migraine to a person who now enjoys a full life with a fantastic mixture of being mum, wife, friend and colleague. No drugs now, just a sensible and practical approach which enables me to respond to my body's needs and the environment around me! I'm still amazed that I'm not getting migraines 2-3 times a week... thank you Angela Stanton!!
-- Helen Herbert

Finally, a solution for migraineurs that doesn't come out of a pill bottle!
-- Bonnie Klaassen

I was a daily chronic migraineur, even with various preventative and abortive meds including Botox. This book and protocol has changed my life to a migraine free existence. I am forever grateful that I decided to give Dr. Stanton's research a try.
-- Cheryl Murphy Schiemer

I highly recommend this book and the Stanton Migraine protocol if you are interested in being migraine free and understanding what your body is telling you it needs and doesn't need. Several doctors, drugs and various scans could not stop the migraines that I was living with on a daily basis but the protocol in the book did and still does.
-- Shelly McReynolds

Hi, just back to report that running the marathon on Sunday was an incredible experience. I felt confident to push harder and took 26 minutes off my previous best time, despite challenges of hills, wind and rain. But the best part was having a clear head and vision afterwards. Sore muscles yes but otherwise I have felt fabulous since then, which is a new experience for me. I am so overwhelmed and ecstatic! Thanks again Angela Stanton, this has been such an amazing journey!
–NM

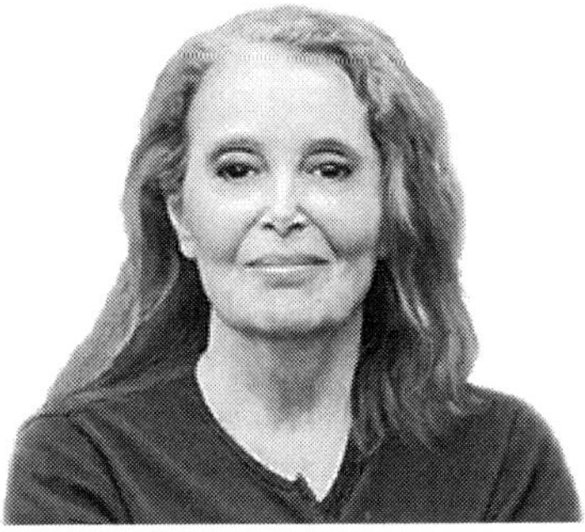

Angela A Stanton, Ph.D.

I am a Neuroeconomist, researching how neuropeptides change us. I live in Southern California; mother of two sons, grandmother of two granddaughters, wife and best friend of a terrific husband and my owner is my cat. A migraineur who got fed up with the lack of meaningful understanding and proven treatment of migraines, my attention has been focused on the cause of migraine, its prevention, and its treatment without the use of medicines for many years. Little did I know that my research will take me from biochemistry ➔ metabolism ➔ genetics ➔ epigenetic forces ➔ and evolution, in this order, to finally identify the "migraine code." Join my ride and decode your migraines on the way.

Member:

American Academy of Neurology, American Diabetic Association, American Physiological Society, Society for Neuroscience, American Association for the Advancement of Science, and International Headache Society

Fighting The Migraine Epidemic: A Complete Guide

Fighting The Migraine Epidemic: A Complete Guide

How To Treat & Prevent Migraines Without Medicine

Angela A Stanton Ph.D.

This book is not intended as a substitute for medical advice by a medical professional. The information given in this book is designed to help you make informed decisions about your health. Before making any changes to your diet or medicines, consult your physician.

ISBN-13: 9781546976370

ISBN-10: 154697637X

Library of Congress Control Number: 2017909074

CreateSpace Independent Publishing Platform
North Charleston, South Carolina

Because of the dynamic nature of the Internet, some links provided in this book may have changed.

Thank you Andy! Without your help, this book would have been impossible!

Special thanks to Kristin Elizabeth Ingram for her critical editing help.

I would also like to express my gratitude to the thousands of past and present migraineurs in my Facebook migraine support group "Migraine Sufferers Who Want to be Cured". They have helped me tremendously in my understanding of migraine by sharing their experiences, symptoms, and pains, and by reporting back on their progress with the Stanton Migraine Protocol®.

Thanks to all the past and present group admins for their amazing work and the countless hours of helping others. Thank you!

Table of Contents

Foreword to the 2nd edition

Since writing the 1st edition of this book in 2013, several new research findings have appeared in academic journals supporting the theories I presented. Besides science advancing in general, I also have published several academic journal articles on the subject, representing the evolution of my own views. This is why I changed the subtitle of this book from 2nd edition to "Complete Guide", indicating that this is not just a simple addition to the 1st edition but it is, in fact, a different book that is complete with current information that is necessary to understand, prevent, and treat all migraines types without the use of medicines. The significant amount of information gained through the years of activities in our dedicated Facebook group has served as a reliable, real life, and indispensable basis for my research and the resulting conclusions of this enhanced edition.

Since migraine can be prevented and controlled without medicines, the question should come up in everyone's mind: is migraine a disease? What if it is a misunderstood condition brought on by a different kind of brain in need of different nourishment, as a result of a set of genetic differences? Does a genetic difference mean disease? The answer to the last question is a definite "no". When approximately 30% of the global population (active or potential migraineurs) has a certain set of genes governing the development and functioning of highly sensitive brains, we have to ask: these genes – while different from that of the general population – are so similar among migraineurs for a reason? Or in other words, which subset of people are "mutated"? The ones with highly sensitive brains (migraineurs) or the rest of the population? Perhaps some time ago all humans had such sensitive brains and as we evolved, a large percent of humanity was better able to adapt to changing lifestyles. Perhaps the migraine-brain was the original default human brain. Did having this special migraine-brain offer any benefits at one time? Why is pain its defining characteristic today? We will work on answering these questions throughout this book.

Following the success of the 1st edition I have received a great amount of constructive input. As a result, this extended edition is created as a comprehensive guide for migraine prevention and treatment. This edition contains my findings based on the experiences of thousands of migraineurs who have used the Stanton Migraine Protocol® and not just my own experience, as it was the case with the 1st edition. There are numerous sections added and old parts updated or deleted, so this is a brand-new book. Enjoy the read and all the new discoveries! If you have any questions or comments, you are welcome to send me a note via the contact form at my website or in the Facebook migraine group.

While the understanding of migraine continues to advance, one thing is for certain: thousands have become completely migraine and medicine free by following the Stanton Migraine Protocol®. As long as you observe and follow the steps outlined in this book, your chances for success – no migraines — are excellent.

http://StantonMigraineProtocol.com

Introduction

I've suffered from migraines for over 25 years. I've seen countless "specialists" all across the country. I've experienced numerous in and out patient "procedures", often as painful as the migraines. I've been on so much medication and wasted so many years drugged and in pain. There is hope... The Stanton Migraine Protocol has changed my life. I'm drug free and living without constant migraines. The relief from pain has been a true miracle in my life. Thank you, Angela.

--Jorie Riesen
Member of the Facebook Migraine Group

I am not an MD, which in this case serves as a blessing. Most MDs' practice is based on what is already known, primarily what they had learned in medical school. It is not part of their job description to research new frontiers. In terms of migraine, they try to stop the pain rather than find how to prevent the cause of that pain. As a PhD, my job is to explore the unexplored. My fate as a migraineur was to suffer along with the millions of fellow migraineurs. Combining my wanting to lead a normal pain-free life with my love for science allowed me to see something that others have missed. I received my doctorate in a then new field – Neuroeconomics – which incorporates several specialties: neuroscience (focusing on manipulating neurotransmitters in live volunteer participants), human decision-making (the subjects change their decisions in response to neurotransmitter fluctuations), and even certain aspects of the law as they relate to experimenting on live humans. I fell in love with neuroscience and have remained focused in this field ever since.

My academic experiments aimed at learning more about decision-making by tinkering with neurotransmitters (hormones in the brain) on volunteers—adding more of a certain type than what they naturally had. Thus, the neurotransmitter variations were caused by me, were very well known for their quantity and for their role in the brain. I used financial games to evaluate decision-changes as influenced by the hormonal changes I administered. Neurotransmitter levels were altered to a known state, so I could see how humans responded to their manipulated hormones by the kind of decisions they made. In migraine research I needed to use a reverse engineering method: I didn't know the causation but I could see the behavioral changes.

Whatever methods I used to manipulate human decision-making could not be used to find the cause of my annoying migraines. I could not find much help in medical books either. Medical books cater to doctors who are made to memorize every single illness and their associated symptoms in great detail. Physicians also must continuously update their knowledge of medications and how those medications alleviate symptoms (not curing the cause). However, medical fields are so specialized today that most doctors – with their focused knowledge – have difficulties seeing connections to other areas of medicine. The human body is organized so that one part can send signals to another seemingly unrelated part when it's in trouble. Pains are treated locally by specialized fields and not in a whole-body-system, or integrated medicinal approach. Because my doctorate is multidisciplinary, the type of thinking my research required helped me to connect disparate dots of information.

It has gradually become more accepted that migraine has a strong genetic foundation and there are several online human genome databases that can be searched specifically for migraine associated genes. Many researchers are heading in various directions in their efforts to comprehend the genetic connection. Most research has been in the direction of finding the pain-source in order to dampen the symptoms of pain, rather than trying to understand what that pain-source may mean. Imaging scanners can show the ongoing process of migraine and even the causal mechanism. However, it seems that the correct interpretation of these findings is lacking. It is analogous to seeing that "there is a black hole there" but not understanding why the hole is black and why it is there.

I have come to resolve my migraines by the prevention mechanisms defined in this book: the Stanton Migraine Protocol®, which is based on my initial self-experimentation as a volunteer guinea pig. Given that some of my efforts consistently proved to be successful for migraine prevention while other steps turned out to be futile, I can consider myself to be a one person "clinical trial". While some of my sensitivity toward getting migraines remained over the years of prevention, they are at a much lower level, and others have completely vanished. Thus, if not careful, migraines may return but by paying attention to signals and taking the necessary preventive steps, all migraines can be averted.

Based on my initial findings from online migraine groups and the more significant ongoing discoveries in my own migraine group, I am now nudging science toward a different understanding of migraines with a new direction for their true cause. This new direction I call "tri-migraine complex." The term refers to the three conditions that seem to go hand in hand for migraineurs. These have evolutionary origins.

The tri-migraine complex contains:

1. Heightened sensory sensitivity years before migraines start;
2. Fight-or-flight response as a result of the heightened sensory input that leads to stress hormone release with negative consequences;

3. Biochemical imbalance caused by the hypersensitive, excitable brain, glucose intolerance[1], and the suboptimal concentration of minerals that are needed for proper electrolyte homeostasis.

The hyper sensory feature of the migraine-brain has been recognized by other scientists as well[1-3]. It is caused by several factors connected to the increased number of sensory neuron receptor connections and to the fact that a migraineur's neurons fire differently from non-migraineurs[4-6], leading to depleted energy resources. Glucose intolerance is not usually discussed but it is a genetic signature of the migraine-brain, as is the inability to maintain optimally balanced electrolyte homeostasis. The three factors of the tri-migraine complex are based on an ancient evolutionary advantage that is not needed in our contemporary lives. Today, it is exceedingly rare that we would have a need for this hypersensitivity but it still makes us react to less-than-life-threatening environmental signals. The hyper sensory neurons[3] of a migraineur are much more active than that of a non-afflicted person[4]. The nutritional demands of a migraineur's brain are correspondingly higher to support all of the increased electrical[4,6] and neurotransmitter activity[7]. The most important nutrition components for the brain are those that facilitate the creation of proper voltage and proper voltage gated channel functions,

1 Officially *glucose intolerance* refers to hyperinsulinemia, insulin resistance, or type 2 diabetes. In the case of migraineurs, I use this term (for lack of a better term) to express that migraineurs have an exaggerated reaction to eating glucose even if they have no hyperinsulinemia, insulin resistance, or type 2 diabetes. It refers to migraineurs genetic variances in their inability to use glucose the way others do.

including the prevention of voltage leaks. These, in turn, establish the conditions necessary for the appropriate level neuronal communication by neurotransmitter exchange. For migraineurs, their genetically different brain has modified ionic channels and pumps that render them unable to efficiently utilize carbohydrates, leading to negative consequences, such as metabolic syndrome to which migraineurs are strongly connected[8-14]. Migraine is a consequence of a set of gene variances whose evolutionary benefits are not called upon in our modern lives.

Our typical diet is guided by various considerations; trouble-free neural functioning is not one of them. It does not seem to have reached the consciousness of most scientists, let alone the consciousness of the public, how much difference nutrition can make. In this book, I explore the connection between migraines and the necessary conditions for proper neuronal functioning, the factors that influence those conditions, and how things can get out of balance and why. I also show how to regain and maintain balance once it has slipped out of control. The nutrition components needed for neuronal activity play a crucial role in the quest for neuronal health. In this respect, the nutritional method I describe represents a 180-degree turn from the conventional nutritional recommendations of the Standard American Diet (SAD)—the acronym is telling.

There are no magic pills in my book, only magic cellular balance at the biochemical level. It requires the reader to scrutinize her lifestyle—in fact to change her lifestyle—in order to maintain the cellular well-being of her brain. The book is laid out in five parts. Part I describes the circumstances leading to the creation of this book. Part II includes descriptions of "prodromes" for recognizing the possibility of an upcoming migraine, as well as "first aid" help for a migraineur in pain. It guides the migraineur to treat her pain on the spot and also helps her prepare for emergencies, such as hormonal cycles, travel, etc. Part III contains a deeper, though accessible, explanation for migraineurs who want to understand what migraine is, what causes it, how to prevent it, and what is required for maintaining a migraine-free life. Part IV is for scientists, medical professionals, or curious migraineurs with some scientific knowledge, who wish to have a detailed and more technical understanding of migraine, this common and all so human condition. Pat V is a very long list of citations. Don't despair if some of the words in this introduction are unfamiliar. Just read on; you will be an expert on the terminology of the new migraine science in short order.

Part I

THE WORLD OF MIGRAINES

Section I

Originally This Book Was About Me

The beginning is the most important part of the work

Plato

I am a migraineur who got as frustrated as all of you must have gotten about the number of medicines thrown at migraineurs without any lasting relief accomplished. I had belly aches and "headaches" from a very young age but didn't realize they were migraines until I was in my 20s. I think this is very typical. Many children as young as two years of age have migraines and as adults they remember the headaches that no one ever had taken seriously. By the time I received my doctorate, my migraines were five days a week with two days of fog in between. It was time for me to start my journey and find the cause of my migraines.

My doctoral studies did not start out with the goal of understanding migraine but they helped for many, somewhat unrelated, reasons. One of those reasons is that doctoral studies are aimed at research, requiring an open mind to recognize patterns and connections, rather than to gain a deep knowledge in a specific field. Secondly, my studies of the brain and its connection to decision making were so much at the leading edge of this branch of science at the time that to succeed I had to learn to see outside the box. Thirdly, my doctoral studies (and all my studies prior to that) were very heavy in mathematics and so my world is viewed through the eyes of logic and proof. My research could be based on existing knowledge only to a small extent since the field was very new. With hindsight, it is clear to me that the same mindset that was necessary to succeed in academia also helped me see migraine from a perspective of something new, rather than following the logic of prior interpretations. And finally, my doctoral studies involved brain research with live humans who volunteered to neurotransmitter level stimulation so that I could observe connections in novel ways that had previously not been explored. In my research, the neurotransmitter I administered was the known cause of the observed behavioral change. In case of migraine, it is the other way around; I observe a migraine and then have to figure out the cause. My goal became to reverse engineer the migraine process back to its roots.

I now understand what causes my migraines. I can cause or stop a migraine on demand without the use of any medicines and I can prevent any migraine. This immediately suggests a few things:

1. If I can cause it, *I know the cause.*
2. If I can stop it, I do not only know what caused it but *I also know what to do to stop it.*
3. *If I can cause it and stop it, I can prevent it from happening.*

The statements above constitute the logical foundation of this book's central thesis. With them I have demonstrated that migraine is not a mental illness (apparently, many people and doctors believe it is); it is not a physiological disease (just about every doctor and migraineur believes it is); and it needs no medicines for prevention or treatment (virtually every doctor and migraineur believes that medicinal treatment is necessary).

Connecting seemingly disparate dots is a prerequisite of any breakthrough in science. This book provides a radically new view by looking at migraine as a symptom, uses the term migraine-brain, explores associated genetic variances, and describes migraine's connection to lifestyle. Besides getting relief from my migraines, by now I have helped over four-thousand migraine sufferers around the world to accomplish the same.

> *When something hurts, there is always a cellular reason for the pain.*

Cellular imbalance is always the cause of every pain, while the pain is the symptom we feel. Cellular imbalance in most cases refers to a state in which some crucial minerals or energy sources are not available to the cell for its optimal functioning. To repeat, in this book we don't treat symptoms but offer an understanding of the cause based on the cells' chemical interactions with their environment and each other, the cells' genetic limitations, and the roles of a few vital chemicals that are crucial to satisfying the cells' energy needs and proper functioning. It needs to be also understood that a migraine-brain is anatomically different from a non-migraine brain. Thus, we are not in search of the cause of an illness! Instead we are in search of the underlying anatomical differences that trigger a pain response. What this means will become clear in later sections of the book. Once we understand the where and the how, the possibility of migraine prevention and pain abortion is close at hand. The knowledge that all migraine problems start at the cellular level has been the guiding light during my research. All migraine symptoms, including pain, auras, and paralysis in the case of hemiplegic migraines, originate at the cellular (neuronal) level.

The subject of migraine was thrust upon me not as my choice but by having been a migraine sufferer since my 20s, including through the years of my doctoral studies. My first *aha* moment happened during the doctoral studies, as I was able to modify behavior by applied hormones. Changes to the environment of neurons can cause changes in people's decision making, moods, and their way of thinking, feeling, and being. At this point the goal became clear: connect migraine to the environmental changes of neurons. If pain is based on neurons and how they feel in their environment, then the pain associated with migraine must be the consequence of some chemical change in the neurons' environment.

My Migraine Family

I am designating a special section to my Facebook Migraine Family, who stood by me through fire and ice until most flames were put out; flames caused by those trying to taint the reputation of the group without ever trying the recommended steps. Who is my migraine family? They are members of the migraine group I started in February of 2014. I opened the group at the time the 1st edition of this book was published. The goal was to help those with questions and problems, and to take on special cases that are harder than the norm. I did not realize what an incredible group this was going to become over the following several years. Because so many members have put their hearts and souls into helping others selflessly, perfect strangers in the somewhat detached environment of the internet, and also because they dedicated themselves to helping my understanding of the various types of migraines they suffered, I owe very special thanks to them. Therefore, it is important to acknowledge that this book is *not only by me*. Although I am the sole author, I am not the only *contributor*. The many stories shared and the many questions asked helped me see a broader picture. I also received permission from many members to share their stories on my blog and in the book as well. Albeit names are not always provided, all stories are true and can be verified in the Facebook migraine group.

This extended edition would not be possible without such immense help by the migraine group members. With their input, it is well attuned to deal with all the nuances and road blocks that many of them have experienced in their recovery process. The total number of participating members has been more than 4000 over the several years of the group's existence, many joining and leaving, some staying permanently. I still have some members in the group who were with me when I opened the digital doors on Facebook for the first time.

Prior to starting my migraine group on Facebook, I had initially joined some already existing migraine groups. I asked questions and tried to participate in an open exchange of ideas. Some of the ideas I wanted to discuss were unheard of in these groups. For some reason, many migraineurs seem to have feared the discussion of new ideas and they preferred to operate in their well-travelled mental grooves, to the extent that I ended up being banned from many migraine groups. Thus, migraineurs were closed off from gaining any benefit that comes with looking at a subject from new angles. Only pain management and related information was welcomed and shared in these groups. The importance of communication was completely lost—no one was used to it and no one wanted it. They had no means of exchanging any information other than how much they hurt and what medicines they had tried or were trying at that time and how much a certain medication did not work and made them sicker. They also shared the stories of their misfortunes and sorrows, how they had lost their jobs and had attempted to gain disability assistance.

In fact, I have a recent story to tell you. I received a plea on my Facebook page from a mother who has a young migraineur child—I invited the mother to join my migraine group. She was utterly dismayed what she found there. In the message she sent to me she was focusing on her child (slightly modified here for clarity):

> *I'm not sure if I'm in the correct group. My child is a migraine sufferer and I was looking to find a migraine group that discusses the journeys migraineurs have to take to become migraine free. In your group, I've read about chia seeds, vanilla beans, and various recipes. If this is what the group discussions are generally about, I will leave the group. I'm looking for a cure for my child's chronic pain, and not a chit-chat group on irrelevant subjects. My child's health is not a laughing matter.*

Note how this mother thought that a migraine group, by definition, must be a somber assembly, where members talk only about pain, and medicines. It never occurred to her that perhaps while migraineurs in pain do talk only about their pains, migraineurs can also end up pain free! Migraineurs who are no longer in pain like to enjoy life, learn about different recipes that are migraine prevention friendly, talk about events they could attend without migraine (Thanksgiving, Christmas, weddings, birthdays, football games, heavy metal concerts, just to name a few). On occasion when a migraine does break through, for some usually known reason (such as eating a cookie), many group members instantly rush in to help and support. This is how a real migraine group has to operate. This mother decided to leave the group. Although she wanted to see her child become migraine free, she just could not relate to the possibility that a migraineur can exist without permanent migraine.

My goal is to prevent the pain without the use of medicines by understanding what causes it. I accepted that I could not talk to everyone in other migraine groups about anything other than medicines, so I stopped visiting them. In my migraine group, one of the most important rules is: talking about medicines is not permitted! Thousands of migraineurs have joined, and with no possibility for discussing their drugs, they have found they could finally discuss their problems, solutions, and experiences. I also developed a questionnaire that serves as the basis of my personalized analysis and guidance for each new member at the start of their journey toward recovery.

At the beginning, the book and my entire concept of migraine cause and treatment were received with great skepticism. This I could totally understand since doctors, research scientists, and pharmaceutical companies had all been trying to break the mystery of migraine without success; who was I to say they are getting it all wrong? And I said that loud and clear: they do get it wrong. Migraine sufferers who have tried everything available by both Western and Eastern medicines, had their teeth perfectly aligned, spent their money on chiropractors and weekly acupuncture, received massages regularly, got Botox shots, had neuronal stimulators surgically implanted into their bodies, daith pierced their ears, and took a long list of preventive and abortive medicines, were still hurting every day. And then this "nobody" tells them that migraine can be prevented and treated and on top of that without medicines? Nah! She cannot be for real, for sure.

Yet, all through these trying times some members of the group tried my method and stayed with it through thick and thin because they noticed that my suggestions were actually working for them. Together we came out as winners because we have no migraines and we stopped all medicines as well! Today we no longer have such attacks in the group because by now those who join and stay know that the program works. Even many doctors have come to recommend it. I am pleased to see a lot of cooperation and that people have joined the protocol from all corners of the world.

Here is an example from a UK member who has been with us almost from the very beginning; she calls all migraine group members "flower", which I think is really sweet. She is welcoming a new member here and urging her to stick with the program:

> *"...the thing is flower it is with anything in life when things are going ok we think it's ok to let other things slip; that it will be ok and that's how things creep back slowly in. Fortunately for us our brains are so tuned in, they know they are not good for us. Not just because [the brain] will give us a migraine, but just Angela's post the other day explaining how sugar messes with our bodies' insulin messages. So in some ways once we learn to*

read our bodies they are pretty awesome, (eventually) but yes, our whole life is a work in progress and even those a year down the line on protocol, or longer, still learn much valuable lessons. Learn we can't afford not to be vigilant. I have a brain that likes to talk myself in and out of all sorts of things fooling myself with great reasons why I'm doing it. Wow, if I put that energy into the right things I'd be smarter. Lol. But I'm also very much always giving myself a hard time when I get things wrong, pre-accident, a perfectionist, academic, I tore myself apart making sure things were right, I don't have the same thinking ability but still able to give myself a hard time for getting things wrong. I realise it's wasted energy, doesn't help anyone especially me, so I chose to go back to motivating myself. [Remember] the lesson, and [know that] when things are good that's when I seem to try and sabotage things, trick myself into: I'm sure just one will be ok. This protocol [of] learning to listen to my body, to even admit it is my body, has been a big deal. But I've found it has uses. [It] can help me, inform me. That I can handle.

So one day at a time, and it does get easier. As I've said I was a sugar addict, fruit gums were my thing, the thought of one makes me feel as though I could be sick. Lol

You are doing great. Being honest allows the team to really help you.

Proud of you flower…"

This member had a major car accident and was bed ridden with mini strokes every day when she first joined our group (I could see the slurred words on her phone writing). She has made the most incredible recovery, now walking a tad, medicines reduced from 40 to about 20, no more mini strokes, and despite her amazing difficulties she is there to cheer everyone on. She is our group's mascot. Such incredible support within the migraine group from all members toward each other makes the group strong, helping all migraineurs succeed no matter what their original issues may have been.

Recently I was also able to publish several academic articles and as a result I am enjoying worldwide interest and support. These days it is not unusual to receive a call from a doctor for a consultation or a call from a hospital that a migraineur is not getting any better with their treatment, would they be allowed to pass on my information. Interesting how things change!

There is more to cooperation than meets the eye. As the section's title says, originally the 1st edition of this book was about me; only about me, my migraines, and how I got rid of them. My understanding was based on only my experience and the available research at that time. It seemed to me that no one in the research arena really knew what it was like to be a migraineur. Now, in the extended edition of the book, it is about and for all migraineurs, since the Migraine Family made me understand that the cause of all migraines is the same. Let me repeat: the cause of all migraines is the same, although the manifestations of the actual migraine (the symptoms) can greatly differ.

To be a migraineur is to have many different symptoms but most researchers and doctors only focus on the pain. There are migraine types where there is no pain at all (silent migraines). How do you look for a solution when there is no pain? This already suggests something important: migraine without pain implies that pain is only one of its symptoms and is not its necessary condition. There is no clear understanding of what a migraine really is in medical communities. To diagnose a person as a migraineur, the medical practice still consists of eliminating all other possible illnesses. When nothing may explain the pain, the "catch all" category is migraine. In other words, there is no specific diagnosis for migraine (except for those cases in which aura is also present).

The right questions are still never asked. Migraineurs are only looked at as sufferers of pain. The pain has to be extinguished and the solution must lie with a pain killer or a pain prevention method, even though medical science does not know what migraine is and what causes it. Migraine was (and still is in many places) looked at as some mental disease, a downright nuisance, or even as an excuse for drug seeking. There still are husbands who yell at their wives for ruining their day if the wife comes down with a migraine. There are families where the migraineur gets punished for having a migraine. There are doctors who pat their patient's hand and tell them to "go home and rest", as if rest cured migraines. Migraineurs are often ignored by their families and doctors alike and frequently lose their jobs. As I was picking up on these and other details of migraineurs' lives, it has become obvious to me that the book cannot be about me anymore. So this time, while the book still includes my story, it also represents the stories of other migraineurs, as well as the solution for how to prevent and terminate all migraines. My approach seems to be universally working for all types of migraines (except for vegans—more about that later), so what works for me, works for all. Many of the stories I will share in the book are not my personal stories. These are real life – sometimes shocking – stories of other migraineurs, the stories of pain, anguish, and agony prior to joining our program as well as joy once they are able to enjoy a migraine-free life.

The following list of advices migraineurs receive demonstrates how they are treated by their family, friends, and doctors. These are examples of what migraineurs in the Facebook group were told to do to stop their migraines:

- Have sex. It will take your headache away
- Drink some wine. It always helps my headaches
- Have a soda pop. You probably have a caffeine headache
- Have a cup of tea and put your feet up
- Get some exercise
- Just lay down, it will go away
- It's all in your head and cannot possibly be as bad as you claim
- Don't think about it...it will go away

- Get Daith piercing (a very painful ear piercing)
- Place onions in your socks
- Put a frog on the top of your head! (Alive or dead? Not sure it matters)
- Take an aspirin.
- Take a bath.
- Eat something (said to me while vomiting).
- Go outside in bright sunlight.
- Focus on something happy and it will go away
- Here's some Advil that helps mine
- Rub essential oils on your scalp
- Stop stressing out
- You shouldn't let life bother you so much. You make yourself sick
- Drink some water and go for a jog. Endorphins will take it away
- You must have learned this from your mother, she used to have these
- It's hereditary so nothing you can do about it
- Maybe your neck is out!!
- Cayenne pepper up the nose
- Ginger water up the nose
- Fresh air and sunlight
- Cupping... (hot glasses are put on you that suck the skin up as the air cools)
- Breast reduction!
- Spiritual healing

- OMG! I had acupuncture and the doctor left a little needle behind my ears. He said to press it whenever I feel the migraine coming
- Just get out of the house and spend some time around people
- My husband wasn't all that great about them… he just left me alone
- My husband generally blames me for ruining his day/week/life and reminds me he has things to do
- Place lemons on head and try to balance them
- Coffee enemas...
- We've come a long way from the Greeks drilling holes in our skulls!!!! Oh yeah – a clay crocodile wrapped around the forehead with a cloth…
- Relax and take deep breaths
- Place your feet in ice water
- "Not another migraine, I'm sick of hearing about them…"

As you can see, family members are not very supportive, friends even less so, and doctors can sometimes be downright hurtful and ignorant. Migraine is a very serious condition that is swept under the rug due to lack of understanding. I feel very fortunate because I never had this type of bad experience. My family always supported me, tip-toed around me and helped me in every which way they could. Reading how much anguish others went through made me realize that the Facebook migraine group I created was not a group. It was a family for all afflicted with this condition; we understood each other and we could relate and provide the support needed—in addition to what we have come to realize: we are nearly siblings in terms of our traits, abilities, and symptoms.

In the process of being part of this group, we often initiated discussions that made us realize how similar we all were! We could have passed for sisters and brothers! We had identical symptoms, identical funny things that no one would believe or could identify with. For example, we all had special abilities that non-migraineurs did not have: we could smell certain unusual odors and from longer distances—this has been called phantom odors by the scientific community because they cannot smell them[15,16]. We would hear noises and people think we are crazy but we could hear people whispering several rooms away. We realized we all were sensitive to light. Most of us were walking electrical outlets, shocking everything we touched, and killing batteries in our watches and cell phones. We had better vision in the dark than other people, and pupil dilation at the ophthalmologist caused major problems. In other words, we had very similar abilities and problems, all relating to something special about our sensory organ associated regions in the brain. Our group turned out to have members from all parts of the world, possessing very similar brains that are different from the brains of non-migraineurs. We were related in some way. This recognition created a shared identity; a better understanding about what migraine really is. Since all migraineurs seem so similar, a genetic connection is a reasonable assumption. Having a genetically different brain in a large percent of the population indicates another possibility. Perhaps this particular brain had some evolutionary advantage at a relatively recent time; it might still be an advantage in certain parts of the world and, hence, the gene variances are still with us. So rather than look for a way to get rid of such a different brain, why not embrace it and learn how to live with it in harmony? It is possible and we are doing just that in our migraine group.

THANK YOU, FELLOW MIGRAINE-SUFFERERS OF THE FACEBOOK MIGRAINE GROUP! ♥

My Motivation

My migraines got me angry, impatient, but also curious, and I needed answers that no one had. I wanted to learn but what should I look at? Where do I start looking for the cause? I decided to talk to other migraineurs. I did not focus on their pains but tried to gather information on their personality type, daily habits, and whatever else that may distinguish us migraineurs from the rest of the population. My discussions with other migraineurs made a very big difference in my understanding!

Pain is pain. It can range on the scale of from 1 to 10… and then what. What can we learn from that? Not much.

Pain is not an indication for the brain-location in distress, since the brain has no pain sensing nerves. All pain is felt by the meninges, a layer of very thin tissue between the brain and the skull. Thus, if I hurt over my right ear it says absolutely nothing about where exactly the pain originates in my brain or what causes it. It seemed impossible to identify the originating location of the pain in migraine-brains and I also wondered if the pain or its location really mattered at all. My first area of study centered on prodromes, the precursors to migraines. While prodrome types vary from person to person, and also sometimes from migraine to migraine for the same person, their significance and their relationship to certain types of migraines should have been comprehensively explored but to date this has not happened. It is important to note that migraines are always preceded by at least one prodrome. Pains that appear without any prodrome are not migraines.

The list of prodromes provided by medical manuals and institutional web sites has little meaning because there is no explanation how, for example, the prodromes *nausea* or *anxiety* are connected to migraine and why. Through my discussions with other migraineurs, and based on my own migraine experience, it has become clear that prodrome variations are connected to the type of migraine that is about to hit, and that prodromes may change depending on the stage to which migraines have progressed. Prodromes can – in some cases – even point to the brain location of the migraine's source. Many prodromes are identical for migraineurs and these have specific functions that can lead to a better understanding of migraines[17].

Most doctors only learn about those prodromes that migraineurs recall during a visit, assuming that a doctor actually asks (I have yet to meet a doctor in person who does). When patients do report their prodromes: aura, sensitivity to bright light, symptoms of IBS, RLS, dizziness, etc., these are considered to be independent diseases and are medicated separately by most physicians (except for aura, which is always associated with migraine by medical science). Treating prodromes is quite meaningless and shows lack of understanding of the migraine condition. A prodrome is a sign that something is out of whack and a migraine will follow. Treating the sign removes the warning so the migraineur does not know she is about to come down with a migraine. It also neither deals with the migraine pain nor with the migraine cause.

I know that if you are a real migraineur you are already intrigued. Read on! I will teach you how to connect your prodromes to your migraines and how to prevent your migraines based on the information your prodromes are telling you.

My Migraines and How I Got Angry About Them

As you are reading this section see if any of this is familiar to you. I started getting migraines in my late 20's. They have increased in their frequency, duration, and intensity over the years. By the time I was 50, I had migraines every week for several days.

When I was in my 20's, I was told that women get more migraines than men do (still seems to be true according to statistics) and that there is a female hormonal connection. I was told I was going to have fewer migraines after I had children. I had children at age 28 and 29, had no migraines while pregnant but boy did they ever return. In fact, the migraines increased both in frequency and intensity after I stopped nursing. As the years went by, I was told that after I hit menopause I should have no migraines at all because the female hormones will have left my system. Then at age 42 I had a complete hysterectomy (radical hysterectomy with oophorectomy, in which the ovaries and the uterus are taken out), removing all traces of female hormones from my body. The hormones that could be causing monthly fluctuations and causing migraines as a result of "being a female" were all gone. My migraines not only did not stop, they got worse. I was put on estrogen shortly after surgery, since at age 42 I suddenly entered full menopause with no female hormones at all. That was really nerve-racking. But this hormone was a stable and steady intake, same amount every day, no hormonal variations, no menstrual cycles. Still migraines persisted and got worse as I got older.

At about age 52 I finally went to see a migraine specialist. My specialist put me through several tests to ensure that I had no health conditions that would cause migraine—in other words, I had to be completely healthy and only have migraine for no other explainable reason. Since it is caused by "nothing," this type of migraine is defined as "primary headache." After I passed all of those tests with flying colors, she said: "yep, you've got migraines." Great, I thought. Confirmed! So now what?! She started to put me on a variety of medications, changing them time to time to see if any of them would work. One medication worked for a short time (about 30% of the time), one got me sick, another did not do a thing at all, and so on—all of these were triptans. I went through all possible types, each with different dose, some as spray in the nose because the tablets got me sick, etc. I also tried some narcotic medicines and barbiturates but none worked—they made me feel stupid with pain; not what I was looking for. Then we finally reached one particular medication that she said I will have to take for the rest of my life and "it seems to help a lot of patients preventing migraines" but I can never stop taking it. I could no longer take any other migraine medications either because I may end up with "serotonin toxicity". Being a scientist myself, it was at that time when I realized I'd better take this seriously. This was a preventive medicine making my brain into a serotonin machine 24/7 (an SSRI), and which had nothing to do with the pain cause. A dangerous symptom treatment if there was ever one. I said "no thank you" and left.

Serotonin is an essential hormone of life that keeps you "feeling good" among other very important things. It has a large role in moving food through your intestines and some other functions as well—in fact 90% of serotonin is made in and used by your intestines and only 10% by your brain. Serotonin is not a pain killer; though it will make you feel good enough (or bad enough) that you don't feel the migraine as much as you did before taking the medicine but rest assured, the pain – and the underlying neurological disturbance – is still there. In the brain, serotonin is a neurotransmitter that is derived from a chemical called "tryptophan."

Medicines in the triptan or reuptake inhibitor families are all either adding more serotonin or shut down the neuron's knowledge that enough serotonin is already made, so the neurons end up with more serotonin or keep on making more and more and more. Many people take serotonin reuptake inhibitors without migraine for various other conditions like anxiety, bipolar disorder, depression, fibromyalgia, diabetic neuralgia, and many more. You may have heard of some variants as SSRI (Selective Serotonin Reuptake Inhibitors) or SNRI (Serotonin-Norepinephrine Reuptake Inhibitors) or SARIs (Serotonin Antagonist and Reuptake Inhibitors), etc. They may dull the patients' senses but they don't function as true pain killers, and as a result many migraineurs continue to have migraines but now with a host of side effects they didn't have without these drugs.

When the same medicine is prescribed to treat many distinct and unrelated conditions, you can bet it is only a symptom treatment; a Band-Aid® approach, without any guarantee that it will work for even the symptoms.

Many migraineurs get even more dangerous medicines that block the neurotransmitters from being released completely: voltage gated calcium channel blockers. These are more harmful because while the medicines let the neurons make neurotransmitters, the neurons fill up with them but cannot release them. This can cause a neuron to commit apoptosis (cell suicide). Alternatively, or simultaneously, a reduction in the number of receptors in those neurons that would have received neurotransmitters can occur (synaptic pruning). In the brain when something is not used, it gets removed. Thus, these drugs are neurodegenerative drugs. Stopping their use may not leave you with the same brain as the one you started out with (depending on the length of time taken and your age). Many migraineurs take both SSRIs and voltage gated calcium channel blockers. This is major trouble for their neurons because on the one hand they are ordered to continuously manufacture serotonin but on the other they are blocked from releasing them.

Some doctors believe that migraines are vascular and prescribe heart medicines that often block voltage gated sodium channels or L-type voltage gated calcium channels. These channels of the cell membrane have crucial roles in hydrating the cell. In addition, since most migraineurs have low blood pressure[18-20], a beta blocker or any type of blood pressure reducing medicine can be truly harmful.

I just wanted to give you a partial picture of the appalling lack of understanding and treatment standards I encountered early on in my investigation. This is why I started my own research, using myself as a lab rat, to find out about my body, my habits, and my aches and pains. Most importantly this is what led me to recognize the cause of my migraines, eventually eliminating it and stopping my pain completely.

Why is This Book Different from Other Books?

There are many migraine books available. So why choose this one? This book blossomed into representing several thousand migraineurs' experiences; the ones who have sent me messages, emails, or talked to me in person either on Facebook, or by email, Skype, phone. These migraineurs are from many countries from all over the world. In the writing process, this has become a book of and for migraine sufferers, in general. It is a *complete manual* for migraine prevention and management. However, an important fact remains: this is still an insider's story. The story of someone who actually had migraines and managed to get rid of them without using any medicines, and remained migraine and medicine free for many years by now, as I'm finishing the writing of this book—indeed, it still is an insider's story. Thus rather than advising you about what to do, here I describe what I did and if you follow in my footsteps you can become migraine free as well. Each person is different; my migraine solutions may slightly differ from what will work for you. Because of this, I created a service under the name Stanton Migraine Protocol®, as mentioned earlier.

Using the Stanton Migraine Protocol® I will not be the one to take your migraines away; you will be! You will learn how to do it if you choose to follow what I did. There is more than one way to abort migraines. I present a simplified quick-relief version in Part II and a thorough explanation in Part III. These methods are not simple, they require full attention at the beginning and adherence later on. Since a migraine-brain is a special brain for life, whatever changes you need to make to stay pain free will have to be applied for life as well, though this does not mean that you cannot switch methods; you can. You will find that some of your sensitivities will lessen and triggers will not be as frequent (if any at all) once you settle into your correct balance and stick with it. The changes you need to make are based on the understanding of the neurons' need for biochemical stability, the essential condition for their proper functioning. The changes in my diet were based on the understanding that many foods I ate (and likely you eat) contained an inappropriate balance of chemicals for my neurons to work with. I recognized that my migraines had been caused by the biochemical imbalance I had created by not providing the proper energy for my brain. I will not always mention genetics but every time I mention biochemical imbalance as the cause of migraines, it automatically implies that such imbalance is possible because of the attributes of our genetically different brains.

There are a good number of migraine books in the market advertising many food categories or types to be taken out of your diet, like chocolate, dairy, and nightshades (examples are: peppers, tomatoes, eggplant, potatoes, etc.,). This book is not one of them. Some foods will become taboo but with the full understanding of why they cause migraines and why that cause cannot be resolved. You will learn why certain foods may trigger your migraines, as well as how to cancel those triggers by mixing and matching foods in a way that their combined effect is supportive of a migraine-brain. The books that recommend that you cut families of foods do so without understanding why those foods trigger in the first place. In this book, I also cover how to eat known trigger foods.

While this is not a medical or an academic book, it contains a thorough biochemical explanation of what the brain needs on a neuronal level. I provide a basic summary in a way that is understandable without complex biochemical knowledge. There is nothing in this book that can hurt you and you may find that my suggestions will be working for you quite rapidly!

Because each migraine episode is independent from the one before, you need to treat each one separately. You brush your teeth and have them cleaned regularly in order to prevent dental issues. You prevent the occurrence of future migraines by applying preventive maintenance to the migraine-brain, and avoid the need for further treatment. This places YOU in control!

The brain is like a giant "hormonal gland", as one of my professors was fond of saying. No one wants to think of the brain as a yucky hormonal gland but in fact it is just that. It functions by sending messages from neuron to neuron using electrical currents that zap the neurons to release their neurotransmitters. This book shows and explains, both in words and also with simple illustrations, how neurons work and what the cause of migraine is. Again, the best thing to do is to prevent all pain. Prevention requires the migraineur's full and constant awareness of what she is doing. I use "she" for the simple reason that statistically most migraine sufferers are female.

Of course, there is a very large group of male migraineurs who I am sure will find this book just as useful. In fact, I believe there are a lot more male migraineurs than is typically assumed; men are less likely to visit a doctor for a "headache". I find that males tend to be diagnosed more as having cluster headaches and women more as having migraines. I find a disproportionately large misdiagnosis by gender.

I want to be sure you know: this book is not about hormones, although that is my field of specialty, and I also know many people believe that migraines are caused by hormones. I will demonstrate that they are not, although there is some indirect hormone connection to migraines and it applies to people of both genders and all ages. The hormonal connection to the female reproductive cycle has a separate biochemical explanation as well. We cover that in Part III.

You should be skeptical of anything you read, including this book. What you find in this book worked for me and for thousands of other migraineurs. The solution in this book is intended for those with primary migraines. For some, whose migraines are caused by certain underlying factors (e.g., stroke, brain injury, pinched nerves, or brain damage), this method may not be as effective. However, even if your migraines are secondary headaches, you have nothing to lose by trying! One thing is for certain, you will not achieve a migraine free or a pain-free life without action. It took me 6 months of constant maintenance before I could say I was pain and migraine-fog free but even now, years later, I can get kicked out of balance if I am not being vigilant to my needs as a migraineur! Although the migraine-brain is a permanent part of you, the sensitivity lessens with the use of the protocol over the years. Similarly to a broken bone, it is your own body that must heal itself with your nurturing and vigilance. It may have taken one second to break a bone but at least 6 weeks for your body to completely heal it with the support of a cast. The cast does not cure: your body does. Just as there is no instant cure for broken bone, so it is with migraine.

What You Will and Will Not Find in this Book

I went through some tough slugging in my search to find the cause of my own migraine. I found my solution by looking at the biochemical balance provided by what I ate or drank and how important elements, such as water, sodium, potassium, calcium, etc., behave at the cellular level; how that glass of water I drank had changed the chemical environment in my brain and body. Did the beverage I had just drunk, the food I had just eaten, kick the perfect chemical equilibrium in my brain out of balance with the minerals it provided to the neurons? And if it did, and I came down with a migraine as a result, what do I need to eat or drink to provide the missing chemicals to re-establish the lost equilibrium? In other words, how do I re-establish homeostasis again and why did I get knocked out of that homeostasis in the first place?

There is a need for understanding the chemistry of our nourishment and for understanding why some nutrients behave differently in a migraine-brain versus in a non-migraine-brain. For example, for a migraineur eating a large piece of dark chocolate is a known migraine-pain trigger. The exact same piece of dark chocolate does not trigger any pain in a non-migraineur. Why is that? Has anyone asked? Is there something special about a migraine-brain that makes it more sensitive to dark chocolate? What may that be? And is the trigger the "whole food", or something within the food that may be commonly found in other foods as well? My approach is based on scientifically developing an answer to questions like this, so that we can learn to avoid or mitigate the effect of the specific food, or component of the food, and thereby disarm the trigger. By knowing which chemical trigger exists in a certain food, we may *un-trigger* it by pairing it with another food that addresses the particular imbalance. One goal of this book is to help you recognize why and under what conditions a particular food becomes a trigger so we can prevent it from becoming one.

When everything is in balance, there are no food triggers to cause migraines. However, migraineurs have some genetic predispositions and a unique metabolism. As a result, some foods (an entire macronutrient group) remain a trigger in such a way that by consuming them, migraineurs are not only going to get a migraine but they are much more likely to end up with metabolic disorders, particularly type 2 diabetes. This is discussed in great detail later in the book. I formulated a specific section for the explanation of the connection; it is vital to keep migraineurs not only migraine free but healthy in general. Everything I suggest in this book is based on chemical interactions at the cellular level, as well as matching the foods and drinks in a way that they provide a biochemical balance for the health of every cell. You will not likely to find any food or drink item mentioned in this book that you have not already eaten or drunk. Crucially, absolutely no medicines of any kind are recommended to be added—if you are taking any, that is fine but there are no recommendations for you to add more. As your migraines start reducing in frequency and intensity, some of your medicines will block your advancement. While you can certainly keep using your medicines, you will find, as all migraineurs I have ever dealt with have, that medicines are only for pain. Once you have no pain, you have no need for medication. This book is thus "The holy grail of non-medicinal migraine prevention."

I am a scientist and have access to all kinds of scientific research in various medical journals. These are not likely to be available to most of the migraineur readers of this book. For this reason, in the 1st edition I was not citing authors whose work was not available to the general public. After the publication of the 1st edition, however, I received several comments from scientists and doctors (and also from many migraineurs) who wanted to see the original findings. Therefore, this edition is sprinkled throughout with citations. Their source information is included at the very end of the book as notes.

You will not find in this book any recommendations for any alternative medicine such as naturopathic or homeopathic. I am not a believer in either and I do not consider my approach to have anything to do with them. I am a member of many academic associations and follow their teachings (for the most part) but modified for migraineurs. If I were asked where I belong with my knowledge, my answer would be that I am a student of electrolytes, the maintenance methodologies of electrolyte homeostasis, the relevant genetic effects in the migraineur's brain, and the associated nutritional components and metabolic health. Thus, don't expect recommendations from me for cleansing, detox, herbs or magic pills. This book is about healthy eating, *eating for the sake of homeostasis in your brain*. This previous sentence is truly the heart of my message to you.

Purpose and Function of this book

The purpose of this book is for you to understand the cause of migraines, but it does not stop there. This is a practical book, and now in the extended edition it is more of a "user manual" with greatly enhanced knowledge and experience. It is meant to help you in your daily struggle and give you directions on how to handle tricky situations. It is a workbook too! You need to work to get rid of your own migraines. Reading the book, and nodding "yes" and "I see," will not make your migraines go away. You need to move into action and follow up when sections that need work on your part are provided. This book should be used as a self-help guide with directions and suggestions on what to do and when to do them. Please take an active role in your migraine-pain-free life! My goal is that every single person with a migraine-brain becomes migraine and pain free without the use of any medicines by learning what it takes to manage her migraine-brain.

This is not an academic book although the many citations may lead you to believe it is. It is first and foremost a book for practical use by those who suffer migraines and are willing to work continuously to maintain the lifestyle necessary for providing a pain-free life. My approach is not based on lab tests; there are no medications, no brain stimulation, no yoga or relaxations, no acupuncture or massage. My method is based on one thing: the understanding of the cell, the basic unit of life in the body and the brain. I employ biochemistry and its rules. Since we are made up of cells, it's logical that keeping them as healthy as possible is the key to a healthy and pain free life!

Section 2

Are You Sure You Have Migraines?

Hiding my migraines on the set may have been my toughest challenge as an actor. There were times when the pain from migraine headaches was so severe that I literally had to crawl across my dressing room floor. But I couldn't let anyone know. If they thought I might slow production, I figured that would end my career.

Morgan Fairchild

There are many types of headaches that people (and doctors) mistake for migraines. Migraines are not the most severe of pains—cluster headaches are a lot worse. Nevertheless, migraines come with many debilitating symptoms that are not common to other headache types (except for some overlap between cluster headaches and migraines). Interestingly, some people who have cluster headaches often also have migraines and respond well to the Stanton Migraine Protocol®. The other way around, many migraineurs may come down with an occasional cluster headache. The connection is unclear at this point; clearly more work is needed along this line. I must also add that while for primary migraines the Stanton Migraine Protocol® works without exception, for cluster headaches, it only reduces the severity and the duration of the pain; it neither prevents nor stops cluster headaches. This book is thus very specific to primary migraines. Primary migraines are migraines not caused by tumors, head injuries, neck injuries, etc., and while the Stanton Migraine Protocol® seems to help secondary migraines as well, the level to which it helps depends on the nature and the severity of the condition.

Below is a picture of the pain regions that are affected by the most common headache types.

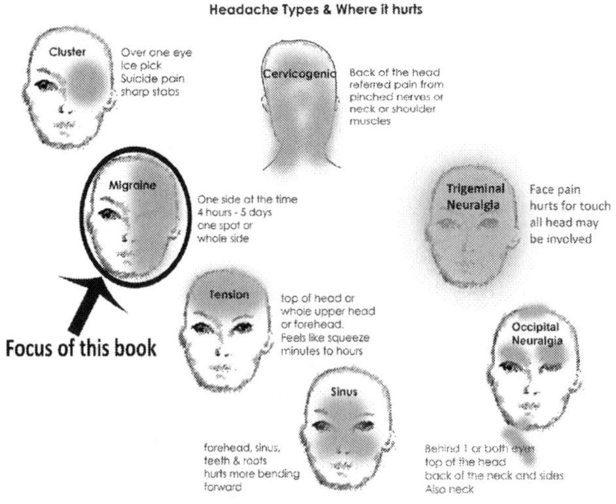

Figure 1. Most common headache type pain locations

Note that Migraine is always on one side of the head. It need not always be on the same side, though usually it is. It can be either side and may move from one side to the other under certain conditions (like when your body is fighting a bug) but it is never on both sides at the same time, never in the back and never at the forehead, face, or top of the head, and most importantly, migraine does not throb. These distinctions are significant, not only for the sake of a better diagnosis but also because different treatments work for different types of headaches. Migraine is the only type of headache condition in which there may not be any pain at all in the head—thus technically a migraine need not even be a headache. Migraines without pain, silent migraines, are common and are usually accompanied by aura. Let's discuss the different types of headaches and see what they are made of (if known) and how to treat them (if possible). The list of headache descriptions below can guide you about what to do when you have something other than migraines.

Rebound Pains

Rebound pains are very common for all types of headaches, including migraines, and are caused by medicines or caffeine. Rebound headaches are without migraine prodromes, they can show up in various parts of your head, and may move around during the day. In other words, a rebound headache may feel like a migraine but it is not a migraine. Rebound headaches are caused by the absence of pain medications or caffeine the brain has adapted to—this includes many of the most common medication types prescribed to migraineurs, like triptans, and also OTC medications, and any caffeinated beverage. Many doctors call rebounds from medicines "medication overuse headache." That is an incorrect definition because the medication is not used more than it is prescribed or recommended but the prescribed dose or frequency is inappropriate in the first place. Thus, medication rebound headache is caused by doctors who prescribed the medicine the wrong way, rather than being the fault of the migraineur who is dutifully following instructions. Many doctors call migraineurs "drug seekers" because of this "drug overuse" problem, which the doctors have created themselves. If this happens to you, know that it is not your fault, neither are you alone! Nearly all migraineurs struggle with rebound pain when they decide to reduce and eliminate their medications.

Rebound headache is not caused by opiates or barbiturates. Those medicines cause *addiction* not rebound headaches. Rebound pain is a consequence of your brain having gotten used to some of the effects of the medicine; for example, triptans increase blood pressure by constricting blood vessels—similarly to caffeine. When you have a triptan rebound headache, a cup of coffee may be in order. Some medicines make your brain forget how to kick in its own painkillers so your brain becomes *dependent* on them. The pain is caused by the *lack of neurotransmitters* that previously have always been provided by the medicine—the reduction of SSRIs (Selective Serotonin Reuptake Inhibitors) is well-known to cause this type of pain. Pain caused by your brain's inability to make a neurotransmitter because of the lack of a medicine will not respond to treatments other than taking more of that medicine. To get rid of this sort of a rebound pain, one needs to grit her teeth and go through a few very harsh pain-days or even weeks before one is free from the rebound effects[21]. It is not an easy thing to do. The Stanton Migraine Protocol® was devised with rebound pain prevention in mind: it is medicine-free and can help hasten rebound recovery but cannot remove the suffering associated with the rebound pain.

There are rebound pains that all people can experience, all people who are habituated to drinking coffee or tea or caffeinated sodas. They have nothing to do with pain medicine, they are prompted by not drinking coffee or tea or caffeinated sodas. Caffeine is a vasoconstrictor (constricts blood vessels), thereby increasing the pressure with which your blood travels in your arteries and blood vessels. In plain English: caffeine increases your blood pressure. When you forget to have your daily dose of caffeine you may suffer a headache. This headache is a rebound pain from the *lack of caffeine*. Your blood pressure is not increasing and may even drop lower than normal as a result of your body's realization that the anticipated caffeine is not arriving.

It is not just your taste buds or alertness that is going to miss the caffeine. When you drink caffeine, your heart changes! With caffeine, you tighten up the pipes (arteries and veins). The heart gets used to having to press hard against the narrowed pipes through which it has to pump the blood. Now consider a day when you don't drink any caffeinated beverages. Suddenly the arteries and blood vessels are relaxed. Your blood volume has not changed but you appear to have less volume as the existing blood volume takes up less space in a wider artery. With wider arteries and veins than before and the unchanged amount of blood, your heart has a harder time to get blood equally everywhere with the lower blood pressure. This is a common reason for feeling dizzy! If you have only been drinking one coffee a day, your heart will have an easier time to return to its normal operation because it has not adapted to a big change. However, if you drink coffee, caffeinated tea, or soda all day long, rest assured that your heart has adapted and changed. If you suddenly stop all caffeine, your blood pressure will drop significantly, enough to perhaps land you in the hospital.

Even from occasional caffeine, when you stop drinking it, your heart will be in trouble for a short time and will mess your blood pressure up, which then could lead to a headache. When we are talking about rebound headaches, it is not just one thing that causes the problem but it is a chain of events, like dominos falling one by one until they all fall, resulting in a rebound pain. As painful as a rebound pain is, it need not be dangerous. However, there are rebound effects that are dangerous—this is referred to as "discontinuation syndrome". For example, taking and then stopping medicines that inhibit certain brain neuron sensors (such as SSRIs or others in its family, like SNRIs, and voltage gated sodium or calcium channel blockers), as well as heart medications that are prescribed for migraines, may result in a medical emergency. You will find more on this later in the *Drugs of Shame* section in Part IV.

An additional type of rebound pain can be caused by anti-anxiety medicines. Migraineurs all suffer from anxiety, only the degree to which they suffer differs. The best medicines for anxiety are long-acting benzodiazepines. Doctors often prescribe benzodiazepines incorrectly, causing severe problems. There are many benzodiazepines but only two have long half-lives in the body (the time it takes for half of the medicine to be used up by the body): Valium (Diazepam) and Klonopin (Clonazepam). These medicines have a half-life of between 36 and 50 hours. That means that a prescribing doctor should limit their use to once per day or once per every two days, to avoid a buildup of the medicine in the patient's body. I have found that many doctors have no idea about the half-life of these drugs and prescribe them for use 2 or even 3 times a day. If you consider a 2-per-day dose for a drug with a half-life of 2 days, then your actual dose is 4-6 medicines a day, as the first pill has not reached half its potency before you have already taken 3 or more other pills. Taking benzodiazepines this way will cause major addiction problems. As a matter of fact, benzodiazepines are starting to be restricted because of the misuse (by those addicted as a result of the wrong prescription information) of these medicines. Short half-life benzodiazepines are also often prescribed but since they need to be taken 2-3 times per day, they cause major addiction. These short-acting benzodiazepines usually have a very fast "high" and a very fast "crash" leaving the migraineur both craving and also in anxiety. Lorazepam is an example of such short acting benzodiazepines.

Can you tell when you have a rebound pain or a genuine migraine? Most people cannot since pain is pain, but remember: a rebound pain is only a bad headache! It is not preceded by a prodrome and is not accompanied by other symptoms of migraine. It is simply a pain resulting from the removal of a drug.

Tension Headache

Tension (or stress) headache, as the name suggests, derives from a tension or stress situation you are exposed to. Stress can have external sources, like your boss, the traffic, or the nightly TV news. It can also have internal sources, like an illness you came down with, or a bug your body is fighting, or skipping a meal, even without your awareness. For example, a party may cause a tension headache due to all of the stress involved—weddings are famous for this for everyone involved in the preparation, especially on the wedding day—including the bride.

Stress or tension headaches are brought on by excitatory hormonal changes, such as increased adrenaline, cortisol and other stress hormones that evolved to respond to things unexpected and dangerous. Whatever the cause, a stress headache is "only" a pain. This is not to minimize the pain but to emphasize that there are no prodromes associated with it. This type of headache, however bad it gets, usually responds to an over the counter medicine, a massage, a relaxing hot bath, calming music, a cold or hot drink, a cold or warm shower, stepping out for some fresh air, or eating in case of a skipped meal. Stress headaches can be caused by hormonal shifts due to emotional trauma. The Stanton Migraine Protocol® has been used successfully to stop these tension headaches. It is possible because hormonal shifts may cause biochemical imbalance via the Renin Angiotensin Aldosterone System, which responds to hormonal shifts and which modulates the body's electrolytes[22,23]. Providing electrolyte support via the Stanton Migraine Protocol® can reverse the imbalance.

This type of pain may be anywhere in the head though typically the entire head feels squeezed—forehead pain is often the start. You may also feel feverish when having no fever, the pain is often throbbing, and can shift its location.

Illnesses such as simple colds, or flu, as well as surgeries and other conditions your body finds stressful can bring on a strong tension or stress headache that can last for days. These headaches may not respond to a pain medicine because the reason for the headache is an internal battle by the body's immune system. In cases like this, particularly if a tummy bug is involved, Gramma's legendary chicken soup is your best treatment; it is a perfect electrolyte. I usually have some kept frozen as single-serving broths, with all the wholesome goodness of a full chicken soup that I have prepared myself—forget about the canned, pre-cooked variety; that's just salty and sugary water with a lot of fillers and preservatives.

Sinus Headache

Sinus infection can cause a major headache as well as face pain. Sinus headaches are hard to distinguish from trigeminal neuralgia (see in a later section) since essentially the same head region hurts.

One of the most typical signs of a sinus headache is that if you bend your head forward toward the ground, the pain gets much worse—this is not so in the case of migraine or trigeminal neuralgia, so if you are confused about what you have, test it. Although the pain can also increase with other headaches if you bend your head down, the pain change in other types of headaches in this downward head position is minor compared with the pain increase of a sinus headache. If you bend down and wish someone would chop your head off, you are having a sinus headache. In case of sinus infection, bending your head down will increase pain in your forehead and sinus cavities, so it will be an all-encompassing face and forehead pain, sometimes even the top of the head will hurt. You may even feel pain in your teeth and wish to have your teeth pulled, it can be so intense. I know some people who ended up at the dentist thinking they needed a root canal; the sinus pain had been so bad.

Although sinus infections often come with stuffed up nose, sometimes your sinuses feel dry in spite of being infected. Just another quirk of sinus infection—a conflict: being stuffed up but no runny nose (at least at the beginning). Use a saline jet (not a regular weak spray) to rinse your nasal cavity. Don't use Neti Pot; it is not sterile unless you are committed to boiling the bottle after every single use. Blow really hard, one nostril at a time after you have soaked your sinus with saline for about 15-30 seconds. You will feel the mucus loosening up. It is gross, so bend over a sink.

Sinus infections can also be caused by allergies. The best way to get rid of sinus infections is to prevent them by frequent use of the saline jet in high allergy season. Keeping your mucous membranes moist traps pollen and thereby prevents sinus inflammation. Use the saline jet upon the first signs of an infection, and use it several times a day as long as it takes and you are in the clear. Many people rely upon antibiotics for a sinus infection; they may kill the bacteria but will not clean your sinuses.

Cervicogenic Headache

Cervicogenic headache is really a referred headache (secondary headache) that is often misdiagnosed as a migraine. A secondary headache means that the physiological source of the pain is somewhere else in the body. The most distinguishing feature of cervicogenic pain is that it starts in the back of the head and neck area.

Cervicogenic headaches are caused either by a pinched nerve in the neck or shoulders or upper back, are the result of tense muscles, or degenerated discs, or are postural. Postural pain can be caused by, for example, slouching in front of the computer too long, having a pillow that doesn't support your head right or positioning the pillow wrong, or a very common cause is exercising (specifically yoga and weight lifting) without holding a "perfect form".

This type of headache may or may not respond to massage or relaxation since the cause may be pinched nerves that require physical therapy and/or surgery. Usually OTC medicines work upon the first sensation of the pain but if that window of opportunity is missed, a major headache will follow. It may even morph into a migraine as a result of not keeping up with proper hydration and nutrition while in pain. I found that using a strong rounded hard object as a tool to press on the area of the spasm can release a cervicogenic pain before it starts. The trick is to find the exact spasm spot.

Cluster headaches

Cluster headaches are the most painful headaches one can have. Cluster headaches are also called "ice pick" headaches in addition to "suicide headaches" (the names are descriptive!). The pain may only last for a short stab but it is repeated with some frequency, from a few seconds to minutes between stabs. The pains from a single episode of cluster headache can go on for a few hours to several weeks. There are many members in my migraine group who also have cluster headaches. They seem to get some relief from the Stanton Migraine Protocol® by reducing the many weeks of hell to a few days of hell, and the pain's intensity is also reduced but not to zero—so far only one cluster headache sufferer achieved full relief.

Cluster headaches are not known to have prodromes or symptoms other than the stabbing pain, usually in or behind one eye, albeit some members of my migraine group report that they also experience some prodromes. I have suffered through what I call mini-cluster headaches a couple of times: to me it felt like someone just put a burning pen in my eye—one eye—with the feeling of a blood vessel in your eye popping open. You cannot help but jump from a pain like that. There is a large overlap between migraine and cluster headache sufferers. Those with prodromes perhaps experience both cluster headaches and migraines at the same time. Some members in my group who get cluster headaches often suffer unnecessarily due to lack of therapeutic oxygen. Oxygen helps, particularly if the pain is caught in time to prevent a cluster headache[24-26]. Regrettably, many healthcare providers lack this knowledge. Often resources are so scarce that fighting for oxygen for home-use (particularly outside of the US) is extremely hard.

Trigeminal Neuralgia

Some headache types are more likely to be misdiagnosed as migraine than others. Trigeminal neuralgia is one of the headaches that is most often misdiagnosed as migraine.

The best way to differentiate migraines from trigeminal neuralgia is by focusing on the direction of the pain. With migraines, the pain is on one side of the head—typically between a temple and a spot above the ear. The pain feels to have originated inside of the head, radiating towards the outside. Placing cold on the affected side of the head feels good.

By contrast, a trigeminal neuralgia event starts as a face pain. It is a pain in which touching your face feels painful—so applying cold is too painful. Unlike migraine, the direction of the pain is from the outside in. In this case, it is the nerve endings on your face (it can involve the entire face causing jaw pain and tooth ache) that hurt. These are nerves that connect to the trigeminal nerve in the brain—it is where the brain stem enters the brain. It is not fully understood what causes this kind of nerve sensitivity—some researchers theorize of a possible nerve pinch in the trigeminal area—hence the name trigeminal neuralgia. In any case, this pain is not a migraine as the cause of the pain is very different from migraines and is not preceded by prodromes.

Occipital Neuralgia

Occipital Neuralgia, or ON as just about everyone refers to it, is an unusual health condition in which the nerve between the eye and the occipital cortex (back of the brain, the visual lobe) is damaged and hurts. This is another form of headache that is frequently misdiagnosed either as migraine or as cluster headache. The damage can be genetic or caused by an illness or brain injury, or even by medicines. The fluoroquinolone class of antibiotics, such as Cipro or Levaquin, and many more, are well-known causes of ON and they are now required to be labeled as being such since ON is a permanent nerve damage[27].

ON can be extremely painful, and since it is a nerve damage, there is no cure as of yet though caught early, the damage may be reversible. It is not a migraine, though many doctors classify it as such because the pain is similar to migraines. Except in addition to a migraine-type pain on one or both sides, over the eyes at the forehead with pain moving toward the back of the head, behind the ears and also in the neck, ON sufferers may experience cluster headache like pain as well. ON has no prodromes but the pain can be excruciating. The only known symptom treatment that works for some individuals is a nerve-block. The damaged nerve is injected from the back of the head with a nerve blocking agent.

Unfortunately, ON can lead to blindness. Although there is no known cure, there is a possibility to prevent further nerve damage by removing major nerve irritants. One of the biggest nerve irritants is sugar. In later sections I discuss diets that help rebuild neurons.

Abdominal Migraine & Cycling Vomiting Syndrome

Although these are called "migraine," they are not "yet". They represent very common signs of the migraine-brain in its development toward being a more sensitive brain with more neuronal connections[28] and it is accompanied by increased serotonin release[29]. I would call abdominal migraine and cycling vomiting syndromes two of the three signals that the person will turn into a migraineur—the others being the onset of anxiety and panic attacks. Therefore, since the migraine-brain is in the process of being "built," abdominal migraine and cyclic vomiting syndrome represent the time when the genetic switch is expressed. I had all of these when I was 10 years old but I didn't yet have migraines. This paragraph will make more and more sense as you continue reading this book.

I have had Hemiplegic, Status, Silent and Chronic Migraines. It took a while before I was even diagnosed as I had two bad Hemiplegic episodes, went to the doctor and they didn't know what it was. They were triggered by women's perfumes at work which caused me to basically be paralyzed. I could hardly talk, walk, think, or move. My brain was impaired; it was crazy. When I explained this to Dr. A she told me what it was and why it is so hard to diagnose. I have Hashimoto's and Hypothyroidism as well of which I just found out about. But when I came in the group I was having 18 migraines or better a month taking 4 or more abort meds plus I was having seizures and blood sugar issues, which she brought up during my Analysis and I remembered it I was hypoglycemic during one seizure when I was taken to the hospital after a series of seizures. When she suggested that I monitor my sugar, I found that it was running high and she helped me with what foods to eat and not eat. The Stanton Migraine Protocol helped me get off of the abort drugs and reduced my daily medicine in half because of Dr. Stanton. Because of my Hashimoto's I did find that iodine and I are not friends and certain foods make me ill and tired so I am still playing around with my foods. But I am so very thankful for Dr. Stanton and her time and her Admins' time as well. This is an Awesome program and group. Thank you for saving me when no one else could... You're the Bomb Diggity Angela..

--Pam Peterson Sayne
Member of the Facebook Migraine Group

Do You Have Other Symptoms Beside Pain?

If you are a migraineur, your symptoms are not just pain. Migraine is not a headache. You may have aura (20% of migraineurs do as per official statistics but I believe that number is an underestimation[30]), or vertigo (which is not the same as dizziness; vertigo means you fall over like a log with everything spinning around you). You could have dizziness (sea legs that may last a long time and may be called Mel de Beurre), irritable bowel syndrome (IBS), anxiety, nausea; you may throw up, cannot talk, stutter suddenly, or forget who or where you are at a given moment. Half of your body may suddenly experience temporary paralysis (people fall off staircases and end up with serious injuries as a result). You may find that one side of your face is droopy or you may slur speech as if you have had a stroke, you may not be able to tolerate lights or sounds or smells (including food smells). You may be yawning non-stop; your blood pressure may suddenly shoot sky high then drop low just a moment later; your pulse may race like you have just run a Marathon, even though you have been sitting in your chair. You may have restless leg syndrome (RLS). You may lose your ability to hear, you may not recognize family or friends, your shoes and rings may become too tight to remove or too loose and they fall off, you may even lose your sight temporarily or may begin hearing sounds and seeing things that only you can hear or see. You may become argumentative or overly happy and energized the day before. You may be vomiting for two days straight without having anything physically wrong with your stomach. This is a partial list of things that may happen, and note I have not even gotten to the headache aspect of migraine. The headache is the last thing the migraineur may experience, and it usually lasts 72 or more hours, non-stop, without responding to any medicine, followed by a postdrome, which is brain fog, forgetfulness, lack of the ability to think clearly, and extreme fatigue.

Unfortunately, the general public is uninformed and believes that migraine is just another headache. Use every opportunity you come across to enlighten people that this is a false belief.

Migraines

Migraines are "one-sided" meaning they hurt only on one side of the head. As mentioned before, migraines typically start between the temple and the area above one ear. Migraines don't start with pain. Migraines always have one or more prodromes and always end with postdromes. There are hundreds of possible prodromes. A list of a few of them I provided earlier; the description of many of them is provided in Section 3 of Part II.

The pain on one side is stationary; it feels like it is pinned there. It may feel like a sore, a reopened wound. The pain is intense but does not pulsate or throb. It is a constant pain with the same strength and at the same location for usually three to five consecutive days. Before the pain period, excess urination, vomiting, diarrhea or constipation, as well as being nauseated by any smell, light, sound, or touch are extremely common. During the pain period eating or drinking is difficult because of constant nausea and frequent vomiting. Dizziness and vertigo may continue all through the pain period. All neurological effects may continue during the pain, such as slurred speech, or paralyzed half body for hemiplegic migraineurs. However, there is usually no aura during the pain period.

After the pain lifts, a major "fog" settles over the migraineur with memory loss, communication troubles, extreme exhaustion, and dehydration—this is postdrome that may last for several days. If during the pain period there was no urination, the first urination is a sign of the migraine letting up. If there was constipation, the first bowel movement is a sign that the pain is over. (Why this is the case is a subject for a later section.)

Therefore, migraine is not a pain but a series of phases that often happen to have a pain phase in the middle—but pain is not a requirement. The prodrome and postdrome periods for a migraine can be more debilitating than the pain itself.

Auras

Auras are only associated with visual disturbances in this book, even though many medical facilities mistakenly include other symptoms in their definition of the word. Not all migraineurs have auras but with the confusing definition of what an aura is many migraineurs are misdiagnosed. This can present a real danger since aura migraineurs have a 10% higher risk of strokes[31-33]. Auras very specifically represent a flow of current across the brain and what you see is what your occipital lobe (the region of the brain that normally recognizes the patterns your eyes see) recognizes as a result of the stimulation by the current flow. What you see is a pattern of activated neurons—this discussed in detail in Part III, Section 4. The blind spot corresponds to a brain region that is without enough voltage to function—hence that is a true blind area. Auras are visible with eyes closed or open. You see what is happening in your brain. Auras are in one eye only but it is really hard to see that since they are visualized with closed or opened eyes. Thus closing one eye to see if it is affected will not help in deciding which eye is affected.

A few more words about the confusing definitions of auras are in order. Auras are strictly visual phenomena. Nevertheless, in many online sites (and even in some academic journal publications) auras also include auditory or other sensations, such as heightened sensitivity to smells, sounds, numbness, tingling, inability to speak, etc. These are not auras but prodromes, just like aura itself is a prodrome. Many migraineurs don't have auras. A study identified 38% of migraineurs with aura[34], while another only 15%-20%[35]. Because so many aura types are not in popular knowledge, the number of aura migraineurs is under-reported and therefore under-estimated. Surveying my migraine group, I found few migraineurs who have never experienced auras, though most don't have auras with all of their migraines.

Part II

How to Anticipate and Stop a Migraine

Section 3

Stop Your Migraine Now

Read in 24 hrs too gripped to take a break. All the things about my migraines that I understood or suspected, together with all those I hadn't understood or considered were pulled together into such clear unmitigated sense that I knew it would work before I even started to test it.

--Fiona Horan
Member of the Facebook Migraine Group

Preventing migraines requires that you recognize and understand the signs your body gives you. Most often your body shows how it feels about the foods you eat and the drinks you drink. It may also react to barometric pressure changes, temperature changes, brightness, noise, places full of people, impatient bosses, unruly kids, traffic on the road with road-rage drivers, etc. By far the most prominent migraine cause is carbohydrate consumption. This is just a sample of the many things that can trigger a migraine. You must develop your own "shortlist" of what you are sensitive to and watch out for them in order to notice what can and will go wrong, upsetting your balance, and causing migraines. Migraine is not an emotional disturbance, although many doctors mistakenly think it is "mental" and it is all "in your head" (heh… it is ... it hurts there...). In reality, it is the result of an overstimulated brain running low on energy. Of course, we cannot stop the noise or kick the traffic in the butt. However, we can change how our body reacts to its surroundings by ensuring that even if we are overstimulated, our brain can keep up with the demand. To accomplish this feat, you will require determination, the mastery of the prevention steps, and some awareness of the people around you. The reasoning behind the necessary measures will be explained in Part III. Here you will find actual, practical steps for how to stop a migraine in its tracks when you are about to come down with one.

How to Abort a Migraine

Upon recognizing the start of a prodrome you need to act quickly:

- **Grab a very little bit of salt**—a few small crystals—and **place it under your tongue**. Do not talk, do not move your tongue, and do not drink. Pay attention to what you feel.

As the salt enters your blood very fast, it will make you feel either better or worse or you will feel no change.

- Hearing cracks, pops, like an old engine is cranking up for the first time in 20 years? Super! You are salt deficient!
- Is your pain easing up a bit or your aura lessening a bit? Super! You are salt deficient!

If your pain is easing after the salt test and if you don't mind the taste of salt, take 1/8th of a teaspoon of salt and drink a sip of water with that, just enough to swallow it. If you dislike the taste of salt eat 10 olives or a salt pickle or take a salt pill—details on salt pills later**.**

- Feeling worse than before from the little bit of salt under your tongue?

Spit out the salt, rinse your mouth, and grab some potassium containing food like avocado, salmon, steak, pistachio nuts, or milk. Don't drink sport drinks and do not take a potassium supplement!

- Feeling neutral? Neither worse nor better? There are 2 possibilities:

1. One is that you have not had enough water, so think back how much water you have drunk today. Most

migraineurs drink too little water. **If you typically drink less than 8 glasses of water (the absolute minimum for standard weight and activity adults), you are not sufficiently hydrated, so drink 1 glass of water now.**

2. The second reason could be that you did not eat enough or skipped a meal for the day. **If you ate next to nothing all day, you may be low in nutrition!** Drink whole milk (it has carbohydrate, protein, and fat to give you a full spectrum of nutrients) or eat a piece of cheese or a bite of fatty meat.

Common Direct Causes of Migraines

You may wonder about some of the items on this list; all of them will be thoroughly explained in the rest of the book.

1. Not drinking enough water. Use any online calculator to evaluate how much water you need a day. If you drink much less than what you calculate, increase your daily water intake at a slow rate, not faster than half a glass per day. If you are not online, determine your daily minimum water intake by calculating 55% of your weight in pounds. This is the minimum amount of water in fluid ounces you need. So if you weigh 150 pounds, your minimum water need is 82.5 oz or upon dividing by 8 (8 oz per glass) it is 10.3 glasses of water

(this formula is generally used by all in the migraine groups and it seems to give optimal results).

2. Drinking too many cups of coffee. Coffee's caffeine constricts blood vessels and increases blood pressure. It also dehydrates and with the urine salt also leaves your body. Drink no more than one small cup of coffee a day. If you drink more than that, reduce gradually. Don't quit cold turkey as that may drop your blood pressure too quickly, making you feel ill.
3. Drinking teas. Teas (even herbals and decaf) are diuretic plus the caffeine in teas lasts longer in your blood that that of the caffeine in coffee, constricting your blood vessels longer than coffee. Migraineurs should avoid all teas. If you drink herbal or decaf, just quit. If you drink regular, reduce slowly by half a cup a day max.
4. Eating or drinking sweetened foods or beverages. Sweeteners, whether real, artificial, or natural, are migraine trouble.
5. Eating a diet high in carbohydrates—carbohydrates are not just sugary stuff but also fruits, vegetables, grains, nuts, and seeds.
6. Drinking water before, with, or after carbohydrates.
7. Not having enough salt or potassium in your diet.
8. Drinking smoothies, shakes, juices, sodas, or alcohol.
9. A low fat diet.

Various Migraine Emergencies

Common migraine emergencies, you may encounter:

3:30 AM Wakeup Call with Migraine

Many migraineurs awake in the wee hours of the morning to a migraine. This is so common you should know what to do about it.

Why: Migraineurs' brains have a very busy night while they sleep, with vivid dreams and often nightmares. These subconscious events interrupt a critical "brain cleaning" service that removes debris, protein fragments, glucose remnants, etc., from the brain[36,37]. Not getting a good night's sleep prevents this brain-cleaning function, which can predispose you to metabolic syndrome[38] that is prevalent among migraineurs. All this extra brain activity makes your brain run out of voltage in the middle of the night, usually between 3:30 am and 4: 30 am.

What to do: To prevent such an early morning migraine, before you go to sleep you need to give a dose of energy to your brain that lasts through your regular sleeping time. In the Stanton Migraine Protocol® this consists of two such elements:

1) **A glass of whole milk (can be mixed with a little heavy cream for extra fat) or cheese or some protein, such as a few bites of meat or an egg if sensitive to milk, taken about an hour before bed.**
2) **15 – 30 minutes before you lie horizontal take 1/8th of a teaspoon of salt or a salt pill with an entire glass of water (8 oz).**

Salt pill: there are many reasons why you need to increase salt in your diet, which will be detailed in later sections. I have found that, on average, the best dose of salt to take to prevent the morning migraine is 1/8th of a teaspoon of fine grade table salt with a glass of water. This works very well if you like the taste of salt. While there are many migraineurs who enjoy eating salt, most migraineurs seem to dislike the taste (including me) and welcome a pill or a capsule that we can just swallow instead. You have many options for salt pills. Some are pressed pure salt (1 gr sodium chloride), which is totally fine. However, iodine is a very important element added to some salt types for improved thyroid function (assuming you don't have Hashimoto's or Grave's disease). Iodine is not commonly found in salt supplements. I designed a salt supplement that includes iodine. It is available through a company with which I am not financially affiliated:

https://www.healthbyprinciple.com/. Should you be on low budget, you can create your own salt pills by purchasing empty capsules and grinding table salt (with iodine) down to powder. Fill up each capsule. This may be time consuming but is certainly the least expensive method other than simply eating salt.

Taking a salt pill at night definitely beats having to measure out 1/8th of a teaspoon of salt and then choke on its (to me) horrible taste! If you cannot have iodine, there are many options for you. At the time I write this book, the only salt supplement available with iodine is the one I designed. It contains 360 mg sodium and 15 mcg iodine.

This special nutrient cocktail of milk, followed by salt with water before sleep, will support your nutritional needs throughout the night. Many migraineurs have followed my example by adding heavy cream (whipping cream without sugar or any sweetener) to their evening milk to enrich the brain support—about 1-2 oz cream added to 6-7 oz whole milk is great. Also, since you take salt before sleep as well, you will not need to get up – or at least not as frequently – to urinate in the middle of the night. Try it, this really works!

Morning Hydration

One of the most important steps in migraine prevention is proper hydration in the morning. Take a salt pill, or 1/8th of a teaspoon of salt, and a glass (8 oz) of water the moment you open your eyes, even while you are still in bed (keep salt and water on your night stand). By the time you head for breakfast, your brain is fully energized and hydrated with salt and water. These steps — evening milk and salt with water, and morning salt with water — are foundational elements of the Stanton Migraine Protocol®.

Special note: Always drink up 8 oz of water at once, and do not sip. Never drink more than one 8 oz glass of water at a time. If your water need is high, please drink a glass of water more frequently but never drink 2 glasses at once. The only exception to this rule is after an endurance workout, where you may need to quickly replenish your water and salt. In that case you can drink up to 3 glasses of water maximum at once with 2 salt pills or ¼ teaspoon salt. The added salt is essential, otherwise you leach nutrients out of your electrolyte and end up getting hurt. There are many phone apps to help you measure how much water you have already drunk and how much more you still need to drink the rest of the day.

Ate Sweets

You had a party last night for your child's birthday, you were at a wedding, or you simply could not resist that cookie or that tub of ice cream. You may have had too much champagne, a giant bowl of pasta, or some similar food "adventure". Now you have a migraine. What to do?

What you cannot afford to do after eating too much carbohydrates – sweets and desserts, alcoholic beverages, fruits, starchy vegetables, and grains are all carbs – is drinking water and waiting until the pain starts. Never drink water right before, with, or after a meal with carbohydrates in it. Be prepared and have salt pills or salt packets with you all the time. **After eating or drinking carbohydrates, you will be thirsty: DON'T DRINK! Take a salt pill with just a sip of water, but no more than a sip, and wait.** Within 5-10 minutes of taking salt, your thirst will vanish. After the salt pill, after you stopped urinating, as your thirst vanishes you can return to drinking water.

Myth: they always tell you to drink when you are thirsty. This is not true for migraineurs. Do not follow this advice!

In future sections I explain this in much more detail but here it is in short: migraineurs have an exacerbated response to carbohydrate consumption. Carbohydrates, as they turn to glucose, remove water and sodium from the cells[39] and that's why you feel thirsty. However, since sodium was also removed, the water you drink cannot stay inside the cells so you will remain thirsty. Drinking water at this time can leach more nutrients out of your cells and actually increases your chances for a migraine. In extreme cases people even get water toxicity. When you are thirsty you should take a little salt to bring the water removed by carbohydrates back into your cells. Your thirst will stop.

Hormonal Migraines

You are about to get your menstrual period and you always get a migraine several days before. Detailed explanation about how and why this happens comes later; here just learn what to do. About 5 days before your period, you enter the premenstrual phase (PMS). Signs are moodiness, unreasonable stubbornness, craving sweets, feeling bloated, and a migraine may start any minute.

Prevention: about 5 days before your period, and all through your period, increase your hydration by one glass of water and one salt pill a day. Do not eat sugar, no matter how much you crave it. This will provide the energy for your brain throughout your period.

Perimenopausal Hormonal Migraines

Myth: when you reach menopause, your migraines will vanish. This is exactly as true as when you were told that your migraines will vanish after you had children. It isn't true at all. Not only will you not have your migraines reduce in intensity or frequency, they may increase instead. With perimenopause also comes irregularity in the timing of your cycle. Therefore, you may not know when your period is about to start, causing a problem. In the previous paragraph I explained how 5 days prior to your period you need to start to prepare. However, if your cycle becomes irregular, how do you know which day exactly you have to start the prevention process?

The problem is easier to solve than you think. The female body—especially the face—changes in attractiveness during the fertile period (around ovulation); it becomes more symmetrical, eyes appear bigger and wider apart, cheeks a little rosier, neck thinner and longer, pimples magically disappear, lips appear a bit fuller[40,41], etc. Men notice this change[42] and so if you cannot see the difference, ask a male friend, relative, or spouse to observe your face. **The best way to do this is to take selfies for a month every day, upload the pictures to your computer, date them, and place them side by side.** If you cannot see any difference, your friends can. Alternatively, you can also check your own preference for male faces! Many studies show that females change their preference and are attracted to more masculine and higher testosterone males during their ovulation and less masculine and lower testosterone males prior to and during their period[43]. To see some sample images, search the web for the sentence "facial asymmetry during menstrual cycles" and observe the hundreds of images placed side by side—both men and women—so you can check where you stand. The most well-known female and male images for demonstrating the differences can be found here:

http://d1vn86fw4xmcz1.cloudfront.net/content/royptb/366/1571/1638/F3.large.jpg

You really can find out when your cycles start even if they are irregular.

Travel Migraine

Migraineurs fear travel and for good reasons. Airplanes are depressurized for high altitude flight and re-pressurized to low altitude prior to landing. Coping with these sudden changes gives migraineurs a very difficult time. At 3000-5000 feet (the altitudes for which many commercial flights are depressurized) you have somewhat less oxygen to breathe. Your blood vessels expand in the reduced pressure. The increase in diameter of your blood vessels means vasodilation, so the blood volume that filled your blood vessels up perfectly while still on the ground, no longer does so. The result is lower blood pressure. Since the blood pressure of most migraineurs is already low; further reduction is undesired. The goal then is to increase the volume of your blood for the duration of the flight. The procedure is as follows:

- After you have passed through security – where you had to get rid of all your water – purchase a big bottle of water before you get to the gate. Take a salt pill or salt packet and drink 8 oz of water with it. If you have more than an hour before your flight takes off, drink another glass of water without salt before the plane takes off, and then one more, with salt, while the plane is taking off.

- During the flight drink a glass of water and take a small amount of salt approximately every two hours. If you have salt pills take one with every 2nd or 3rd glass of water—depending on flight length. Every 4th hour also take potassium, as food and not supplement, with salt (salted nuts will do) and a glass of water. You need to be drinking a glass of water every 2 hours and with each glass alternate between just salt or salt plus potassium.
- If you have food served, choose cheese, leafy greens, and low carb options like nuts; avoid starchy veggies and fruits because of their high carb content. Drink only water or milk and maximum a single cup of coffee. Coffee helps in constricting your blood vessels, thereby increasing your blood pressure. Just remember that caffeine has a half-life of 6 hours, so if you are going for a 2-hour flight, don't drink coffee!
- About an hour before landing, stop drinking, stop taking salt, and eat only potassium (e.g., unsalted raw nuts of any kind). Do not drink more water. When you land, you will have to run to the toilet since your body is now releasing the extra water. All will be fine!

Sometimes you travel by car. The procedure is the same: driving up the hill you need to drink water and take salt and coming down the hill you need to eat potassium rich nuts. The difference is the speed with which the pressure changes given your altitude changes. You may drive through smaller hills or larger hills. You need to pay close attention to your altitude. The higher the altitude, the lower the pressure and the more hydration you will need.

In The Sun

Migraineurs do not tolerate heat and light as well as non-migraineurs do. Thus, whenever you go in the sun, wet your head, wear a hat, sit under an umbrella for shade, wear dark sun glasses, and always have salt and water ready. Hydrate frequently but do not sip water; that will only hydrate your tongue. Drink a glass of water every time you drink, and only sip if the humidity is very low but also drink your glass of water on schedule in addition to sipping.

Exercise and Migraine

Myth: Exercise will avert a migraine. Although most migraineurs do not even dare thinking of exercise before they start the Stanton Migraine Protocol®, as they start feeling better they also start to get back to real life and the temptation to exercise grows stronger. Exercise causes sweating and migraineurs are sensitive to dehydration. Notice how after exercise even your blood vessels move closer to your skin and are more prominently visible—this assists the body in cooling. Therefore, it is vital to have plenty of water and salt with you, both before and after exercise, depending on how much you sweat. There is also a potential issue with low blood pressure as most migraineurs have sub-normal blood pressure. Blood carries vital oxygen to the lungs and other organs—including the brain. With low blood pressure, it takes more effort to circulate the blood for the increased oxygen requirement of the exercise. So, start slow and build up gradually to more challenging levels. This allows your body to naturally reach its optimum work-out equilibrium. Taking 1/8th teaspoon salt with a glass of water about 30 minutes **before your exercise** will increase blood volume and enhance your oxygen delivering ability.

Not every exercise is equally good for migraineurs. For instance, yoga and weight lifting are two exercise routines during which holding your head and upper body in proper position is critical. Many migraineurs end up with cervicogenic headaches (not migraines) as a result of bad posture and strain on their neck, upper back, or shoulders. This type of pain starts in the neck and the back of the head and moves forward. This is not a migraine but can turn into one. Prevent it by focusing on the correct "form" as you exercise—and try different exercises.

One of the first things a migraineur should do is to train her heart and head to be able to adjust to the changes in blood pressure that occur before, during, and after exercise. Since migraineurs have a more intricate circulatory system and lower blood pressure than normal, their pulse can run too high for comfort. A higher pulse is exactly how the body compensates for low blood pressure in order to ensure the availability of adequate oxygen levels. You need to calculate your maximum heart rate and take between 70% - 85% of that value to arrive at the pulse rate you should have for aerobic training. This is age dependent so use this formula: 220 – your age = maximum heart rate for men and 202 – 80% of your age = maximum heart rate for women. During aerobic activity for training your heart, you want to start your pulse at about 70% of your maximum heart rate and increase it gradually up to 85%. To illustrate: for a female age 40: 202 - 80% of 40 = 202 – 32 = 170 is your maximum heart rate. For the recommended aerobic rate calculate 70% and 85% of your maximum heart rate ➔ 170 x 0.7 = 119; 170 x 0.85 = 144.5. So for a woman of age 40 the aerobic heart rate should be between 119 and 145. As you start your exercise program, make sure to have salt and water or milk with you for the after-exercise recovery. Many high school sport programs offer pickle juice to athletes on hot days—if you like pickle juice, make sure it is brine and not vinegar based pickle juice!

During the workout you don't want to drink a whole glass of water since it may give you discomfort, so sip salted water but only if it is very hot or you are an endurance athlete. If you run or row or bicycle outdoors, put 1/8th of a teaspoon of salt into a bottle of 24 oz water and sip that during your run or outdoor sweating activity. Drink up after you are finished as you are cooling off. Never forget to take salt with you! You will always need it!

Protein Shakes

Never drink a protein shake or any shake or smoothie. They all convert to glucose quickly kicking you out of electrolyte homeostasis.

You may end up with a migraine before, during, or after your exercise. If you want to take protein before workout, have some meat or fish (canned tuna is one of the highest in protein so have some). Always eat whole foods instead of powder, liquid, or supplement equivalents because their metabolic pathway is different.

Full Moon and Migraine

While I have a big section with full explanation on this elsewhere in the book, here is a brief intro: a full moon causes your sensory organs to overreact, and so you need to prepare similarly to how you prepare for your PMS. Start with extra hydration at least 3 days prior to the full moon and continue through the full moon plus one day. The extra hydration is $1/8^{th}$ teaspoon salt (or a salt pill) and one extra glass of water. It helps if you wear an eye mask during the night of the full moon to be sure your alertness is reduced.

Stomach Bug or Food Poisoning

It is often hard to distinguish a migraine prodrome from a tummy bug or food poisoning since they come with very similar symptoms. If you are vomiting and have diarrhea, your fluid loss is large. It really doesn't matter if you ended up losing all that fluid as a result of a tummy bug, or food poisoning, or a migraine prodrome. The fact is you are dehydrated. This can happen very fast so pay attention. If you cannot hold any fluid down for more than 4 hours and you are still having diarrhea (by this time it is clear like water) and still vomiting, however little, it is time to head to the ER for IV supplementation. This happened to me during a bout of stomach flu, and within 4 hours I was so dehydrated that I needed two IV bags (half a gallon or 8 glasses of electrolytes). This indicates how much fluid is actually lost—it's more than most people would imagine—and the loss is not just water but also sodium, potassium, magnesium, calcium, and glucose!

A Quick test of your fluid loss: Press one of your nails down with a finger to make the blood run out of it. If you have on nail polish, press a finger into your skin on your arm anywhere where you can see it. Press in deep until you see all the blood running out of it. Now lift your finger and count until the blood returns. **If the speed with which the blood returns is 2 seconds or less, you are fine. If it is 3 seconds or more, head to the ER. If it is more than 5 second, have a friend take you to ER or call the paramedics since you are severely dehydrated.**

It is time for glucose, magnesium, and calcium, in addition to potassium, salt and water—in other words full electrolyte—so a full IV is warranted. If you cannot head to the ER, this is the only time I recommend a sport drink but diluted 4:1 with salt added. That means: grab a bottle of regular sugary (not sugar substitutes!! Read labels!) sport drink that contains all of the ingredients I listed above and pour a glass a quarter full. Fill the rest of the glass up with water, **AND**, add two salt-shaker dashes of salt. **DO NOT DRINK UP!!!** It will come right back up if you do. Instead, drink one tablespoon of this electrolyte and wait 5-10 minutes. If you manage to hold that tablespoon of electrolyte down, take another and wait for a bit shorter time. When you are reliably holding the fluid down after several tablespoons and over a period of at least 20 minutes, increase your dose to 2 tablespoons and repeat what you just did. If that, too, is staying down after 20 minutes, drink 2-3 sips and wait again. Slowly increase the number of sips until you start feeling better. Your migraine will also ease. You want to drink 3 more 8 oz glasses of the above described mixture at the minimum. You will start feeling better after that.

If you have no sport drinks at home you can prepare your own emergency electrolyte drink: mix a tall 10-oz glass of water with $1/16^{th}$ of a teaspoon of salt and 2 tablespoons of a freshly squeezed orange juice with pulp. Start with spoon-drinking as described above.

Surgery Preparation

Surgery preparation requires you to go without food and often water for at least 8 hours. That kind of time frame will cause you a migraine if you don't prepare in advance. Therefore, 4-5 days before the procedure increase your water and salt by a glass a day and also drink lots of home-made bone broth or chicken soup in addition to what you eat when solid food is allowed. When you get to the time that only liquids are allowed, keep on drinking the broth—strain off all particles and drink only the liquid. You can make chicken or beef bone broth and freeze single serving sizes; they will be ready when you need them. Although you can buy broth cubes, powder, or liquid, remember that some of those have MSG in them, a headache trigger for many. Furthermore, store bought broth has no fat. When fasting, fat provides nutrition that your body can burn.

Homemade broth has fat, and this will help keep you from feeling hungry. When you get to the day that only water is allowed, put salt into your water and drink as instructed (salted water, like saline IV fluid, is OK since it absorbs). When you are prepped for the surgery, you get an IV and that will continue to hydrate you. Once your procedure is over, as hospital food is not usually migraine friendly, have a relative or friend bring you salt, high potassium nuts, and whole milk if possible. Having these instead of sugar-crazy hospital food will save you from migraines.

Note to Self (and You)

Migraine is not a disease. Only a person with a migraine-brain can get a migraine. Having a migraine-brain is not a disease, but an anatomical difference that must be understood, accepted, and appropriately nurtured. Every migraine is an independent migraine from the previous one—it need not be on the same spot or the same side of the head. A person may have different symptoms for each migraine. Nevertheless, each and every migraine you experience is caused by the same fundamental reality: an electrolyte imbalance has occurred which was brought about by one or more of the many factors we cover in this book. Although electrolyte imbalance may be caused by a variety of factors, the outcome is always a migraine for those with a migraine-brain. As we age and the migraine-brain develops, more and more distinguishing changes take place, with the result of increased migraine frequency and intensity. When one migraine goes away, if care is not taken, another migraine may just be around the corner.

Part III

Deeper Understanding of Migraines

Section 4

The Basics of Migraines

If you can't describe what you are doing as a process, you don't know what you're doing.

W. Edwards Deming

This section assumes that you – the migraineur – are not in pain, are able to concentrate, and are interested in learning more about your condition. Here I describe in layman's terms, as much as possible, both the cause and prevention of migraine. This is a very long section of the book—the heart of the book—and requires slow reading and full focus. I provide a guide to terminology where it is necessary. In this section, you will also learn about food triggers and how to prevent migraines while still eating the trigger food. I also cover various nutritional approaches, some that are counterproductive or harmful and some that are beneficial to you. This part also distinguishes between migraines for kids, men, and women of all ages, including post-menopausal women. I discuss some classes of drugs and provide a few sample brands for each class so that you can learn to identify them in the future. Full information for the most frequently prescribed drugs can be found in part IV of the book in Section 13. There are no effective migraine medicines. All medicines are thrown at migraineurs to see if they reduce the pain. Knowing in advance what you may be offered, and why you never want to take them, or if you are already taking some, knowing why you should reduce or stop the medicines altogether, is essential information. The decision to start or stop a particular medicine should always be made with the guidance of your doctor. Of course, when you are migraine free, you will have no need for any medicine. You can become completely migraine free for the rest of your life, provided you follow the guidance of this book.

Having gone to school for art and art education I remember very little from all those sciences classes I took prior to higher education. After reading the book and following the protocol for almost a year, I am grateful to finally understand what this migraine journey actually is all about from a factual and scientific view point. More importantly, I understand how to combat it in a way that makes sense and works!

--Kimberley Smith-Kovacs
A Member of the Facebook Migraine Group

Terminology

To help the reader with the scientific terminology scattered throughout the book, a few basic definitions are in order. You are not going to hurt my feelings if you decide to skim or skip this – a bit technical – section; you can always refer back to it and find a word you need help with.

Ions

Ions are atoms or molecules that are electrically charged – meaning they have an electron imbalance compared to their standard, neutral, state. If an atom or molecule lacks electron(s), it is positively charged, and if it has extra electron(s), it is a negatively charged ion. Identical polarity (+ to +) or (– to —) ions repel each other, while opposite polarity (+ to -) ions attract each other. This is very important to understand for electrolyte homeostasis, the goal of migraine prevention.

The best way to think of voltage transport is by considering an ion, either positively or negatively charged. This ion will attract an oppositely charged ion. Thus, salt can be created easily by mixing sodium: Na^+ and chloride: Cl^- ions together. The two ions will attract each other and form a neutral state salt molecule NaCl — without either positive or negative charge.

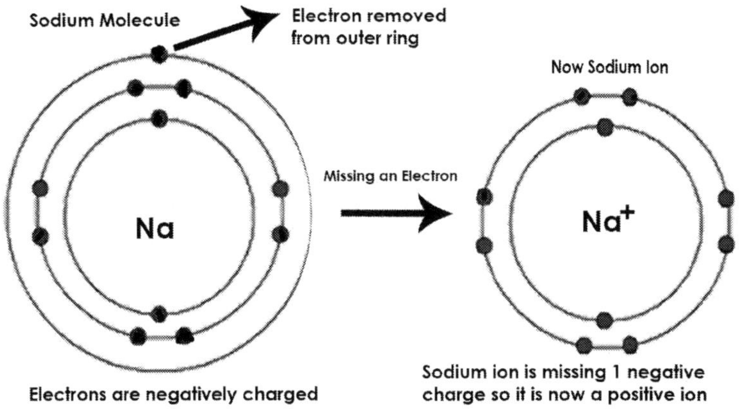

Figure 2. From neutral to ion

Ions having more than one electron differences are designated by a number and a + or – sign. The number shows how many electrons the ion needs to attract to reach a neutral state. For example, magnesium ion is Mg^{2+} indicating that it is short of 2 electrons. To neutralize a magnesium ion, another ion must be found that has 2 extra electrons or two ions, each having one extra electron charge.

In cells, ions, such as sodium ion, can only move across cell walls through voltage gated pumps or channels (special protein structures), in which the channel's opening with a negative charge will attract ions with a positive charge. However, each channel's opening gate is very specific in shape and size to what may go through it. A voltage gated potassium channel cannot let a sodium ion through since a sodium ion is bigger and has a different shape even though both sodium and potassium are positively charged. Thus, voltage transport is selective by not only polarity but also by the size and shape of the ion.

Interstitial Fluid

Interstitial fluid surrounds each cell's extracellular space. It is filled with nutrition for the sustenance of the cell. It also contains electrolyte, in addition to fats and other vital nutrients. Cells utilize the nutrition (including electrolyte, glucose, fats, etc.,) from the interstitial fluid.

Capillary

The fine, thin as a hair, network of final branching of the veins, which delivers elements like blood, triglycerides, glucose, insulin, electrolyte, etc., to the interstitial fluid. The capillary system is connected to cells by the interstitial fluid, so electrolyte, fats, glucose, and other nutrition are available to the cells from the capillary via the interstitial fluid.

Electrolyte

In biology (as opposed to physics) electrolyte is the fluid full of ionized or ionizable elements within and surrounding cells in most parts of the body, and most importantly for our subject, in the brain. Electrolyte is a solution, meaning it is water (solvent) with chemical elements (solutes) dissolved in it. In everyday parlance, the term "electrolyte" represents only salt (NaCl, sodium chloride) added to water. Therefore, salt supplements on the market are often sold as electrolyte supplements, even if there is nothing else in them just pure salt. Hospitals provide intravenous saline (salt and water mix) solution to hydrate as electrolyte.

However, just placing salt in a glass of water is not a true biological electrolyte—it is just saline. For a functionally useful electrolyte the constituent ions, the solutes in the water, must become "active" and dynamic components. So, while adding salt to water visibly creates salt-water or saline, salt can also be broken up into ions using voltage, rearranging water and salt into a dynamic substance. In this substance, salt breaks up into sodium Na^+ and chloride Cl^- ions with polarity which then can move through voltage gated channels of a cell's wall (membrane) from the interstitial fluid.

The complete profile of an "active" electrolyte contains the following elements: sodium (Na^+), potassium (K^+), chloride (Cl^-), magnesium (Mg^{2+}), calcium (Ca^{2+}), hydrogen phosphate (HPO_4^{2-}), and hydrogen carbonate (HCO_3^-) dissolved in water (H_2O). Potassium is abundant in intracellular space, while sodium and chloride in the interstitial fluid in extracellular space, though all can be found inside and outside of the cells in constant motion. Fluid balance, which I refer to as electrolyte homeostasis, is the balance between sodium, potassium, and chloride ions as they are transported between intra and extra cellular space with a specific rhythm. Neurons function by maintaining electrolyte homeostasis using non-ionic transfer by *osmotic gradient* and ionic transfer by *voltage transport*.

Osmosis & Osmotic Gradient

Osmosis is a process by which elements in fluids flow from high concentration to low concentration through barriers – like cell membranes – to equalize intracellular and extracellular non-ionic concentrations. An example of such non-ionic element is water. The movement from higher to lower concentration is called the osmotic gradient. Water molecules and some other elements with very small molecules (typically not ions, with a few exceptions) can move in and out of cells via such osmotic gradient utilizing tiny channels that are not voltage dependent. Potassium ions can sometimes use this gradient because they are very tiny and their polarity isn't powerful enough to be blocked. The larger sodium ions cannot use the osmotic gradient and must use voltage transport to get into or out of the cells. When solutes cannot pass without voltage help, rather than fluid equalization, solvent equalization is the result of the osmotic gradient. This means that the solutes' *concentration* needs to be equal, even though there may be different amounts of fluids inside and outside of the cell, and the solute (essential mineral) concentration will be the same both inside and outside in the liquid even if the *volume* of the liquids differs. This has serious implications with respect to fluid volume differences between the inside and the outside of the cell membrane—and is specifically important to migraineurs.

Voltage Assisted Transport

Some ions, minerals, and nutrients need assistance to get inside or out of the cells. As noted earlier, sodium, for example, is too large to pass any channels of the cell using osmosis. Voltage assisted transport (also called voltage gated or voltage dependent transport) is one of the most important functions that must work in cells. Voltage assisted transport is a tad complex. Voltage assisted transport gates are proteins whose folds dictate what shape and polarity ion may go through them. The gates that permit sodium to enter, for example, are shaped specifically such that only sodium can enter. The folding of the protein creates polarity such that when a sodium enters, it is handed down into the cell via what can be visualized as a step ladder. Each step ladder is short so the sodium ion can pass next to it but each ladder is polarized to guide the sodium deeper into the cell and not let it turn around to leave the cell.

There are many nutrients that must be carried into cells by the guidance of ions that have the proper polarity and shape to enter a cell. Glucose is one such nutrient. Glucose is carried into the cell by sodium ions. Smooth and consistent voltage assisted transport is one of the most prominent features of a properly functioning brain. The migraine-brain has genetic variations associated with voltage assisted transport of many ions with serious implications for migraineurs.

Neuron

A neuron is a cell type in the central nervous system (CNS). Although the spinal cord is also part of the CNS, in this book I deal only with the brain because the brain is the location of migraines. The distinctive name *neuron* describes cells with their specialized appearances and functions; they are very different from other cells of the body.

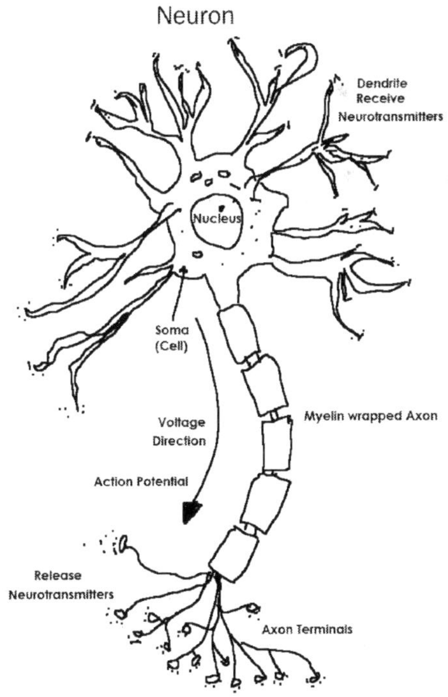

Figure 3. A neuron

Although neurons have only one nucleus (control center) they can be very long. The longest neuron can be three feet long—it is a neuron that starts at the base of the spine and ends at the end of the little toe (see any anatomy books or this link:

http://www.intropsych.com/ch02_human_nervous_system/neurons.html).

Neurons communicate using neurotransmitters that they create and pass on to other neurons. They push the neurotransmitters from vesicles (storage containers) into a little space called synapse between neurons via axon terminals (look like many legs in Figure 3). The act of spilling the neurotransmitters out of the vesicles into the synapse requires high voltage at functioning voltage-dependent calcium channels. A neuron that lacks vital nutrients or proper energy to generate action potential may not be able to release neurotransmitters.

Neurotransmitters & Neuropeptides

Neurotransmitters and neuropeptides are short-chain polypeptides made from amino acids (protein). The supply of neurotransmitters is replenished in nerve terminals by local synthesis, and many conventional neurotransmitters are recaptured after secretion. In contrast, neuropeptides are initially synthesized in the cell soma (main part of the cell) and transported down the axon and are used only once[44]. Neurotransmitters are more commonly known and are used as communication messengers—they are signaling molecules[45]. Anything and everything you do, think, dream, or choose, is governed by neurons communicating by means of these neurotransmitters or neuropeptides. They are biochemically identical to hormones but when they operate within the brain we call them neurotransmitters. When neurons are not able to release neurotransmitters, communication between neurons may be cut (synaptic pruning). Synaptic pruning is the leading indicator in many diseases and is also part of ageing[46]; its prevention is the goal of many drugs and research.

Neuronal Electrical Charge

Neurons receive signals from other neurons via neurotransmitter transmission. Neurons can message other neurons with shared connections to amplify or inhibit (dampen) the signal. In the case of amplification the receiving neuron will pass the signal on to the next neuron(s), and so on, and at the end the body performs the desired action, such as the release of a hormone or standing up from the chair. If inhibited, nothing happens. The electrical charge of neurons is essential for taking in nutrients and generating and releasing neurotransmitters. The charge or voltage amplitude differs for each of these functions. The largest voltage is generated for the release of neurotransmitters from the neuron by voltage gated calcium channels. Many anticonvulsant medicines prevent the function of voltage gated calcium channels.

Myelin Sheath

The myelin sheath, a very important part of the neuron, is made from fat and cholesterol and is located in what we refer to as the white matter. Other than the areas at the Nodes of Ranvier (ionic exchange areas), the entire length of the neuron's axon is coated with myelin, which acts as the insulation against voltage leaks. In many health conditions it is damage to this myelin sheath that causes trouble. For example, Parkinson's, Multiple Sclerosis, and also seizures are known to be connected to and exacerbated by damage to the myelin sheath. It is now understood that this region is also damaged on account of migraines[47-51].

Voltage Gated Sodium & Potassium Pumps

A specific voltage gated pump type is the sodium-potassium pump that is aggregated around the Nodes of Ranvier where there is no myelin sheath. It is at these areas where concentrations of ions may initiate the build-up of action potentials, resting potentials, and refractory periods.

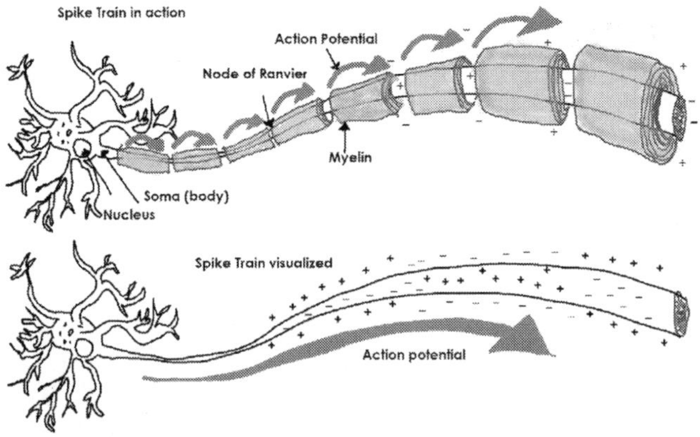

Figure 4. Spike Train: voltage transmission through an axon

The Nodes of Ranvier have a vital role in the propagation of voltage through the axon, region by region—meaning pump area to pump area. At each node the influx of sodium increases as the gates of the pumps open. Sodium ions flow into the neuron (positive charge fills the neuron at that node) and potassium ions leave at the same time as action potential is generated. Subsequently, potassium ions start flowing back into the neuron and sodium ions leave, generating a resting potential. These are local, discrete events at each node and don't happen at all nodes at the full length of the axon at once. Therefore, each pump helps to generate voltage when sodium enters (action potential), then reverses when potassium enters (resting potential), followed by a rest (refractory period) when the pump cannot open in any direction, while there is a slight negative charge inside the axon at that point. The voltage itself forces the next series of pumps to open where the action potential, resting potential, and refractory period are recreated. It appears that the voltage jumps from node to node but it really never leaves the axon, only the pumps act sequentially from node to node and the positive and negative ions enter and exit in and out of the pumps at each node. The voltage is recreated and stopped at each pump—visualize this as Newton's Cradle: one ball is hit on one side, it hits the next ball, and so forth, and out pops the last ball at the other end. Because the pumps are so small relative to the axon, to us it appears that the voltage is one continuous flow but it is not. It can be stopped at any point along the line of the axon if the pumps in one location don't function in adequate numbers and not enough voltage amplitude is reached—this is pump failure (see figure 5 below). Pump failure is the initiating precondition of a migraine prodrome and is also the target of many medicines that stop the voltage from passing all the way through the axons' length in hopes of preventing a migraine.

Action Potential

Action potential is a very short event in which the electrical charge difference between the inside and the outside of the membrane rises very fast—from node to node as described above. Many cell types generate action potentials, such as muscle cells and heart cells, as well as neurons. Action potentials are electric impulses that can be recorded and that look like rounded spikes (sinusoidal) on a graph.

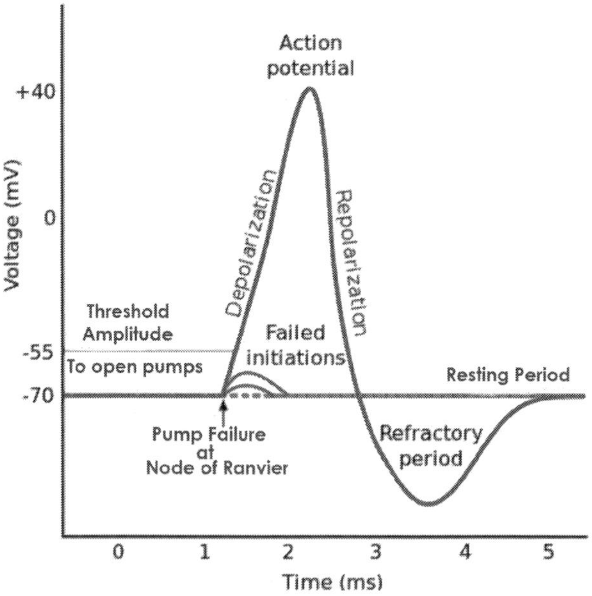

Figure 5. Voltage curve

The ability to generate action potential is the most important function of all cells that operate via voltage. As we have seen, the process by which an action potential is generated is purely based on polarity and charge differences between intra and extracellular space. Action potential is said to be an "all or nothing" event, meaning that if the charge difference between intracellular and extracellular polarity is not sufficient, action potential will not happen—the pump fails.

Resting Potential

In resting state, the charge difference between intra and extracellular space is below a certain threshold, as potassium ions rush in, sodium ions rush out. The inside of the neuron at the pump is now filled up with potassium ions and is slightly negatively charged, while the outside space at the pump is slightly positively charged. Similarly to action potential, this too is a local event and doesn't cover the entire axon at once but hops from node to node.

Refractory Period

After the pump "fires" (action potential) then reaches resting potential, it quickly returns to a state of rest via a refractory period. During a refractory period, voltage dependent gates and pumps at nodes of the axon membrane are closed. Just like action and resting potentials are local events, so is the refractory period. In this way, just as the action and resting potential is moving through the neuron's axon in a wave like manner, so is the refractory period. The refractory period controls both the size and the frequency of an action potential a cell is capable of generating. The magnitude and frequency of action potentials need to be in synchrony with neural respiratory functions and the energy available for the neuron. Absolute refractory period is one in which no stimulus, no matter how large, can cause an action potential. The sodium channels are inactivated and cannot open. In a relative refractory period the pumps can open but they require a larger stimulus to do so. The length of refractory periods has serious implications for migraine.

Cortical depression

Cortical Depression (CD) characterizes a region of brain cells that are not able to generate voltage—these cells are in an absolute refractory period. That is, the neurons in such a region have too many of their voltage gated pumps and channels closed at a minimum one Node of Ranvier and are unable to function. Think of it as being stuck in an elevator—people outside of the elevator hear your plea for help but the door stays shut.

Cortical Spreading Depression

Think of Cortical Spreading Depression (CSD) as the people outside of the stuck elevator are trying to help by forcing the door open or call for assistance to start the elevator working again. The effort people outside of the elevator exert in their attempt to open the door may or may not help. If the door opens, all passengers inside the elevator can come out and new passengers go in and life returns to normal. If the door does not open, the problem is escalated to the fire department or paramedics or a repair company for assistance. While all this is happening on the outside of the elevator, the people are stuck in the elevator behind closed doors.

All neurons are connected to tens or hundreds of thousands of other neurons. When neurons don't function, we can see a region stuck in absolute refractory mode, the CD, and neurotransmission (communication) stops. Connected neurons know where the trouble is and they send a wave of energy called CSD to try to energize the neurons that are not working by opening their pumps and shocking the affected neurons back to work once again. CSD can be seen by an observer via a scanner and as an aura by those with aura type migraines. The CSD is a wave of energy that moves through the brain one-directionally and slowly—2mm-5mm per minute[52-63]. Those with aura migraines may see a blind spot in their vision; this corresponds to the location in the brain region (visual cortex) stuck in CD. The CSD is visible as the aura itself.

CSD is often believed to be associated only with aura migraines but this is incorrect. As described above, an aura migraineur is aware of her CSD because she can actually see it. However, all migraine types follow the same process. Each type can be identified with a brain region that is in CD. The CSD of all migraine types eventually reach the meninges if the brain's attempts at restarting the refractory region to normal functionality fail[52,64-86]. Because the meninges (dura) is the layer where the pain sensors are located, many medicines are aimed at blocking the high voltage gated calcium channels to prevent the firing of voltage by the neurons that would initiate a CSD[87-97].

Cells and Neurons

Look down at your hand with a magnifying glass and you will see little odd shaped forms that are your skin cells. Every single body part is made of cells; they look somewhat different and have different functions. Their sizes are also different. If you were to look at the cells in your brain, you would see completely differently shaped cells—neurons. While on the visible parts of the body cells vary relatively little in shape and size and don't seem to move, neuron sizes vary greatly and neurons can move[98-100]. Neurons move[101] and reformulate by elongating their dendrites (growth "cones"), their axons (where the voltage travels), and repositioning their feet — the "buttons" (the neurotransmitter projecting ends, axon terminals)[102] – forming new connections or trimming old connections via synaptic pruning[103,104]. Growth cones can be envisioned like bricks being laid end to end. The more bricks are laid, the longer the wall becomes. Growth cones allow the lengthening of the dendrites in search of new neurons. When more and more growth cones are deposited, giving the dendrite-length a boost, the dendrite is directed toward another neuron. Neurons have little arms whose job is to "reach out and touch someone" (other neurons) via microtubule dynamics[101,103-105]. Most neurons form tens of thousands of connections. But these connections are not permanent for life.

If one neuron moves or dies for whatever reason, or if it stops signaling, all those neurons connected to it must find connections with other neurons in the brain; the connections to the non-functioning neuron will be pruned[106,107]. If you want to see how neurons move, search YouTube for "moving neurons in a Petri dish" and you will get many videos where you can see what the neurons look like and how they move. I have found a descent one:

https://www.youtube.com/watch?v=GBIa8G3gBH0

or another one:

https://www.youtube.com/watch?v=Nmvk3zlyQ2w

They show how neurons are looking for new connections as well as how connections get trimmed. Because neurons move, some treatments aiming at hitting the exact spot where a nerve ending is supposed to be—such as with acupuncture or Botox—may backfire as a migraine (or anything else) treatment, since the nerve ending of a particular nerve may have moved!

Brain Anatomy

The brain's anatomy is very complex, full of little up-hills and down-ditches and little crevices with complicated names. When a migraine pain sufferer points and says "it hurts just over the left temple sort of behind", it could be in over 150,000 different places within a cubic millimeter of brain matter; the usual sized "voxel." Voxel means "box" in medical jargon. It is the measuring unit in fMRI (functional Magnetic Resonance Imaging) analysis. Finding the migraine pain centers is great but remember: the pain is not the cause of migraines; the pain is the symptom. Finding the pain centers using fMRI is like finding a drip in a dripping nose using fMRI… we can see the nose is dripping; we may even find which nostril is dripping or which part of the nose is dripping, but we cannot find the cause of the drip this way. The cause may be a reaction to a virus or some allergen. Similarly, locating which part of the meninges corresponds to the migraine pain tells us nothing about the real causes of the migraine.

Sodium in Neuron Holding Water

Throughout the book, I often mention that sodium holds onto water inside the neuron or cell. This is a gross oversimplification since sodium holds onto water in the interstitial fluid and not inside the cell. Interstitial fluid surrounds every single cell all through the body—think of it as a fluid filled with supply of energy and nutrients. Sodium holds onto water here rather than inside the cells but short of having to explain this every time, I simply note that sodium holds water inside the cell—though technically incorrect, it is simple to relate to. It is very true that since sodium retains water in interstitial fluid and water can go in and out of cells according to the osmotic gradient, water content of the cells is solely supplied and managed by the availability of retained water (by sodium) in the interstitial fluid.

I call supplementing with electrolytes and metals:
The Electrical Chemistry of the Human

Steven Magee, Health Forensics

Challenges

Migraines are very much misunderstood by scientists, physicians, and everyday people. I have met people who told me that they had one migraine 10 years ago—one migraine. That is not possible. Why that is so will become clear as I detail what a migraine-brain is—but you can already get the gist of it: migraine can only be had by those with a migraine-brain that comes as a permanent anatomical feature, measurable in many ways. Those without such a brain cannot experience a migraine. Unfortunately, most doctors, scientists, and people in general (including migraineurs), have no idea about this very important distinction. This can clearly be seen by the many definitions of migraine. Note the lack of causation and the confusion in the following definitions:

Dictionary Definition of migraine

> *"a condition that is marked by recurrent usually unilateral severe headache often accompanied by nausea and vomiting and followed by sleep, that tends to occur in more than one member of a family, and that is of uncertain origin though attacks appear to be precipitated by dilatation of intracranial blood vessels"* [108]

Another Dictionary Definition of migraine

"Recurrent vascular headache, usually on one side of the head. Severe throbbing pain is sometimes accompanied by nausea and vomiting. Some migraine patients have warning symptoms (an "aura") before the headache, including visual disturbance, weakness, numbness, or dizziness. If a stimulus (e.g., a particular food or drink) is found to trigger attacks, avoidance can prevent them. Medicines may be taken as an attack begins (to abort it) or daily by patients with very frequent attacks (to prevent them or reduce their severity)"[109].

Another (confused) Definition of Headache and Migraine

"Headache: A pain in the head with the pain being above the eyes or the ears, behind the head (occipital), or in the back of the upper neck. Headache, like chest pain or back ache, has many causes. All headaches are considered primary headaches or secondary headaches. Primary headaches are not associated with other diseases. Examples of primary headaches are migraine headaches, tension headaches, and cluster headaches. Secondary headaches are caused by other diseases… Migraine headaches are the second most common type of primary headache. An estimated 28 million people in the US have migraine headaches. Migraine headaches affect children as well as adults. Before puberty, boys and girls are affected equally by migraine headaches, but after puberty more women than men have them. Migraine

often goes undiagnosed or is misdiagnosed as tension or sinus headaches"[110].

Several migraine types are usually missing in most definitions, most importantly *Hemiplegic Migraines,* which are also accompanied by temporary partial paralysis of the body as a prodrome, typically on one side, that sometimes cause serious injuries, such as falling down the stairs[111]. Also, many of the prodromes and sensations prior to and during migraines fall under my definition of "functional prodromes" that are really the falling dominoes in the cascade of events toward a migraine[17]. I can also point out some incorrect elements in the usual definition of migraines. For example, migraines never throb and are always only on one side of the head. There is quite a bit of confusion in official definitions, so what might be our expectations from lesser "experts".

Not surprisingly, the lack of clarity in scientific circles about the nature of migraines extends to society in general. There is a stigma attached to migraines in our culture and among many care-givers. Accordingly, migraineurs are "people who just complain too much" or - as per many doctors and hospitals - "migraineurs are drug seekers." In this section of the book, my goal is to shed light on what a migraine really is in terms of symptoms and cause, highlighting the differences between the two. When it comes to migraines, the most important part – just to be able to begin our conversation – is to recognize that a migraine-brain is a genetically different brain[112-119] that comes with high levels of neurological sensitivity, associated with hyper sensitive sensory organs with a variety of anatomical differences from a non-migraine-brain[120-122]. I should state that the statement "Migraines can alter brain structure permanently" should instead be: "Permanently altered brain structure is the hallmark of a migraine-brain."

(see: http://www.medicalnewstoday.com/articles/265345.php)

I believe that the migraine-brain is an ancient brain with anatomically different features that evolved differently for a reason. There are too many migraineurs and too many completely identical prodromes, migraines, and postdromes (with very identical genetic variances) to suggest that they are the results of recent, chance genetic mutations. A migraine-brain is a different brain that develops differently with different features from regular brains. There is nothing wrong with having a different brain but there is very much wrong with considering a different brain a sick brain and trying to reduce its capacity or modify its ability by medicines. Understanding what a migraine-brain is, is essential to understanding why we have migraines, who can have migraines, and how we can prevent migraines without the use of any medicines.

The first recording of a migraine was by Willis, in which he describes the migraines of Anne, Countess of Conway in great detail and accuracy in 1672[123]. Interestingly, his account of migraine prodromes and his description of migraine pain were more accurate in some ways, written nearly 450 years ago, than what many scientists and medical institutions list as prodromes and define as migraines today.

Not all migraines come with pain in the head, thus not all migraines can be classified just by pain alone; the head need not hurt to have a migraine! Yet today's migraine research is exclusively beholden to pain. This is the main reason why the understanding of what a migraine is lacking. Migraine is not understood well in the research community because researchers are looking at pain or aura, neither of which is necessary to suffer a migraine and neither of which informs us about the cause of migraine; they both are symptoms.

If migraine is not a disease, then what is it? Here is my hypothesis for the existence of migraine-brain: Migraine-brain is an evolutionary adaptation, an advantage—or at least it was for a long time. Migraineurs have hyper sensory organ sensitivity in the brain (sight, sound, scent, touch, taste). This sensitivity is genetic. In a later section I explain the details of the *migraine-brain paradox* from a biochemical point of view, showing why a migraine-brain runs out of voltage energy faster than a non-migraine-brain and why migraine is a symptom of the brain, an energy crisis rather than a disease. A migraine-brain is in a state of constant struggle to find enough energy for its biochemical balance in order to maintain electrolyte homeostasis. Once you understand what I have just written in the previous sentence, your life will change, so read on.

The Lack of Understanding by Others

Having a migraine is the most impossible situation for many migraineurs. Those around us who have no migraines have no idea what a migraine is all about. After all, they've never had a migraine, so how would they know? The problem is that they *think* they know, and this determines their behavior toward those of us who have migraines, and our ability to interact with them becomes all the more difficult. As a migraine group member said, "If I had a dollar for every time someone had something 'smart' to say about my migraine, I'd be rich." And this is so true. Many migraineurs lose their jobs because of such ignorance. I don't recall other people with different kinds of chronic pain being in as much trouble based on ignorance as migraineurs are. I suppose the problem is that for most migraines (not all), it is the head that hurts, and those around us associate that with common headaches, which they are familiar with. But just as an arm can hurt from hitting it, breaking it, burning it, having it chopped off, or having it bitten by a snake, all of these "hurting arms" have very different histories, pain types, and require different treatment, similarly, we cannot say that every pain in the head is simply a headache! Head pain can indicate many things, including cancer, aneurysm, stroke, a head injury, or a migraine! Why is a migraine any less serious in the eye of the world than other conditions?

We cannot blame people for their lack of understanding but we certainly can do so when they refuse to learn, and this is true whether they are friends, family, or medical professionals. Unfortunately for many migraineurs, there are people in their lives who are not only ignorant but also lack compassion to the point of being downright rude. Some of the stories I hear bring tears to my eyes.

In some families migraineurs are punished for having migraines; in some they are called lazy or complainers; and in others they just lose their families altogether. I feel very sorry for these migraineurs, and frankly – before I got involved with the migraine group – I had no idea the situation was this dire. However, family is not the biggest problem. Instead, it is the medical community that looks at migraineurs as if they were little green people from outer space. The majority of physicians have no idea what migraine is. They probably learned what it should be from their text books many years ago, and hence they believe they know what migraine is but the reality is quite different. Most have never had a migraine themselves, and never had to use the medicines they give to migraineurs, so they really have no firsthand experience with the medications, and are completely unaware of the nature of the migraine-experience and the harm these medications cause! One of the migraineurs in the group wrote this:

> *"I sincerely hate walking out of a doctor's office in tears!! (Happens to me so often). I believe in reasons and solutions.... not [in] being a Guinea pig or being shunned for refusing shitty drugs that will only mess one up further. I find that a lot of doctors go through trouble and hard work of getting their [doctor] degree then they totally stop learning or educating themselves!! I*

guess the saying 'the most expensive thing you can own is a closed mind' is so very true!!"

Indeed! There is nothing worse than a closed mind.

It isn't only doctors who exhibit narrow visions and closed minds. I asked one of my long ago doctoral advisors – a scientist of supposedly open mind – if I could use his hospital lab for running some experiments. I was going to work with people who have migraine. He responded with this: "these are mental issues and in any case, no one takes them seriously." Mental? So those who have a pain with an unexplained or not yet understood cause are mental cases? Really? If this is how a research scientist looks at migraine, our expectations from the medical profession, not to mention the general public, cannot be too high.

Still, we are dealing with chronically ill patients. Assume it is mental for a second: schizophrenia is a mental disease but no one is refusing to try to work making schizophrenic patients' life experience better. Being bipolar is also a mental condition, as is depression, Parkinson's, autism, multiple sclerosis (MS), epileptic seizures, and many more. Yet, even though these illnesses affect mental abilities, they are regarded as illnesses deserving of treatment, whereas migraines are dismissed as insignificant. Since migraines come with a headache, which is often the only visible symptom for an outsider, it likely evokes the sense that migraine is not a real disease – everybody comes down with a headache once in a while – and thus it can be discounted.

The Migraine Epidemic And Its Challenges

The migraine epidemic is just being recognized. Our generation enjoys a platform for truly high-level communication – the internet – and thus the prevalence of migraines can be measured by means other than reports by doctors who happen to encounter and diagnose patients with migraines. With the help of the Facebook migraine group I have learned that many people who have been diagnosed with migraine later find out they don't have it at all, and many who have been diagnosed with something other than migraines, in fact, do have them. The communication platform allows for information sharing about health conditions at an unprecedented level of detail and personalization, which in turn facilitates the useful discovery of patterns with diagnoses and misdiagnoses.

For example, it is believed that men outgrow their migraines after puberty and females don't get cluster headaches nearly as often as men do[124,125]. When members join my migraine group, I ask them to fill out a questionnaire. One of the obvious questions I ask is "Where does your head hurt when you get a migraine and what symptoms and prodromes do you have?". Interestingly, I find that many female members have been diagnosed with migraines when they have either cluster headaches or a combination of cluster headaches and migraines, and that many men have been diagnosed with cluster headaches who actually have migraines — some acquiring it prior to puberty and some in adulthood. Some who have been diagnosed with migraine ask me "what are prodromes?", so clearly, they are not migraineurs at all. I can at least speculate that previously held beliefs and statistics are highly questionable, simply because the differentiation of headache types is not an easy matter.

It is well documented that migraines are one-sided, meaning only one side of the head hurts—not behind the eye(s), never throb, and are not all over the head. Yet some well-known and respected medical facilities still explain migraines as an all-over the head throbbing pain. Not only is migraine one-sided, but most migraineurs have the same side hurt all the time and for many it is the very same spot—it nearly feels like a sore[17]. Migraines last minimum 24-72 hours with many symptoms that appear unrelated, such as nausea, vomiting, diarrhea, vertigo, IBS, RLS, and a host of others; aura migraineurs have aura; hemiplegic migraineurs end up with one side of the body temporarily paralyzed. Migraines end with a postdrome that can last for several days during which the migraineur is worn out, in a "flat" mood, weak, forgetful, cannot focus—we call it a *fog* but "feeling like a floating vegetable" maybe a better description. Most migraineurs who are aura migraineurs are not aware that they are. In a later section I provide a list of 34 types of auras as reported by actual migraineurs. They are not listed anywhere and most doctors are not familiar with them. This makes me also question the statistics about the percentage of aura migraineurs.

There are no tests that are specific to migraines — tests today aim at the exclusion of any other diagnostic cause of the pain. As I have stated repeatedly, there are no medicines for migraines, at least none that works! Take triptans, for example, a favorite drug prescribed for migraines by perhaps the majority of doctors. Triptans only work sometimes[126] and the reason why they don't always work is grossly misunderstood[127]. The problem is that the accepted current medical consensus is based on incomplete and often false premises for defining what migraine is. When doctors lack a basic understanding of the migraine condition, the use of any medication cannot hope to target anything but symptoms. Why triptans are not effective all the time is quite simple: triptans act on receptors to release serotonin. If the brain region in Cortical Depression (unable to generate voltage) happens to be the one responsible for serotonin production, triptans will work. However, the brain region in CD may be responsible for something else! If it happens to produce dopamine, one can take as many triptans as one wants but the migraine will not budge. Unfortunately, many migraineurs don't know this and will continue taking triptans despite the fact that they don't work. Not only can this be very harmful—it can also be life threatening. This problem then reverts back to the prescribing doctor because the migraineur—at the very least—complains that the medicine doesn't always work, or presents a new, "unforeseen" medical condition generated by the misapplication of serotonin.

Recent scientific reports show that migraines, seizures and strokes all relate to ionic imbalance of sodium, potassium, chloride, magnesium, calcium, and water. One particular model looked at how changing potassium ion concentration affects brain activity and how seizures and migraines have similar underlying mechanisms[128].

Migraines and strokes have a very similar underlying "dramatic failure" that is captured well in the following quote:

> *"Cortical spreading depression (CSD) and depolarization waves are associated with dramatic failure of brain ion homeostasis, efflux of excitatory amino acids from nerve cells, increased energy metabolism and changes in cerebral blood flow (CBF). There is strong clinical and experimental evidence to suggest that CSD is involved in the mechanism of migraine, stroke, subarachnoid hemorrhage and traumatic brain injury"*[129].

Focusing on neurons, an overabundance of intracellular potassium ions and depletion of extra-cellular sodium and chloride ions will expel water from the affected brain region[130]. Electrolyte homeostasis is the most important requirement for a healthy nervous system and body[131]. The over-supply of potassium ions coupled with the lack of sodium ions will trigger migraines because the neurons are not able to generate action potential or retain water, and may also trigger seizures and epilepsy[132,133]. In my article: Dehydration and Salt Deficiency Trigger Migraines[134], I talk about the importance of hydration and explain how it works at the cellular level.

A major challenge migraineurs face is their physicians' lack of interest in updating their knowledge. This is an across-the-board problem but in the specific medical fields where doctors are tasked with diagnosing headache conditions, the situation is especially gloomy. A considerable percent of new members entering my migraine group are not migraineurs at all, but instead have cervicogenic headaches, tension headaches, cluster headaches, trigeminal neuralgia, occipital neuralgia, and some even chronic sinus headaches; yet all of them had been diagnosed with having migraines. To state the challenge differently, migraineurs don't have an easy time finding a doctor who recognizes a migraine when she sees one.

Another trial for migraineurs is to find a physician who understands that migraineurs have low blood pressure and giving them blood pressure lowering medications (still believing that migraine is cardiovascular) can easily make things worse[19,20]. This situation, of course, is just another facet of the "not keeping up with the latest scientific developments" shortcoming of many doctors but it is also part of the problem that doctors don't see migraineurs when they are not in pain and pain increases blood pressure.

Frequently, when a migraineur is referred to see a psychiatrist or neurologist, she is pretty much doomed. These experts have a strong economic interest in suggesting that migraine is a mental condition. Many migraineurs end up with mean doctors who treat them as damaged goods. Physicians will have to gradually recognize the defects in their knowledge about migraines (which is frequently based on a long-ago education), and the ones with an open mind will come around to the true cause of the migraine epidemic. Good science will prevail.

All migraineurs have special abilities courtesy of their enhanced sensory organ sensitivities. As a migraineur myself, the topic of migraines has always been between me and my doctor and perhaps my closest of family members, and usually remained on the subject of pain rather than the benefits a migraine-brain can provide. Migraine is not usually something one desires to talk about beyond complaining about the pain. Furthermore, no one cares about a migraineur's special abilities, the migraineur doesn't think of bringing them up and the medical professional has not been trained to ask about them. This causes a huge challenge; doctors only learn about the pain but miss the whole picture of what a migraine-brain is all about. The lack of information they receive from migraineurs is real but even if migraineurs were to tell their whole migraine story, doctors are not trained to recognize the significance of statements that reveal the existence of a different brain type.

Migraineurs have not been talking to each other in the context of special abilities and so a consistent and coherent picture of migraine has not emerged outside of my migraine group. In my group migraineurs are now learning how similar they are to each other in terms of their special abilities, although this type of open discussion took quite some time to establish. Migraineurs take to sharing pain and medicine information naturally, but not curious things, like "do you all hear noises and think you are crazy, then you discover that people are whispering in a far room?". Since my group requires frequent participation, and the chatter must be about something other than medicines, the discussions have become less restrained and suddenly a new world has opened up about the identical benefits, problems, and stories migraineurs encounter.

In the first few months of the migraine group's existence I realized the reason why medicines had made migraineurs sicker. It is because current medical treatments for migraine decrease the sensitivity of the migraine-brain to a *less functional* state by downregulating all of these special abilities[135-137]. In other words, medicines *dumb down* the brains of migraineurs to the point that these special abilities as well as their standard abilities are diminished. The cost to migraineurs is huge. Beyond losing their special abilities, they also lose brain power, are on a bullet train to dementia, begin stuttering, experience strokes, and are at risk for type 2 diabetes[8-11,138-140]. Migraineurs usually get sick during and after taking medicines. These medicines don't work; if they did work there would be no migraine groups on Facebook—yet there are hundreds and some with a membership of over 50 thousand migraineurs.

Let us also remember that a migraine-brain is anatomically different. Thus, reducing a migraine-brain to the capacity (in sensitivity) to a regular brain is akin to forcing on a pair of shoes that are a couple of sizes too small.

Here are just a few of my special abilities that medicines would *dumb down* if I allowed it to happen:

- I can smell if someone has a bacterial infection versus a viral one (a very important distinction!);

- I can smell type 2 diabetes;
- I am also our home's personal *sniffer* for food spoilage;
- I can hear very far faint noises. I do not have better hearing but I can separate "white noise" from unusual sounds and can sense vibration as a sound;
- My pupils do not close completely; consequently, what is regular light to a non-migraineur may be intolerably bright light to me (particularly so when I am out of electrolyte homeostasis). However, I see better in the dark than most non-migraineurs do;
- I also have extreme peripheral vision for sudden changes – my general vision is poor but boy, one leaf moves out of place in the corner of my eyes and I am on that faster than how a non-migraineur would even notice that there is a tree full of leaves there;
- I am a super taster as well. Try to get a Brussels sprout near me—I tried but failed. Many vegetables contain chemicals that – in increased amounts – can be dangerous or even lethal. Being a super taster allows one to sense such chemicals. Did you know that Brazil nuts can poison you with selenium? Or that broccoli has two chemicals that combined can harm you if you eat a lot of it? Dried beans, raw olives (off the tree), and raw peanuts (immediately after harvest) are toxic without preparation. A super taster likely has trouble eating Brazil nuts, broccoli, spinach, peanuts, bananas, olives, some beans, cilantro, and other "healthy" foods because the taste gives away their toxin.

There are also negatives of being a migraineur—other than pain. Here are a few examples (some also representing other migraineurs not just me) some of which diminish with the protocol's use:

- I am charged like a power outlet! There is a very strong possibility that with a hand shake you will be shocked by my static electricity as if I were an electric eel.
- I physically hurt if I must hold something cold—like taking ice cubes from the freezer. Forget about playing with snow balls or building a snowman with a migraineur. This is something the majority of migraineurs also complain about—it is Raynaud's disease that is discussed later. (It doesn't respond to the protocol.)
- I itch when cold air touches my body. Even fully clothed, when going for a walk, if the wind hits my thighs through my pants I will scratch like a mad person up until my thighs finally warmed up—my thighs look totally burned red from the cold. This is allergic urticaria. (It doesn't change either with the protocol.)
- I have perfect pitch (you may think this is an advantage but it is a curse). I cannot attend a live concert because if one instrument or singer is out of tune a tiny bit, I am in physical pain and must get out of there.
- I sometimes get dizzy from moving my head too fast. Most migraineurs do.
- I am hyper jointed—meaning I am extremely flexible. When I was young I could rotate my shoulders 360 degrees all over

my body holding a small towel (over the head and then step over it and back up where I started) without my shoulder popping out of place. Over 70% of the migraineurs in the migraine group have Ehlers-Danlos Syndrome (EDS)[141]. Some can hyper-extend their joints and others can pull their skins quite a distance from their body. Many of us have nearly transparently thin skin with veins showing through everywhere. (It is not a painful condition and doesn't get better with the protocol in all of its components but there is some improvement).

- I also have hypermobile eardrums! My eardrums start to vibrate to sounds no one can hear — not even me. I simply "sense" the sound without hearing it[142]. While doctors like to suggest that hypermobile eardrums are the result of frequent ear infections (I had one as a child), it is a relic of the extra sensitive hearing migraineurs have. Many migraineurs can still turn their ears—some can flap them like an elephant. I can wiggle ear plugs out of my ears on demand—clearly moving my ear drums and rotating my inner ears like a cat, even though my outer ear lobes may not move.
- I have low blood pressure (like 99.99999% of other migraineurs, often sub-clinically low), but in one instant I can get into a fight-or-flight mode with extreme high blood pressure from the slightest disturbance—again like all migraineurs. This anxiety has some benefits, such as increased reaction speed while driving a car or walking on the street, but overall it is a negative in modern life. It also means that

> if I monitor my pulse or blood pressure, I will get very different readings from one minute to the next—and in a doctor's office the reading may also be all over the place. (It is not a painful condition and is not affected by the protocol.)

Migraineurs have such sensitive sensory organs that they hear things others don't, smell things other don't, and feel things others don't. This often invites various unpleasant "mental case" categorizations by doctors as well as friends and family that are unwarranted and ignorant. Children with migraines are often told they are faking migraines because they see their mom or dad having them and they want attention. They are often told to just stop it or that "no you don't have a migraine" when indeed they do. Thus, while in an emergency the extra sensitivity of migraineurs' sensory organs is beneficial, in everyday life it is misunderstood, medicated wrong, and ridiculed.

Place a migraineur on medicines that block electrical activities of the brain (like voltage gated sodium and calcium channel blockers do) and all these super skills go away and horrible side effects replace them! The question we need to answer is this: do we need to reduce a highly-sensitized migraine-brain, amazingly adapted to survival in the eye of danger, to a level of lower sensitivity and ability? If there is an alternative path to pain prevention by providing the right nutrition and still maintaining a migraine-brain at its highly sensitive state without pain, isn't that a better solution? Are we sure that a migraine-brain, just because it is different, is a sick brain that needs medicinal treatment? I think by now you agree with me on the desirability of better alternatives for saving the high-level functionalities of a migraine-brain and doing so without causing pain, without the use of any medicines at all.

Stumbling Block

I met with one of my favorite doctors about 6 months before the 1st edition of my book was published and told him about my migraine-cause hypothesis. He listened very patiently and then said: "You do know that you are blowing against the trade winds, don't you?" After I nodded he said: "good, because you will need to learn to fly against the wind." He was right in more ways than he thought. We must remember that birds and planes can only take off against the wind!

I fly against many trade winds in my attempts in convincing migraineurs, doctors, and scientists to consider my approach. It was very hard to get the first few migraineurs to commit to what I recommended but as they became migraine free, the information spread. As of writing this book, I have treated over 4000 migraineurs who are now migraine and medicine free. However, academic journals always want clinical trials, and so I am having a hard time publishing my findings. Not everything is possible to set up in clinical trials. Why can't I have a clinical trial?

The first problem is that all subjects in the clinical trial must be migraineurs and that introduces a selection bias. Since only migraineurs have migraines, it is quite pointless to examine how non-migraineurs respond to treatment—thus as per statistical rules, the population is homogeneous rather than random. Next, of course, we need to engage those migraineurs who have the most frequent migraines but these are mothers with families. For a true clinical trial, the researcher must place these patients under full observation and provide food and water according to the protocol of the trial for over the course of several months, since their body must adjust. Unfortunately, it is not possible to lock mothers up in a hospital for a month or more, separating them from their families.

It is also necessary to have a control group (no change) and a placebo group (fake treatment). The control group has no intervention in their daily lives at all, though they would have to be regularly examined in the hospital. The placebo group would have to stay in the hospital and receive a treatment that looks and tastes like the real one, except it is not the treatment. They would also have to come off of all their preventive medicines. Ethical boards must approve any experiment. Knowingly causing pain by providing placebo (or worse, a known trigger) to a migraineur while removing them from all medicines would not be something I personally would agree to and I am sure all ethical boards would refuse as well. Here I summarize the reasons for the lack of clinical trials:

1. Only a genetically predetermined migraine-brain has all the properties that identify it as a migraine-brain. Clinical trials for migraines, therefore, can only be tested on migraine-brains

and that involves a genetic testing of candidates before the trial even starts. There are way too many misdiagnosed migraineurs to take previous diagnoses as facts.

2. Migraine itself is a symptom of an underlying, unmet voltage requirement. The prevention is not medicinal but dietary. Clinical trials of new medications have well established routines but of dietary changes less so. And while dietary changes can be implemented, the time period for a clinical trial in which medicines are removed and the diet is changed would be a long one.
3. Any clinical trial for evaluating the cause of migraines requires migraineurs to be locked up in a fully controlled environment and provided fully accounted-for meals. This may be possible but at an enormous cost and with lots of practical difficulties.
4. Since most migraineurs take medicines that often interfere with the absorption of the very minerals that provide the necessary energy for the brain, migraineurs also need to be removed from their medicines for full success. However, some of the medicines migraineurs are prescribed can take over a year to slowly reduce. Reduction must start at the time the dietary controls reached baseline, indicating that migraineurs currently on medicines may require upwards of a year in a clinically locked-up condition.
5. The question remains about the placebo group that would also have to titrate off of all their medicines but would receive fake dietary changes. This already sounds bad but what

exactly is a placebo for cheese? For a slice of fish? For a glass of milk? For a salt pill? Etc.?

6. As there is nothing to sell, there is no direct commercial incentive in proving my theory. This results in lack of funds to complete clinical trials.

Symptoms, then are in reality nothing
but the cry from suffering organs.

Jean-Martin Charcot, translated from French

Migraine Cause

Having pain when something is not working right evolved for a reason. Migraine can be considered a delayed pain, a warning that a brain region is in trouble, it is in a biochemical imbalance. The biochemical imbalance calls for biochemical rebalancing instead of pain management. Scientists have been asking the wrong questions, although there have been many scientific experiments proving or disproving certain important migraine related details and associations. Once I zoomed in on the right questions, I managed to find a decent number of relevant studies supporting my approach, as well as filling in some gaps (see the many citations and the end of the book). Nevertheless, asking the wrong questions and – as a consequence – not finding actionable conclusions has had an unfortunate effect. Physicians who see migraine patients can only apply the solutions that scientists provide and insurance permits. No solutions have been provided based on the causes of migraines, only symptom treatments. Thus, doctors treat migraineurs without understanding how those treatments relate to migraine causes. For example, when I last time saw my migraine specialist (I think in 2010) she handed me a prescription for preventive medicines. When I asked her why they would help me, she said "some migraineurs report they work". She could not explain why or how it worked. This is unacceptable.

Migraine starts with prodromes that are signals of an impending migraine. These prodromes are elements of a cascade of events that lead to the pain, which starts with the initiation of an alarm status that leads to a fight-or-flight-like response. A migraineur can easily be triggered into a migraine by noise, odor, a specific light intensity, and even some tastes that are above her norm. Migraineurs have hyper sensory organ sensitivities[3] and more sensory neuronal connections than that of the general population[7]. The "falsely" triggered cascade of events uses up available energy, depleting the available voltage. A migraineur will start a migraine unless voltage is re-established. Migraineurs use more voltage energy[4,5] as a result of their hyper sensitive sensory organs. Voltage is the driving force of the ionic electrolyte pumps[143] that are located in neuronal membranes, facilitating ionic exchanges between the inside and the outside of the neuron. Since more voltage use requires more sodium, migraineurs need to consume more salt. Migraineurs tend to pass about 50% more sodium in their urine, showing the extra use[144]. The modern Western diet is forever reducing its salt amount recommendations for the general population, ignoring that a large percentage of the population has specific needs. In general, I found that migraineurs need 50% to 100% more salt in their diet than non-migraineurs do.

While we have covered a lot of ground so far in discussing migraine cause, there is much more to the story. Take a deep breath, onward we go. The next sections are based on everything you learned so far and represent all current knowledge available by science and by my findings combined. I start off with what I call a "simple explanation" to what migraine is. The more complex version (Part IV) is a combination of three published academic articles and additional work. There will be many new definitions and descriptions as well. This part of the book is the most challenging so take notes or grab a highlighter. Tighten your seatbelt.

It's All About the Ions

The hyper-excitability of neurons in certain brain regions and the resulting ionic homeostasis imbalance are responsible for the onset of a migraine. The inability of the ionic channels to respond to electrolyte imbalances are often referred to as ionic channelopathy, albeit this has not yet reached the research community in association with migraines[2,145-148]. The vasoconstriction or vasodilation often blamed for migraines are symptoms rather than causes of migraines. Moreover, migraineurs become deficient in those neurotransmitters that the CD regions cannot make. Most migraine medicines are serotonin based. Only by sheer luck will the affected CD region be responsible for serotonin manufacturing. In these rare cases, there is no CSD reaction by surrounding regions, and so no migraine pain will follow. However, it is important to emphasize that even in these instances the drugs do not have any effect on the true cause of migraines. This explains why triptans and SSRIs don't work for migraineurs all the time, why the pain comes back when these medicines wear off if they worked, and why for some they never work at all[127,149].

An over or under supply of electrolyte ions sets off changes in the brain's electrical activity that can lead to migraines or seizures. Where in the brain those changes occur determines the type of symptoms a migraineur experiences. For example, in the case of aura migraine the initiating migraine location is in the visual cortex. The migraineur also sees the aura with eyes closed. What the migraineur sees is the CSD's wavelike movement in the visual cortex of the brain. The visual cortex's function is to translate the signals it receives into meaningful images. The CSD is a slow moving electrical wave that the visual cortex interprets and presents to the migraineur as an image. The aura often starts with a blind spot. It is my theory that the blind spot represents the neuronal region in CD, the region responsible for the migraine.

The overall neural physiology is very complex but we can say that:

- Migraines are caused by malfunctioning neurons as a result of ionic imbalances that prevent the development of action potentials along their axons.
- Ionic imbalance can be visualized as CD regions without polarity (extended absolute refractory mode).
- CD regions are anatomical representations of a brain in trouble.
- Maintenance of proper ionic balance is critical for migraineurs.

The Role of Glucose

Prior to continuing the explanation of migraine cause, I would like to explain a term I often use to make sure you can relate to it: glucose intolerance. While our body always needs and uses glucose, it can get glucose more than one way in two broad categories:

- Eating carbs that easily convert to glucose (sweets, fruits, starches, vegetables, sweetened food and drink, etc.,), or
- Eating protein that the liver converts into glucose.

Glucose intolerance (remember in Part II I explained that in this book it means the inability to metabolize glucose properly) refers to carbohydrate intolerance—meaning getting "exogenous glucose" from eating carbohydrates. The genetic profile of migraineurs suggests serious problems with consuming glucose, and carbs with their easy conversion to glucose. Hence glucose intolerance doesn't mean you need to stop eating everything that converts to glucose and that you must do everything in your power to avoid all foods that convert to glucose but it does mean that a migraineur should avoid all foods that are "easy glucose pickings" for reasons that will become clear.

Migraine itself is the manifestation of some parts of your brain running low on voltage energy. Not having enough energy robs neurons from being able to communicate and participate in necessary brain activities. The energy needed is not glucose, though that is likely what you crave—glucose is only able to enter the cells with sodium carrying each glucose molecule into the cell. Thus you crave sweets because the available glucose cannot enter the cells without sodium, so eating more sweets will only make things worse—what you really need is more sodium. Voltage requires 4 key elements to be present in ample amounts in your electrolyte: salt, potassium, calcium, and magnesium. Salt is the most critical of the four and, of course, water must also be present in the right amount.

Sugar or any form of carbohydrate is the biggest enemy of electrolyte homeostasis for the brain of a migraineur[2]. The more sugar and carbohydrates you eat the worse your migraine will get because while glucose needs sodium to get into the cell, once in, it removes sodium and water from your cells, disrupting electrolyte homeostasis[39]. While glucose removes salt and water from everyone's cells, migraineurs are much more sensitive to the ensuing imbalance.

Migraineurs need to accept that they possess a migraine-brain, which means they have highly sensitive sensory organs, and this makes them highly sensitive to certain external stimuli. These facts cannot change and are with us for life. The amount of voltage used by a migraine-brain is greater than what is used by a non-migraineur's brain[82,150]. Therefore, migraineurs need more voltage for providing energy. By supplying plenty of energy for extra voltage, the pain can be prevented. A brain in need of more energy is not a sick brain; it merely needs a different nutritional regimen.

2 Since the brain of migraineurs is different, there will be a genetic explanation provided to support this statement later.

Functional Prodromes

To understand the notion of functional prodrome, we must understand the cascade of steps related to a migraine. Since migraine may or may not come with pain, pain is clearly not a prerequisite in the causation of migraines. Similarly, visual auras may or may not appear and so auras are also not revealing. The cascading steps of the migraine process are crucial pieces of information in our pursuit of understanding migraines. As a scientist, who is also a migraineur, I am in a very unusual position of being able to describe this cascade of events and find its relationship to migraine, as I have had the "pleasure" of observing the proceedings of my migraines over and over again—including visual auras sometimes. We have covered prodromes extensively already; here I want to place them in a different context.

Often people comment that "what works for you may not work for me because people are different." While this is very true in many areas of human experience, based on my years of investigation of thousands of migraineurs, I can state that the above comment does not hold for migraineurs. We often get messages in the Facebook group about how members thought that some specific step in the cascade of migraines or a personality trait (such as hurting and itching from cold or turning on the car seat warmer even in 70F (21C)) was just a crazy thing unique to them. To their greatest surprise, they receive hundreds of responses from other migraineurs, announcing that they also have experienced the same thing. It appears that the genetic markers that set the stage for migraine-brains produce nearly identical differences to brains beholden to migraines, to the point that we can characterize our migraine group as a group of siblings. This extreme similarity is also reinforced by how all migraineurs seem to respond to the same thing the same way.

A migraine, be it with aura or not, or with pain or not, always starts with one particular event and proceeds from there like the proverbial falling dominos, one event initiating the next all the way until the outcome is a migraine. In hyper alert mode[3], the slightest odor difference, sound difference, motion of a leaf, etc., imply the possibility of danger. Thus, the first thing a migraineur feels is *anxiety,* and she feels it often. Anxiety (for a migraineur) is not a separate disease but has the function of alerting the body to start increasing oxygen, so the heart starts pumping faster with increased pulse rate, and the migraineur starts yawning in order to get more air into her lungs. As the lungs fill with more air and the heart pumps more and richer oxygenated blood, unnecessary body functions shut down. This implies that digestion stops too, so if there is anything undigested in the stomach, it may be vomited up, or if there is anything in the intestinal tract, a very urgent bowel movement (perhaps diarrhea) may follow. This is the IBS-like step in the cascade of steps in functional prodromes leading to a migraine. Next, given the impeding danger ahead, the released adrenaline and the increased heartbeat and oxygen supply enhance the ability for either a confrontation with the perceived danger or for running away from it. This is the panic attack step—the "fight or flight" response—in the cascade of events. Since a migraineur today does not proceed to run during a prodrome, restless legs syndrome (RLS), dizziness, and irritability are the typical consequences. As you can see, everything I have just described is an integral part of "getting away from danger"[151].

The adrenaline release of the fight-or-flight response is an evolutionary response to some real danger. In our modern world, this emergency reaction is most often elicited by a perceived danger. When a migraineur senses a perceived danger, it is not any different in her brain's reaction to that of a long-ago danger from a real predator lurking nearby. Given the very large percent of the population with migraines[152], the evolutionary nature of this special brain is likely the genetic foundation of migraines. All prodromes fit within the "fight-or-flight" stress response formation. Therefore, anxiety, IBS, RLS, yawning, increased pulse and palpitations, nausea, vomiting, diarrhea, irritability, etc., are not individual diseases or even individual prodromes, but a precisely choreographed chain of events with the functional goal of "getting ready to defend yourself or flee". All of these prodromes are present in migraineurs before a migraine appears—though not all are noticed by them all the time and an individual migraineur may be conscious of only a certain pattern of prodromes. Sadly, many migraineurs are medicated for each independent condition as if these were independent diseases[153-156].

Food craving (without hunger) is another classic example of a functional prodrome. Many migraineurs crave sweets before a migraine, even if they feel fully stuffed—only a few crave salty food.

The brain, in most cases, uses glucose for energy but glucose cannot get into the neurons without functioning voltage gates and sodium. Voltage gates by definition require a minimum voltage to operate. Therefore, while the brain's first instruction to the migraineur (in the form of cravings) is to get more glucose, the brain really needs more sodium-dense electrolyte. This craving represents that some of the brain regions are about to run out of voltage energy, and if no electrolyte minerals are provided, some neurons will run out of fuel and stop working. Instead of glucose, the brain needs a proper balance of potassium, sodium, and chloride to initiate voltage generation and resupply energy needed for cellular communication[150,157]. Studies point to the importance of magnesium, a critical element providing energy for all cells, including neurons, since it is the "key" to opening the voltage gated pumps[158,159]. Voltage gated calcium channels are high voltage channels that require even more sodium rich electrolyte and also more calcium. Since glucose is also required for the neurons to meet their increased energy need due to the heightened sensory organ sensitivity of migraineurs, it is clear that sweet craving is also a functional prodrome.

There are many prodromes that scientists and physicians have never heard of. Migraineurs themselves are not aware of all of them either. As mentioned before, migraineurs in the migraine group experience a change in the size of one of their eyes several hours prior to their migraine. Many migraineurs cannot see the differences—we tend to ignore minute changes and details of something we are very familiar with.

When migraineurs send me timestamped selfies taken several times during the day, I am able to tell them how their day progressed (in terms of migraine). In a few instances a migraineur mother would join the group and would have her child's photo as her icon. I can see that her child will be or already is a migraineur. I sometimes find that after mentioning this to the mother, she will remark that her child has "frequent headaches" but she never realized they may have been migraines. Preventing migraines at an early age helps avoiding them in the future, plus it teaches the child good eating habits for her or his migraine-brain. The change of the size of one eye is not listed in any literature other than my publication[17] and so no migraineur, doctor, or researcher ever pays attention to this as a prodrome. There are many more of these "secret" little prodromes that are typically not noticed but represent telling signals of an impending doom!

Let's examine what the eye size change tells us about the migraine. In the brain, the connections are crossed, and so if the right eye gets smaller it implies that changes are occurring in the left hemisphere of the brain that controls the muscles of that eye. Some migraineurs get as far as not even being able to open that eye. Clearly this is informative of the location of the migraine-causing area and so this is considered to be a functional prodrome. One needs to ask why a particular prodrome is happening to understand the cause of migraine. Here is a very seriously misinterpreted example: all migraineurs are sensitive to bright light, and while it is listed in the literature as a frequent characteristic of people with migraines, no one seems to have asked why they are sensitive, and what "bright light" means relative to light in general.

- Are migraineurs sensitive to the same light when not in prodrome?
- Are non-migraineurs sensitive to the same bright light?
- Are migraineurs always sensitive to the same brightness of that light or does the sensitivity change as a result of passing a threshold?
- And does this have any function in terms of the migraine-brain?

As it turns out, migraineurs are not sensitive to *bright light,* but rather they perceive light as brighter than non-migraineurs do because of two reasons:

1) Given that migraineurs have hyper sensitive sensory organs with more neuronal receptor connections, the minimum amount of light needed for stimulating the brain of a migraineur is lower than the amount of light a non-migraineur would require.
2) Their pupils cannot close so tight, therefore more "unwanted" light reaches the visual brain system; a true one-two punch.

Sensitivity to "bright light" triggers a prodrome only if the migraineur is low in voltage energy. If a migraineur suddenly becomes sensitive to a light, even though the light has not changed and previously she was not sensitive to it, she has exceeded a stimulus threshold and entered alert mode, and her hyper sensory neurons have used up her available voltage faster than the energy was being made available for them.

It is this *change in the perception* of light that matters and not light in general. Similarly, increased loudness of someone talking and sudden sensitivity to this loudness implies that the migraineur's brain is running low on voltage energy. Sudden sensitivity to a scent also represents energy deficit. All these point to an evolutionarily different brain—discussed later in this section.

The Most Typical Prodromes

Let us learn the most common functional prodromes, what they mean, and when they should be a bigger concern or indication of an oncoming emergency. Since there is so much confusion in literature about prodromes, this long section is dedicated entirely to prodrome types—this is not an exhaustive list; you may have additional prodromes not discussed here.

Vertigo and Dizziness

Migraine associated dizziness feels like having sea legs. With dizziness it is possible to walk. Migraine associated vertigo (MAV) is not dizziness at all. It is not possible to walk with MAV. I describe dizziness and MAV—both are migraine prodromes and both are associated with possible insulin resistance[160].

Dizziness is a loss of balance, and is a common sign of low blood pressure or a sudden change in blood pressure. It can represent low blood volume—i.e. dehydration. Dizziness itself doesn't cause a migraine but may represent electrolyte imbalance; it is a migraine prodrome. Suddenly getting up from sitting and feeling lightheaded and unbalanced is a typical migraine prodrome. Dizziness is often experienced during a migraine as well, can cause falls, walking into doors, etc.

Some migraineurs report vertigo as their migraine prodrome. While dizziness is the loss of one's balance, triggered by the ears' balance sensing mechanism, vertigo is the sensation of one's surroundings spinning. Check out this video of how a vertigo-eye looks like as it follows the non-existent spin:

http://upload.wikimedia.org/wikipedia/commons/b/b6/Optokinetic_nystagmus.gif

Medical warning: both dizziness and vertigo can be signs of other, often serious, health conditions. If you experience sudden dizziness or vertigo and have never previously had either symptom, call 911 or have someone take you to an emergency room. Do not drive!

Tingling in the face, hands, feet

While these are very typical migraine prodromes—they may also represent other serious conditions, such as heart trouble, an impending stroke, pinched nerves in the back or neck, and even complications associated with type 2 diabetes, such as neuralgia. Some migraineurs feel tingling either on their face or their hands or their feet, some feel more than one of these but not all, and others all of them together. Tingling anywhere in the body is associated with a nerve ending signaling that the originating neuron is irritated. Some tingling feels like unscratchable itch, some as burning heat, and some as if ants were running all over the body or parts of it. It may feel like pins and needles. In all of these cases the neurons that send the sensation are signaling trouble in their environment. The message you receive prior to your migraine means the neurons are demanding something they lack.

Medical warning: some serious health conditions can be associated with tingling and burning sensations such as pins and needles. If you have never previously experienced them and now do, contact your doctor. They may not be migraine related.

Ataxia, Coma, Convulsion

These are terms most people don't associate with migraines, and thus we don't hear of them often in this context but some form of migraines, such as hemiplegic migraines, can come with ataxia (loss of body control), convulsions (uncontrolled body movements), and even coma (being unconscious for a period of time). Convulsions can also be seizures. Sometimes a migraine can morph into a seizure. While most hemiplegic migraineurs (often called familial hemiplegic migraine type 1 or 2) lose sensitivity in an arm or leg or the entire body on one side, we must remember that organs and tissues contained in the body controlled by the side of the brain in distress are also affected by the migraine. It is entirely possible to lose bladder control, bowel control, muscle control, and migraineurs can even fall into coma since the loss of control can also affect the lungs, the heart, and other vital organs. In the majority of cases they are affected for only a short time. This "short time" doesn't mean seconds. It may mean hours or days. Hemiplegic migraines are a special concern because they can cause serious permanent damage.

Medical warning: other serious health conditions can be associated with ataxia, convulsion, and coma—this is obvious. If you find yourself in this situation, or you know that this may happen to you, please wear a medical information bracelet or similar to alert paramedics and other medical personnel to your condition, so that you are not automatically treated as if you have had a cardiac failure or a stroke. Please consult with your relatives and friends as well, and advise them to tell the paramedics that you have hemiplegic migraines.

Electrical Nightmare of a Magnetic Personality

A woman got in touch with me one day in one of the migraine forums, and she even asked her husband to "testify on her behalf" because she felt her symptom was so unusual that nobody would believe her. Her body is so full of electrical charge that she kills the battery in every watch she wears within three months; her cell phones meet a similar fate with the same frequency. This was the first time I had heard about such an extreme symptom by others, and I was left speechless. I am just like her and then some. I have yet to have a day of opening my car door without being zapped, yet the same car will not zap anyone else in my family. I have a cat that used to like to brush against me, but after so many unexpected zaps, she no longer does. I am full of electrical charge. I kill my keyboard regularly and turn my computer off in the process from simply sitting down at my computer. I decided to "ground" myself and touch a metal shelf on which I keep my printers—yep, I killed my printers. My husband kindly offered shackles for my ankles in order to ground me.

After this electric migraineur told her story, I felt confident enough to ask about the subject in migraine groups and forums and found many other migraineurs who reported being similarly charged. In my Facebook migraine group the question of electrostatic personalities has come up regularly with similar stories of charged migraineurs. This finding is stunning! Upon reflection, it makes a lot of sense. Migraineurs generate different voltage magnitude from the norm, and their modern surroundings offer plenty of possibilities for "unplanned" discharge events. While this may sound funny and weird to someone who is not a migraineur, for a migraineur this is a warning: being so overly charged hints at being overstimulated and using much more voltage power than at other times. Please consider this a prodrome! When full of charge like this, you need to prepare to prevent a migraine.

Auras

Although aura alone, with or without pain, is discussed in migraine literature, I found that many migraineurs who have had aura (me included) had no idea that they were having one. That is because the textbook description of what an aura is supposed to be is not what many migraineurs see. Aura is quite misunderstood. Here I want to take the opportunity to clarify what falls into the category of an aura.

If you search in literature for descriptions of the word "aura" you predominantly will find only two types:

1. Colorful aura that is similar to the Northern Lights
2. Black and white or colored aura that looks similar to a semi-curved chain saw

For both you may get a gray or white or black spot in an area, a blind spot, where you cannot see. Auras are usually one-sided, so only one eye is affected. The lack of general knowledge of all forms of auras is understandable, given the lack of understanding of what an aura actually is and the lack of communication between doctors and migraineurs. Many auras look nothing like the two kinds so well discussed in literature. I list here as many types as I have already heard of or experienced myself:

1. Little shooting stars flying rapidly in half circle, each for a very short time, either color or black and white but they are shiny bright
2. Fireworks flying towards you or away from you in a number of little sparks, normally all at once but each "flare" takes up

only a small space, though the whole fireworks may or may not take up an entire eye's vision

3. Color dots that move out of vision
4. Little twirling light (often red I am told). Interestingly, this aura is typical for those who meditate and may appear during meditation as well
5. Blurry vision as if you would need a windshield-wiper either in one or both eyes
6. Specks like rain drops in your vision that are not floaters
7. Shooting target like circles that may be steady or move—by move I mean become smaller and bigger in constant motion
8. Wavy image as if everything was becoming fluid
9. Scintillating scotoma in which there are little specks in motion making a region of your vision blurry. It can also start as a lightening or a circular irregular shape, or like a bee swarm speckling
10. Many little colored dots coming closer together with a black spot in the middle—the middle is where you cannot see
11. Tunnel vision for a longer period of time
12. Alice in Wonderland phantom movements that make people's faces appear like cartoons or their body parts out of proportion
13. White lines appearing over text (as in crossed out text)
14. Fortification spectrum—similar to scintillating scotoma but a larger "white-out" area
15. "Back lighting" experience where it seems as if there is light shining from behind the eyes

16. Specks that appear and disappear with frequency
17. Peripheral vision blurred
18. Lasers shooting into the view
19. Little white sparkles that drift around in the peripheral vision
20. Haloes around bright objects that are blurred (haloes are generally signs of astigmatism but if you only have them sometimes then they are aura) for a limited time only, not always
21. A circle of purple mini-dots, that morph into a circle with green mini-dots with a black center resembling an eye
22. Headlights or flash lights shining randomly in the peripheral vision
23. A perfectly straight gray line
24. Red and black blotches
25. Like a flip book, showing only every other frame of what is looked at
26. A smudge in the vision
27. Cannot see the middle letters of each word
28. Different color dots that increase in number with vision is fully impaired at the end
29. Picasso--faces appear all broken into segments
30. Similar to daydreaming except for wanting to focus but unable to focus at all—looking at anything specific is impossible
31. Grey watery looking vertical waves that shimmer or move
32. Blurred patches looking like they are bit of fluff or something on the surface. They turn into large black roundish holes with sparkly edges all around

33. Like a smoker's smoke ring moving toward you, changing shape as it moves and changes intensity in waves
34. Sudden bright light for a second several times; bright as if you looked into the sun

Auras very specifically represent a flow of current across the brain and what you see is what your occipital lobe, the region of the brain that tries to make sense of the patterns your eyes see, falsely recognizes as it is being stimulated by the flow. The blind spot corresponds to a brain region experiencing CD and has no voltage to function.

Medical Warning: Transient ischemic attack (TIA), often referred to as mini stroke, also can come with what appears like an aura. It is important for you to be able to distinguish something you have always had as part of your migraine versus something new[161,162]. If you never had an aura before, please call for emergency help.

Blurred vision

Blurred vision is a frequent complaint. I get blurred vision when I enter a crowded store or a very large space or a place with fluorescent lights. I see things a bit fuzzy or foggy, and I often feel dizzy at the same time as well. I can see everything, but I have trouble reading letters and trouble focusing. This is very typical for migraineurs and usually represents an overstimulated brain, consider it a prodrome.

Inability to Read

If suddenly you have trouble reading text messages on your phone, labels at the grocery store, or street signs on the road, you are likely in a prodrome.

Medical Warning: If you have never had the symptom of inability to read as part of your migraine, this can also represent more serious health conditions. Please call 911 or have someone take you to emergency.

Pain in the eye area

One day my right eye started to hurt as if hot burning cigarette ash flew straight into it. I went to my husband for help to find out what was in my eye. He looked at me and instead of searching for what may have been in my eye he said "the hurting eye is half the size of your other eye." In trying to find out what was in my eye, he discovered that I was entering a prodrome. This was a different eye issue from the ones I had previously experienced. In the past they had simply been different sizes; now, the smaller one actually hurt! This was new! Before my husband's observation, I used eye drops and anything else I could think of, but nothing worked.

Cluster headaches are very common for migraineurs—they are extreme eye pains. As migraines increase in numbers (medicine controlled or uncontrolled), at one point cluster headaches may show their ugly face—even if just for a very short time. The cause of cluster headaches is unknown but to some degree they respond to the protocol presented in this book. While cluster headache is a headache condition in its own category, it can often present itself as a migraine prodrome.

Meniere's Disease and Tinnitus

It seems that many migraineurs are "blessed" with Meniere's disease or tinnitus[163]. All migraineurs are sensitive to sounds and many seem to have hypermobile ear drums—meaning their ear drums respond to sounds (vibration in the air) that most people cannot hear or otherwise sense. Meniere's can represent the sound of each little hair in the inner ear being destroyed—this sounds like a bell ringing. Tinnitus is a loud hissing white noise that may come and go or it is there permanently. At this time, no one has yet figured out the reason for tinnitus though it appears that insulin resistance may play a part in it[164]. For some migraineurs Meniere's disease and/or tinnitus is a permanent state but for many it is a prodrome.

Irritable Bowel Syndrome (IBS)

IBS and some types of vomiting (including cyclical vomiting disorders) are prodromes. IBS can take on many forms: diarrhea, constipation, cramping, gassiness, doubling over in pain, etc. IBS can immediately precede the onset of migraine as it morphs into vomiting. Vomiting means that, as your adrenaline is released and your body is ready for the fight-or-flight, you still have undigested food in your stomach—this can morph into cyclical vomiting, which may last for longer than a day. Since digestion stops when adrenaline is released, whatever undigested food is in your stomach will come back up. Those with diarrhea or urgent bowel movement merely empty whatever is in their intestines already partially digested. IBS as migraine prodrome needs no treatment as it stops immediately after your body is fully clear from all food.

Restless Legs Syndrome (RLS)

RLS happens because adrenaline is preparing you for "fight or flight" and your legs are energized in order for you to run away from danger. Prior to RLS your heart rate increases and more oxygen is delivered to your lungs. Everything is prepared for your running but you are sitting, so the adrenaline induced energy is built up in your legs. You would actually benefit from running or at least trying to walk it off. Normally RLS occurs as a prodrome but sometimes as a postdrome as well. As long as you know how to prevent the migraine from materializing, you can walk/jog off the extra adrenaline and remain both pain and RLS free.

Edema

If you wear socks or stockings, or tight-fitting shoes, check out the marks they leave on your legs when you remove them. If you find a deep sock line with puffiness under and over it, you have found the sign of too much water being retained in your body. If you only see this right before a migraine hits, you know this is a sign to pay attention to in the future. This is known as edema, and edema is caused when carbohydrates (any kinds: simple sugars, grains of any kinds, fruits, or vegetables) we eat turn into glucose and enter our cells. Read the following paper for an example:

https://www.hormonesmatter.com/pregnancy-toes-sugar-feet/

Edema like this can show up anywhere on your body. For most people it is around the ankle or toes because of gravity.

Medical Warning: Swollen toes and ankles can also be very common symptoms for people with circulatory problems and blood pressure issues, so if this is constant for you, head to your doctor for a checkup.

Tight or Loose Rings

This often happens to me (and to many women). We enjoy a show, dinner, or party, and go together to the restroom—a standard feature of the female social support system. Before washing hands most of us usually remove our rings—few women ever want soap and water to mess with their rings. Can you remove your rings? If they are pretty much stuck and you need soap and water to remove them, you have retained too much water in the interstitial fluid. This is a prodrome.

If they fall off your finger or keep on turning with the stone facing down by its own weight—assuming they were sized correctly—you have not had enough water and are dehydrated. This is also a prodrome.

Note: both tightness and looseness can be temperature dependent as well. These are prodromes when the temperature remains unchanged.

Urination Frequency

Many migraineurs, women in particular, tell me "oh I can't drink water because all I do is run to the toilet all day long". This is a prodrome! This is a sign that the water is not entering your cells and no matter how much water you drink the water will just pass through. Drinking lots of water is not hydration and can be quite harmful. If you find yourself running to urinate too often (assuming you have no other health conditions that would account for it, like a urinary tract infection) it is a sign that you are entering a prodrome.

Urine Color

A very important sign to judge the health of your hydration level is by the color of your urine. While this isn't something we normally look at, from now on you must. What comes out pretty much represents how you metabolized what went in. It informs you about what is going on inside your body, including your brain. The color of your urine can tell a lot about your hydration level and the health of your kidneys. For most people urine color changes somewhat during the day, so get used to looking at your urine every time before you flush. I reached proper hydration when my urine color is not darker in the morning and does not get lighter as the day progresses—it is always the same color. What this suggests is that my hydration level is ideal and that my kidneys work together in great harmony keeping my cells and organs functioning always at their best. While this may not seem to be a very important issue for a non-migraineur, for a migraineur it is a big deal.

A quick note here for those taking vitamins that color urine. Many migraineurs (if not all) have a certain genetic variation: MTHFR C667T variance, discussed later in greater detail. It is associated with an inability to methylate folate (B9) and to absorb other B vitamins from food. Many migraineurs take synthetic B vitamins and end up with neon color urine. The color implies that you are not absorbing the vitamins; you need to change to a bioactive form! Once you take the right B vitamins, your urine color should not change.

Sound Volume Increase

Here are a few specific examples from my experience and see if you can identify with any of these. One day I was driving the car and my husband was talking to me. We had a nice conversation. Suddenly his voice sounded too loud for me. I asked him several times to lower his voice. He repeatedly told me that he did not change his voice. As I kept on complaining he started to whisper. Obviously, I had become more sensitive to sound. The moment when it seemed that he started to talk louder was my opportunity to recognize that I needed to prevent a migraine—the sound volume tolerance passed my threshold and became a prodrome. It is not that he talked louder; my brain no longer had enough energy to properly handle the incoming sound waves.

Light Sensitivity Increase

Another example comes from a day of bright white skies without sun. I have also heard from many migraineurs that such light often bothers them. Normally, when our brain is not in prodrome, light does not trouble us. But being in such light for an extended period of time causes my brain to be overstimulated – it is working nonstop to deal with such a strong input – and at some point, I will begin squinting. When this occurs, my threshold has been reached and I have transitioned into a state of prodrome.

An example played out while writing this book. My office balcony has white railings that are lit half the day by the sun. They had been lit all morning with a very bright sun but it didn't bother me — the white lit railing wasn't on my radar. Then at one point later that morning I got up to draw the shades to cover that bright white railing, still lit by the sun. It was at this point that I realized I had entered prodrome. Paying attention to your body is extremely important!

Those Awful Odors

Sometimes when I cook a meal, I may get irritated by the smell of what I am cooking. There is nothing wrong with the food and the smell doesn't bother anyone else. However, I am ready to just leave the house I feel so nauseous. This is an indication that I reached my scent threshold—this is my body telling me that I am entering prodrome. If I don't realize it in time and do nothing, within minutes I must rush to open all doors and windows. At this point, I am very close to having passed the prodrome stage and if I don't act, I will come down with a migraine. Others avoid every opportunity to go to the mall because of the spraying of fragrance samples. Air fresheners, cleaning fluids can all cause a prodrome.

Cravings

Cravings are not equivalent to feeling hungry. One can be hungry and not crave anything in particular, or one can be craving something very specific and not be hungry at all. If you have always hated avocados and you suddenly get a craving for one, it is definitely a sign you should pay attention to; it tells you that something has changed. Many migraineurs crave salty snacks before a migraine hits—have some. Craving sugar? Do not have sugar; eat a small piece of low carbohydrate whole fruit or a half a glass of whole milk instead.

Moodiness

In the case of an impending migraine you may also find yourself a little bit short tempered, a bit more nervous or anxious, yawning a lot, and a tad off in general. You may snap at your partner, children, or colleagues without any reason. This is a migraine prodrome so pay attention.

Full of Energy

Some migraineurs report a feeling of being full of energy, nearly at a euphoric level, usually up to the evening prior to a migraine. This is a very hard prodrome to act on since you feel great, better than ever. The last thing you think of is that this is a prodrome but it is. This is also the hardest to control since you feel so great that you feel invincible. However, usually this is a long-lasting prodrome and gives you ample time to prepare.

Yawning

Yawning is the least understood but most common prodrome. It has two functions. One of them is an indication for increased need for oxygen. So take a deep breath more often, or breathe more deeply, sort of yoga style, in order to get your oxygen level increased—your adrenaline and other stress hormones have been released and started the fight-or-flight mode, which requires increased oxygen. The other function is evolutionary. Since migraine itself is a threat and stress response, yawning, to this day, is part of such response in apes and many mammals. It is a sign of power by showing powerful incisors. Notice how when you yawn you show your teeth. This is a prodrome.

Extremely Tired and Beat

Some migraineurs report feeling very tired prior to a migraine. This prodrome is easier to associate with something bad to come.

Thirst

Are you thirsty all the time no matter how much water you drink? If the answer is "yes" (and you don't have type 2 diabetes) then you are dehydrated, despite your drinking lots of water. Dehydration leads to migraine if left untreated. In the migraine group, advanced migraineurs who don't usually come down with migraines anymore may come down with one if they don't hydrate properly.

Prodromes That Others Can See

Lastly, I want to discuss some signs that are visible to others but you may not see them yourself without having them pointed out to you. You need to learn to identify these visible prodromes, so you too can see them without anyone's help. I present them in a way that you should not need another person to tell you what has changed; you can see it for yourself. I'll start with the easiest signs and continue from there. These signs show up as much as four hours before a migraine so you have time to prepare.

In my work with several thousand migraineurs over the past several years, I have discovered some "universal migraine marker prodromes." Most of these prodromes are not documented anywhere else but in this book (and some in my published academic articles).

The Eyes and the Face

Spend some time each day looking at your face and ankles, feel your toes in your shoes, and rotate the rings around your fingers. Look for edema. When we feel really good, we tend to forget our migraine-brain limitations and often find ourselves reaching into that cookie jar without even noticing. Then, hours later—or typically as you wake up in the morning—you look into the mirror and find a puffed-up monster looking back at you with eye lids so enlarged you can barely open your eyes. Or you have nice many-layered pillows or dark rings under your eyes. Or you stand on the scale and overnight you gained a couple of pounds. These are signs of edema that arrived to wake you. Such delayed edema (meaning far removed from the time of the cause) is double trouble.

On the one hand, it means that you ate the forbidden cookie without consideration of what it does to a migraine-brain because you were not even conscious of eating it. This happens to many migraineurs at the beginning. On the other hand, it represents the potentially more serious problem of insulin resistance. A delayed response from glucose moving into your cells and causing havoc means that your glucose transport and insulin were not working efficiently!

Prior to a migraine, there are many minor visual changes in your face, some of which are hard for you to observe unless you have "before" and "after" images to compare. I advise you to take snap shots of your face for a month, every single day—particularly if you are still ovulating, and especially in perimenopause when your cycles become irregular. Your face changes from the forbidden cookie just as much as from your monthly cycles, barometric pressure change, temperature change, full moon, etc. It is important for you to notice when your face changes so you can prepare for all monthly expected and unexpected variables. Your face reflects the condition of your body and the activities of your hormones so pay attention to the signs! Eventually the signs are so recognizable that you no longer need the snap shots.

Either with a tape or a lipstick draw a square on the mirror around your facial image while standing always on the same spot—mark it with a tape on the floor if you have to – to make sure that the size of the square you created on the mirror is such that if you stand at the marked spot you have your entire face (and only your face) in the square and with the same lighting as usual. Take a snap shot of your face with a camera or a cell phone. Save the pictures you create and date/time stamp them. After you have many snap shots of yourself, upload them to your computer and place them all side by side for comparison. You will be surprised to discover some significant changes—but if you cannot see differences, just ask a member of the opposite sex. Your body also changes—pay attention to ankle size, your posture, swollen appearance.

Pay particular attention to your eyes: the size, shape, angle, the size of your pupils, and how far or close your eyes are to each other. Are your eyes open the same way as normally? Are they the same color as always? Are you squinting more than before? Look also at the eye lids. Are they puffier than usual? Do they have the same shape and form as usual? Do your eyes look the same? Do they feel like they are hanging or are they tight like they are ready to crack if you blink? Look also at the area below the eyes: are they as clear and smooth as before? Are they darker? Is the area below the eyes the same on both eyes, or is one puffier or darker than the other? Are the deep lines nearly black? Are they puffed up into several layers of little water-containers? Did you suddenly get more wrinkles under your eyes than you had just a few hours ago?

Eye Size

Your signs may differ but what is important is to look for them. For me, my eye-size change turned out to be the main prodrome. It is the case apparently for an awful lot of migraineurs based on their reports and posted pictures in the migraine group. This change in eye size seems to be an (until now) undocumented universal migraine prodrome phenomenon.

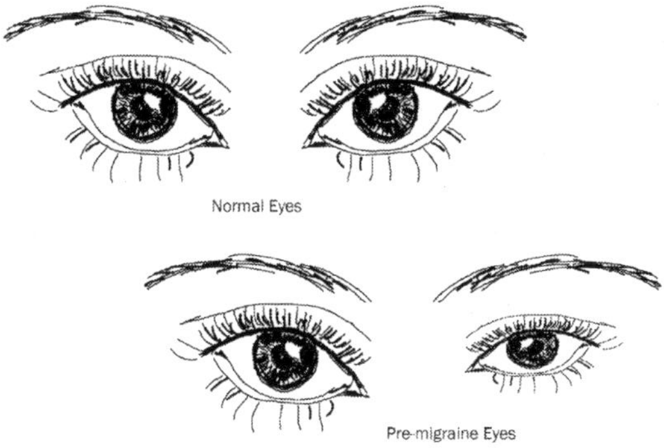

Figure 6. Normal eyes above and prodrome eyes below

For some people one of the eyes can take on a different shape as a result of becoming smaller; it may have a different angle as well.

Eye Lids

Your eyelids may look swollen when you are having a prodrome. I usually see women with puffy eyelids who are vegans or vegetarians, or who drink soft drinks, smoothies, teas, and alcoholic beverages and eat lots of fruits, veggies, or other carbohydrates. Puffy eyelids imply a dehydrated body. Do not drink water only! If you do, your body will make you eliminate that water within 30 minutes and you will only dilute your electrolytes further.

Droopy Eyelids

There are many people of various ages with permanently droopy eyelids. For them droopy eyelids cannot be understood as prodrome. If you don't normally have droopy eyelids, and they suddenly appear, this could be an indication that a migraine is on its way.

Medical Warning: this condition may require medical attention so head to an emergency room if you never had this before as part of your migraine—it can also be a sign of a stroke. Furthermore, this sign is very typical for hemiplegic migraineurs and can be indicative that they are about to lose control of half their body. If you are a hemiplegic migraineur, please lie down and call for help. Do not get up or walk.

Under-Eye Puffs

Under our eyes most of us get a little bulge or puff as we get older. You see yourself every single day in the mirror and it is hard to discover that your bulges or puffs are different from what they were 30 minutes earlier! But knowing what to look for and paying attention helps with realizing that you have identified a prodrome. These signs are indications that you have retained too much water from eating carbohydrates.

Medical Warning: If the under-eye puffiness is constant, it may indicate other health conditions, so please make sure you visit your doctor to exclude any serious cause! Retaining water means your cells are not able to dump their toxins because you have had too much salt relative to potassium—salt loves water, but potassium is needed for that salt and toxic water to leave. It is an unhealthy state and could indicate heart or kidney trouble.

Under-Eye Shallowness

If you are about to get a migraine you may see your under-eye area shallower than usual and may even see dark circles or your existing dark circles get darker and uneven—darker under one eye than under the other. Even if eye size remains the same you may find that your eyes seem "sunken in" and the area under your eyes may have a kind of hollow appearance. If you notice shallowness or darker than normal circles under your eyes, this suggests a condition opposite to the one with puffiness under the eyes: you have too little water in your system and are dehydrated. It is important to note that circles under the eyes can also mean fatigue, lack of sleep, etc. If you did not get enough sleep, chances are you will wake up with dark circles under your eyes. If you had no dark circles when you woke up but develop them later during the day, even if this represents only fatigue, hydration is in order.

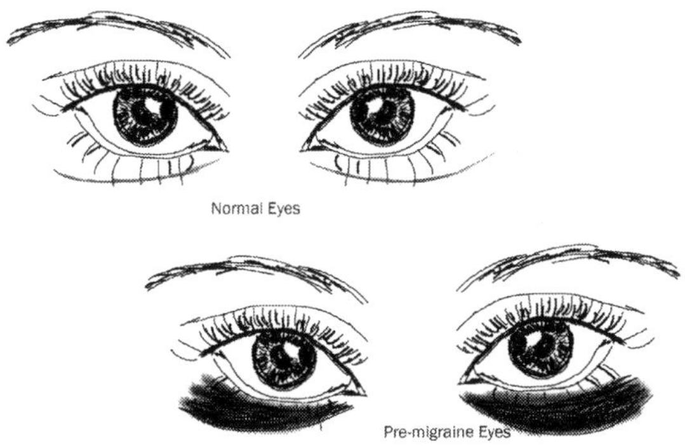

Figure 7. Under eye dark circles, shallowness

Twitching Eyes

Some migraineurs have twitching eyes or a vibrating eye lid or a little nerve jumping under one eye. This is a sign of electrolyte imbalance and is therefore a prodrome.

Speech, hearing, cognition Impairment

"Stumbling over words" was one of the comments posted one day in the Facebook group by a migraine sufferer, and that made me remember how many times I had had difficulty coming up with words and comprehending the meaning of words before the onset of a migraine. I would just internalize it as a "senior moment" and never pay attention to it. Mistake! Pay attention to every little sign that indicates that today may not be like "just another day." Being able to take countermeasures before it is too late makes the difference between coming down with or preventing a migraine.

Some migraineurs expressed concern that having migraines may damage their brains permanently. They are correct, migraines do damage the brain[70,120,165-168]; more on this in later sections. I had "brain fog" one day while working on the first edition of this book. I mean that not only was I searching for words but wrote gibberish—I had trouble comprehending. I prevented the migraine and all was fine but I looked at my writing with fresh eyes the next day and I honestly wondered if I should leave that "foggy paragraph" unchanged so the reader can see how hard it is to fully function while in a brain fog or in any other type of cognitively impairing prodrome. Full of typos, transposed letters, words with missing letters, incomplete sentences, words in the wrong order, bad grammar, etc. Fortunately for me, my recognition of the "fog" as a migraine prodrome allowed me to jump into my prevention routine, and another migraine was averted.

Medical Warning: Signs of a possible stroke

Some of the signs I noted above about speech and hearing impairment are also very typical signs of a stroke. Dizziness, vertigo, Meniere's disease, sudden tinnitus, lack of balance in general, particularly if the body tends to lean toward one side or leans forward too much during casual walking, may signal stroke or even a brain tumor rather than migraine. Lack of flexibility on the face anywhere, like smiling with only half a lip, or blinking with only one eye, etc., are all signs of a possible stroke as well as hemiplegic migraines. If you never had them before as part of a migraine, ask for help to call emergency and get to the ER A.S.A.P! While migraines are not typically followed by strokes, strokes can happen any time; migraineurs have an increased risk for getting strokes[31,169-171].

Symptoms that are new for you should never be ignored!

Too Much Potassium, Too Little Salt

Some signs associated with too much potassium that are prodromes are: heart palpitations, excess urination, feeling cold, rings falling off fingers, feeling faints, cold sweat.

Warning: Too much potassium—hyperkalamia—or too little salt—hyponatremia--can be dangerous to your life.

The Evolution of Migraines: My Hypothesis

As a scientist, I consider evolution to be the most important factor in who we are today. If we look back in time, we can examine certain time periods in our evolutionary past. The particular ones picked by me are arbitrary for presenting a few important points relative to migraines.

Animals in nature are always on alert because if they are not, they become food for a predator. Therefore, for them having a brain on high alert is naturally the default. The migraine-brain is a brain on high alert and as such it fits within the human evolutionary past. Looking at mammals, particularly those with highly evolved social networks, we find that alertness is a shared task. One primate, for example, may be on the lookout while the others forage and rest, and then they take turns so that everyone in the family or tribe can be nourished equally. Primates, our closest relatives in evolutionary terms, likely all have a hyper sensitized brain. I speculate that a brain with hyper sensory organ sensitivities could very well be the default primate brain. If so, and since humans are primates, the ancient human default brain had also likely been the hyper sensory organ brain, i.e. the migraine-brain. If this is true we still have to explain why not all humans sport such a brain today and why such a brain hurts.

As a primate society increases in size and develops stronger social bonds, some primates may retain this hyper sensitive brain and specialize in family or tribe security, while others – who contribute to the social network with other skills – may gradually develop natural talents that are important for their own specific contribution. Slowly they lose the hyper sensitivity whose attributes for them are no longer required.

In early human societies, specialization may have been gender based as well. Archeology and anthropology teach us that the hunters were males and the gatherers females and so their roles required somewhat different brain adaptations. Continuing with my hypothesis, it makes great sense to have more females with migraine-brains because they remained at the home-base but needed to stay alert in order to react to predators of both the animal and human kind. The alertness useful in the males' hunting or raiding activities was quite different, and would have been more active than reactive. The male hunters would be trying to kill pray whereas the females and children were trying to avoid being pray. This would explain why females and children, including males until past their puberty are more likely to be migraineurs.

Now let's look at another scenario under the same evolutionary path hypothesis. In the olden times when our ancestors roamed the savanna and forests which were full of predators, hyper sensitive sensory abilities (i.e. today's migraine-brains) were likely highly prized, and those who had them were valued members of their tribes! Because migraineurs have enhanced sensory organs, and therefore can smell better, hear better, see better in the dark, feel skin stimulus better, and often are super tasters, these special skills must have been very important for every tribe. A special skill like this is a powerful survival advantage that can benefit the entire tribe; it is a definite evolutionary advantage to smell danger from far away rather than when it may be too late. Likely a tribe had only a small number of such highly sensitized males or females and they may have spent the night tending to the fire and the safety of the tribe while the rest slept.

In both of the above scenarios the hyper sensitive sensory organ brain provides a certain survival advantage and this is so beneficial that it is passed on to progeny. This would explain why still today such a large percent of humans have a hyper sensitive sensory organ brain—a migraine-brain. Some advantages associated with having a migraine-brain could still be useful for society. Over the years there have been thousands of migraineurs in the Facebook migraine group. We learned that we all share many of our special sensitivities, and our "skills" are nearly identical. We know that our primate relatives and other mammals have significantly stronger abilities in smelling, hearing, tasting, touching, and often even seeing than humans do. Since we have evolved from primates, it appears likely that many humans have lost their hyper sensory organ sensitivity but not all. This then would place the migraine-brain into the category of an ancient brain rather than a sick brain, and those without migraines into the category of having an "adapted" and more modern brain.

Some humans may adapt faster than others based on epigenetic (environmental) factors. Adaptation happens by genetic changes that are based on natural selection and not on the will of an individual. Looking at primitive human tribes that can still be found today, we find they are perfectly adapted to their "world". Plucking them out of their environment and moving them into modern society makes them ill-adapted and sick. They often perish very fast and not only due to diseases they would not have been subjected to before but also because of the inability to adapt fast enough to the metabolic challenges modern life places upon them. This shows that adaptation is a genetic process and that it takes time. I think you can see where I am heading: a migraine-brain is not a sick brain but a brain that has not been able to fully adapt to modern life—high carbohydrate foods, noise, light on demand, perfumes, and the many brain stimulating tools we use—such as the computer I am writing this book on—cause trouble to a maladapted brain.

Migraineurs tell me that they can hear people whisper even if a floor separates them. Indeed, they can! In the 1994 Northridge earthquake, in which I lost my home, a gas cap popped off some distance away from our house and I could hear the hissing sound from however far it was! It was so faint a sound that my husband could not hear it at all until he was five feet from the damaged pipe. Such skills are life-saving evolutionary skills that can still have definite benefits. When I was in the middle of that earthquake and used my superior senses to possibly prevent a disaster, I did not get a migraine! I used my skills for a purpose, used all my available brain energy and hormones the proper way, and I had no pain. While all these extraordinary things were happening, I went through an entire series of migraine prodromes, such as anxiety, adrenaline rush, fast heartbeat, deep breathing, IBS, and RLS. I had no pain that night because I had reacted to the events in harmony with my abilities, I had even run to help neighbors—and in the process, I had used up all the released adrenalin. I played out the evolutionary role of my skills that permitted the survival (my husband managed to locate and turn off a gas valve upstream of the leak) of many people that night.

> *"My migraine brain probably just saved a whole block of houses, busy road, and businesses! So this morning while driving out of our neighborhood I noticed a gas smell. I call the busses where I first smelled it but they didn't smell anything. I called 911. So now, while driving home...gas company trucks everywhere! My husband went up to talk to them and said, yes, they did find a bad leak from my call!! The owner of the house didn't even smell it! He kept telling my husband thank you over and over! YEAH MIGRAINE BRAIN!"*

Her story is eerily similar to mine during the earthquake.

As noted previously, migraineurs see better in the dark than other people[172-174]. Most migraineurs have very vivid dreams and often restless sleep—not associated with anxiety or depression[175-177]. Migraine sensory organs are always in high drive[3]. These examples show that having a migraine-brain in a dangerous situation, when it can function in the way for which it is uniquely adapted, is a real advantage. The reality of living in our modern, civilized world however, rarely presents a need for this advantage.

Another evolutionary quirk affecting migraineurs is the full moon. It seems to be a puzzle since it simply means that on a clear night we see better under the stronger light of a full moon. Our night environment is better lit. So what is the connection between migraines and a full moon? Predators that used to hunt early humans had an increased probability of success during the bright light of a full moon. Go ahead and stand by a street light as the full moon appears high and bright in the sky and take a photo with your cell phone. Note that the full moon appears brighter than the street light. Understandably, migraineurs with their sensitive brain tend to be more on alert on full moon nights, using up more brain energy in the process. Once this is understood and countermeasures are taken prior to and during the full moon to assure that more energy is available, the curse of the full moon as a migraine cause disappears.

As I have mentioned repeatedly, in the Facebook migraine group we discovered how identical we are in our traits and abilities. We also share many crazy experiences. Here is a message from a member who, having received the 1st edition of my book, wrote to me within days:

> *"Dear Dr. Stanton,*
>
> *I ordered your book and just finished it this past weekend.*
>
> *Within the first 20 pages of your book, I had to put the book down twice because I was crying that finally someone understood me. I felt like you were describing me, either that or you and I are somehow related!"*

As you can see, migraineurs share a lot more than pain! Migraineurs pretty much have nearly identical brains. This means a lot more than you think. Evolution doesn't create genetic variations that stay active in a population in large numbers unless those variations provide some advantage or benefit to the survival of those who carry it and can pass it on. Given that over 15% of the global population has migraines[178], it is too large of a percentage to consider it a *random identical variation by accident.* Rather it is connected to some *advantage* whose importance in modern life is diminished or nonexistent. In evolutionary terms our modern era is a blink of an eye. As a result, genes that used to be advantageous are still passed on, even if they are no longer advantageous to the individual.

The migraine-brain is just one of many similar evolutionary stories. For example, there is a muscle in the arm that is essential for tree climbing (it was in our primate life) but it is no longer necessary. Not being necessary does not mean that the genomes of all people drop instructions for building this particular muscle at once. A certain portion of the population doesn't have this muscle anymore whereas others still do[179]. Such transition is a clear sign that if a trait or characteristic is no longer vital for the survival of a species, it does not disappear overnight but it remains in the genome and it may or may not get expressed during the life of an individual. These no longer "must have" traits and characteristics can sometimes take a very long time to be eliminated from the active functionality of the genome, from the process of a genotype becoming a phenotype. Think of the pinky toe with no acknowledged role or function in modern humans—it has been greatly reduced in its size over our evolutionary history but it is still there[180].

The evolutionary process of elimination is only accelerated in cases when the particular trait or characteristic is disadvantageous for the survival chances of the species. Migraine-brain seems stable in percentage relative to population growth over time—at least for the short time period in which records have been kept, with the exception of one location. A study showed that in the very limited population (6500 persons) of Norfolk Island, whose ancestry for the past 12 generations can be followed back to the same geographical location without the availability of any genetic mix, over 25% of the population is made up of migraineurs[181]. Therefore, in the larger modern world where genetic mixing is possible, the percentage of migraineurs is slowly reducing (currently around 15%). Given the slowness of breeding migraine out of the population, this would indicate that migraine-brains either have not proven to be disadvantageous long enough or that they are not damaging enough in relation to the advantages they can still provide.

If nature has not found the migraine-brain detrimental enough to be eliminated from the genome, it certainly cannot be justified to dull it or to make it ineffective by medications. Rather we should embrace our special skills and figure out what is behind the pain and how to prevent it. To understand what migraine pain is, first we have to understand how we end up with a migraine-brain.

Genetic Inheritance and Migraines

You will find a large amount of confusing – and sometimes misleading – information in the popular media and on the internet regarding this *in vogue* subject. We know that migraine is genetic[119,182-193] and have also discussed that it is not a disease. We have lots of genes that are instructed to turn on (get expressed) at a certain time in our lives by genetic switches. Puberty is a good example for this: certain genes turn on at a certain age to initiate the process of sexual maturity and the release of certain hormones to induce and support those changes. At what exact age the genetic switch turns on the sexual maturation varies based on environmental and cultural factors.

We are now starting to understand that most people by their mid-30's develop at least one nodule that is pre-cancerous from which cancer may develop but need not to[194]. At what point – if ever – it becomes an active cancer depends on the genetic switches that may turn on given the particular environment and lifestyle of a person. A woman may express breast cancer even though she is the first one in her family to do so. For her it does not appear to be inherited but a gene may have been expressed early due to some environmental factor—many cancers, including breast cancers, appear to be metabolic disorders caused by excess carbohydrates[195-200,195,196,201-205]. These researchers are showing the metabolic connection of glucose as a most critical suspect in cancer sustenance and perhaps also as cause. If they are correct about the influence of glucose, and if there is a genetic predisposition to cancer, perhaps the consumption of sugar can be the very stress factor that induces the genetic expression and starts the support of the survival and metastasis of cancerous cells.

While numerous genes are preprogrammed to become active in a certain stage of development or age, many others are expressed due to other factors governed by changes in the cells' environment. Changes in the extracellular environment may generate changes in the intracellular environment, which prompt gene expression in the nucleus of the cell. In many ways, the internal workings of cells are at the mercy of the organism's (in our case: the human's) internal, external, physical and social environmental experiences and challenges. Experiences and challenges get transcribed by various biochemical processes at a molecular-level, influencing cell behavior and genetic development—this is epigenetics. You know one of these biochemical processes, the one that utilizes the "stress" hormones as messengers that trigger an unconscious "fight or flight response". Exposure to repeated high-level stress has been shown to produce permanent changes in the brain, forming PTSD[206].

While this book is not a genetic study of cancer, it is important to understand that everything we do and everything that happens to us has a chance to either help or hinder the expression of certain genes. Therefore, genetic predisposition is just part of the story. This explains why, in some families, migraines seem to be inherited from generation to generation, whereas in other families there is no discernible pattern. "The physiological effects of stress in your body are huge in terms of the power they have in modifying your genetic makeup. [Stress] can turn genetic switches on"[207].

And now we loop back to the genetic predisposition of some people to migraines. I asked migraine sufferers in my Facebook group if they recall having extra sensitive sensory experiences before their migraines first began. About 97% of those who answered the survey clearly recalled having had their heightened senses way before they experienced their first migraine; the rest did not remember because they started migraines at a very young age.

To provide the example of my family: As far as I knew, up until 2014 I had been the first and only member in my family with migraines. No one among my parents, their siblings or my cousins, and neither one of my two sons had migraines. However, my younger son did have the same extra sensitive sensory organs as I did, including smell, hearing, and amazing vision. He had his first migraine in 2014. Now we know that he has inherited his sensitivity from me and his genetic switch for getting migraines was expressed in 2014. Just recently I was given a family photograph by my cousin, which I had never seen before. It shows my mother, my grandmother, and me as a baby on the picture. I was shocked to see that my grandmother was a migraineur. She showed one of the most common migraineur prodromes on her face: one eye smaller than the other, its lid puffy, and under the other eye dark circles. It would be super nice if we could control whether a switch turns on or not; my mother, for example, never had a migraine – I can probably count on one hand how many headaches she had in her entire life. A generation was skipped in the gene expression lottery. A very detailed section with scientific explanation of migraine and its genetic base is provided in Part IV.

Migraine-Brain Development

Migraine-brain development is in some respects identical to, and in other aspects different from, the development of brains in general. Newborn babies do not have migraines, but migraine episodes have been recorded for 2-year-olds. A newborn baby doesn't yet have her neuronal connections and many of her receptors have not yet developed. In fact, the terrible-twos mark the start of the period when connections begin to form in great numbers. The number of brain cells and their connections keep on growing in earnest until adulthood, and then modification continue for the rest of our lives. The migraine-brain has more receptor connections, so it takes longer to develop. Ultimately the brain is turned into a migraine-brain when genetic switches turn on (are expressed).

As a gene becomes expressed, it activates more receptor production for each neuron—receptors form the communication between neurons so more receptor connections increase the amount of "chatter" between neurons. Genetic predisposition to something, including having a migraine-brain, is a probability and not a definite outcome. This explains why some people start their migraines as early as 2 years of age, some in puberty, many as young adults, and some post menopause, while others who inherit the genetics of the migraine-brain may never get migraines at all. At the time this book is written, there are 1069 genes known to be associated with the migraine-brain but this number is a moving target[208]. The development of more connections, more receptors, and more neurons in the sensory organs takes time and it may not be a continuous process. We often find in the history of migraineurs that initially migraines start as episodic migraines, and then migraines increase in number until the level of chronic migraines is reached. A frequency of less than 15 days of migraine per month is defined as episodic, whereas 15 days or more is defined as chronic. It is very likely that the increasing number of migraine days corresponds to the increased complexity of the sensory neuron receptor connections. This is the explanation for the well-known fact that episodic migraine sufferers usually transition into being chronic migraineurs.

I would like to mention here a little survey that popped up unintentionally in the Facebook migraine group. Migraineurs have that one amazingly consistent and little-known prodrome that I mentioned earlier: one eye gets smaller before a migraine with puffy lid over that eye and dark circle under the other eye. Eventually both eyes end up with dark circles. On one of my wedding anniversary days I posted an old photo in the group, taken over 40 years ago. I had never previously noticed that in this picture one of my eyes was smaller than the other—the same eye that would get smaller prior to my migraines in my not too distant past. In response, hundreds of members started to post their photos. Childhood photos showed up of as young as 6-year-olds with migraine eyes. This prompted me to revisit some of my own childhood photos and sure enough, on many shots (not all) I had a smaller right eye. As best I could recall, I didn't begin having migraines until my 20s. However, when I was around 10 years old I started to get major "intestinal infections" I was told with extremely painful IBS periods for no reason. In retrospect, this was likely my period of abdominal migraines. I may or may not have had "headaches" at this time; I cannot recall. Then a few years later, during my teen years, I started experiencing anxiety and panic attacks. So my migraine genes may have started to switch on when I was about 10 years old and the process of building up a migraine-brain began in earnest. The episodic migraine pains showed up when I reached my early twenties.

Because of the gradual changes in the anatomy of the brain, many migraineurs don't even know that they are experiencing migraines during their episodic migraine period. They are often misdiagnosed and ignored.

Episodic migraines can easily be misunderstood, primarily because the pain (if any) is at the end of the actual chain of events that takes place in a migraine-brain. The initial symptoms are often mistaken for conditions that are considered independent diseases themselves, as described earlier.

As the brain develops and more and more extra sensory organ connections are made, the migraine-brain becomes hyper sensitive to sensory stimuli[3] such as light, sound, scent, touch, often taste. Some migraineurs reach a stage of constant migraine-pain, interspersed with a few days of fog without pain, and some have no pain-free days at all. At this stage the migraine-brain is likely at its maximum development of extra connections and the sensory organ sensitivity is at its highest level. A perfume lingering on the street from a person ahead in the crowd may start over-stimulation that can end in a migraine with pain lasting 3+ days. In many cases migraines reduce in number as migraineurs get older. This may be explained by the gradual *degeneration* of the brain; a natural atrophy that causes connection losses (synaptic pruning). The migraine-brain may, at one point, reach a similar brain anatomy to that of a non-migraineur's brain, as it is reduced in its complexity with ageing associated brain atrophy[209]. This way the typical lessening of migraines as migraineurs get older makes sense but not because of hormonal changes--often cited as the explanation of this process. There are many elderly even in their 80s experiencing migraines, well past their female hormonal variation phase and, of course, female hormonal variations cannot explain male migraineurs or children with migraines.

In contemporary life, the ever-present lights, noises, and scents are overly stimulating for migraineurs. Their migraine-brains use up a lot of energy in informing and preparing the body for possible emergencies that never materialize. This increased energy requirement can only be satisfied with an increased level of energy transfer to the neurons, which cannot take place without an increased amount of electrolyte minerals, particularly sodium. In our dietary culture, especially with the reduced-salt and low-fat movements, even non-migraineur brains suffer[210]. It is easy to see that migraine-brains clearly have the cards stacked against them. Proper nutrition is the key to maintaining a healthy body and a healthy brain.

Unfortunately, the advice from nutritionists and others in related fields still conforms to the older guidelines that were formulated in the mid to latter part of the 20th Century, and which do not reflect the current and improved understanding of our metabolic processes and how the foods we eat sustain or harm us. Nutritionists blame the obese for eating too much and not exercising enough but by now we know that an obese person can exercise herself to death and still remain obese if her diet type (not calories!) doesn't change[211,212]. We also now know that for most people the prevention and treatment of obesity and all other metabolic diseases requires low carbohydrate intake, moderate protein intake, and higher amount of animal fats[213-225]. The proper nutritional need is available to migraineurs only from self-education through books, such as this one.

In summary: migraine-brain develops over time with many more neuronal receptor connections than regular brains, and this requires more energy[144,226] since the brain must process far more sensory inputs from hyper sensitive sensory organs[3]. An example is the sensory information that is transmitted by the nose (olfactory bulbs) to the brain. Since there are more sensors associated with the olfactory bulb in a migraine-brain, there are more sensory connections between the nose and brain[7], and with more sensory connections comes a greater need for energy in the brain to handle the processing of all of the additional inputs. When all these receptors and their connections are engaged, the higher energy requirement may not be met, resulting in an energy crisis[17,227,228], and it is this energy crisis that leads to the migraine event.

Nutritional Considerations

Migraines have been recorded since early historical times. Migraines are recorded to have happened most often in those societies where grains became the staple diet[229]. Grains neither provide enough potassium nor enough sodium to support electrolyte homeostasis[230], and they provide way too much carbohydrates[231]. Since grains are even more prominent in our modern life, the potential for a biochemical imbalance today is higher than ever before. Our cells never have the chance to choose between a meal rich in potassium and sodium or one of donuts with sugary soft drinks. These same cells do not have the chance to ask for more salt or magnesium or fat or cholesterol. The accepted wisdom – based on questionable science – suggests that salt, saturated fat, and cholesterol are bad for us because of cardiovascular risk—a discredited theory based on erroneous research[211,232-234].

What is bad about salt, saturated fat, or cholesterol? Nothing actually. The human body contains between 55% (females) to 75% (males) fluid with salt water. Our body cannot make salt so we need to consume this essential mineral. There is not a single human cell that can function without salt. Are we sure that something so vital to our body's functions is capable of causing high blood pressure[235]? And if it is, how does it do that? Most academic publications have something like this as an explanation: "The mechanisms by which dietary salt increases arterial pressure are not fully understood, but they seem related to the inability of the kidneys to excrete large amounts of salt"[236]. There are also very complex explanations[237].

The process by which salt may be connected to elevated blood pressure is exactly the one migraineurs would need for migraine prevention—if the blood pressure increase were true. Practically all migraineurs have low blood pressure[238]. This is because migraineurs are hypovolemic (low blood volume)[239,240], and so for them increased dietary salt and water is essential to maintain appropriate blood volume. Even after years of higher than recommended dietary salt consumption, migraineurs still retain low blood pressure relative to non-migraineurs. In fact, one study showed that migraine itself is inversely related to the amount of salt consumed[241], while two others demonstrated that the more salt a person consumes, the less likely she suffers a cardiac event[242,243]. Based on the inverse relation and that more salt is better—as per the previously cited articles—a migraineur benefits from eating more salt, and my observations from the Facebook group confirms this. Most research on salt and its effects is questionable at best; the reader is encouraged to further explore the cited sources on this subject[226,235,242,244-258].

What about saturated fat and cholesterol? Every single fat type contains saturated fat—including the highly-coveted olive oil. Our body contains a lot of fat. The brain is made up of over 60% fat, and 25% of all our body's cholesterol is in the brain[259-267]. The cholesterol we eat, such as an egg yolk, stays as cholesterol in our body. Our liver makes additional cholesterol as needed in order to provide the amount our body needs for proper functioning. Moreover, cholesterol is more critical for survival of the human body than anything else. Cell membranes are made from fat and cholesterol[268]. Cholesterol facilitates protein synthesis of vitamin D that we absorb with the help of the sun[269]. Cholesterol is also an important substance that helps the body heal and carries fat-soluble vitamins and minerals (such as calcium) to wherever they are needed[270].

Inside our cells are the mitochondria that create most the energy the cells need. Mitochondria can use lipids (fats) or glucose as raw material[271,272], particularly in a healthy metabolic flexibility state[273]. In our modern Western diet, our cells and their mitochondria mostly get their nourishment from glucose. Glucose in large amounts is not only extremely unhealthy, particularly for a migraineur, but it also creates a lot of trouble for our arteries, causing inflammation and high blood pressure[235,254,274-281]. The much-maligned triglycerides too are made from carbohydrates and not from fat[282,283].

I left the worst piece of news for last: voltage leakage. Voltage leaks are a hallmark of many health conditions: seizures, Parkinson's, Multiple Sclerosis, and many others—and migraines as well. What is the physiological explanation for voltage leaks? Voltage leaks occur as a result of damage to the myelin sheath that provides insulation for the electrical communication that occurs between neurons. In the brain, a voltage leak causes a break in neuronal communications, which in turn disrupts normal signaling between neurons and causes our brain to suffer. Due to the increased voltage activity of a migraine-brain, the potential for damage to our myelin sheath – insulation for the electrical communication between neurons – is higher, unless we satisfy the greater cholesterol and fat requirements of our brain[265,266]. What is worse, the damage is caused in large part by glucose[284,285], which is available in large quantities due to the modern diet.

The Anatomy of Migraine

What is the anatomy of a migraine? Do migraines have an anatomy, a location map, in the same way that heart disease does? Migraines have a functional anatomy rather than a simple structural anatomy. Sure, migraine happens in the brain and we feel the pain in our head but does the pain guide us to an anatomical location? No, not in the same way as a blocked artery that points to the cause of heart attack. The symptoms of migraine do not clearly correspond to specific regions of the brain, except in the case of the aura migraine, which points at the visual cortex[286,287]. A study found that migraineurs respond to a particular stimulus differently than non-migraineurs[4,288]. For non-migraineurs the visual stimulus induced neural activity deep in the brain, whereas the same stimulus for migraineurs initiated activation in the occipital lobe and in the lateral frontal cortex, which is the region over and behind the eyebrows all through the forehead to the top and the sides of the head to approximately to the middle of the head over the ears[289,290]. Only 15%-20% of those with migraines have been diagnosed with auras—these are likely the candidates for those migraine locations that are in the occipital lobe[35]. Other than the previously noted article, science has not identified any specific anatomical migraine location, though they have found "maladaptive" stress responses relative to non-migraineurs[291] and altered sensory stimulus responses relative to non-migraineurs[289]. Pain in the brain is not felt in the same way as pain in any other part of the body[292]. It is felt only in the dura or pia (the meninges), the very outer layer that protects the brain under the skull via noniceptors[293]. Thus, where the head hurts during a migraine is independent from the location of the cause.

Most scientists consider aura and non-aura migraines different in cause because they appear to be different in scanners[294]; they are wrong because they are looking at symptoms only, from which the cause cannot be established. If you pay close attention to the prodromes and the symptoms of any type of migraine, you can pretty much tell which brain region is the cause. For example, some migraineurs lose the ability to speak. There is one main region on the left side of the brain that controls language and speaking: the Broca's area. The Wernicke's area region is the posterior speech area, which is connected to speech with different significance. The Broca's area is approximately between the temple and the ear about a half to an inch above the ear, whereas the Wernicke's area is above the visual cortex in the back of the head. Migraineurs who are unable to speak and who are difficult to understand, or the ones who cannot understand speech themselves, are likely having their Broca's and/or Wernicke's areas affected by their migraine. By contrast, those who get vertigo, dizziness, tinnitus, and have a lack of balance while walking likely have their auditory area affected, which is below the Broca's area and is on both sides of the brain. Those with hemiplegic migraine often lose half of their body to temporary paralysis. This can originate in many areas of the brain, including the primary motor area, which wraps around our brain contiguously over our ears on both sides all around the head and the primary sensory area, which is just behind the primary motor area.

Those migraineurs who get confused, or forget where they are and what they are doing have their frontal and prefrontal cortex affected, which would be the entire frontal head area from above the eye brows in the forehead to the top of the head. Those who are left without the ability to make any decisions experience trouble in their orbitofrontal cortex, an area right above the eyes in the depth of the region between the eyebrows and where the eyelid hits the eye-socket bone. These locations are independent from the migraine being aura or non-aura migraine.

Many migraineurs start their migraines with anxiety, symptoms of IBS, and yawning. These prodromes also betray the anatomical location of the disturbance. In the middle of the brain we find the limbic system. It is part of what may be called an "ancient" brain system, responsible for controlling our alertness, feeling scared, fight or flight, and also pleasurable experiences. This region is also directly connected to the outside world via the olfactory bulb, which is deep inside our nose behind the bone ridge. This is the only place where there is a direct connection of a brain nerve to immediate sensory activity. It is not surprising that, for migraineurs, this region is highly endowed with multiple sensory receptor connections, since odor is one of the strongest migraine triggers. Therefore, the limbic system is probably involved in every migraine type[295,296]; it is accountable for the migraineur's hyper alertness and quick reaction for avoiding danger—even if that danger today is associated with a scenting candle or a room freshener.

Biochemical Fundamentals

Hydration is a process in which a substance is "formed when water combines with another substance" (Merriam-Webster). Water is an ideal medium in which minerals can be dissolved and become available to our metabolic processes. In other words, we need two substance types: water (solvent), and minerals that dissolve in the water (solutes). The resulting solution provides nutrition for our cells. With this type of "true" hydration biochemical balance for proper neural operation can be achieved.

In this book, biochemical balance refers to an optimal outcome of hydration that can be verified by the proper functionality of the electrolyte available for the brain's neurons. Electrolytes are fluids in our body, made of a special mix of water and minerals that are also supplied for and utilized in hospitals for emergency hydration. Electrolyte is made from water mixed with: sodium, chloride, potassium, calcium, magnesium, hydrogen phosphate, and hydrogen carbonate. Some electrolytes, such as Pedialyte for babies, also contain small amounts of glucose. You can find more information about this written in a relatively easy-to-understand language on Wikipedia[297].

For migraine prevention, the most important elements in electrolyte are sodium, chloride, and potassium because they help the neurons generate action and resting potential, manage nutrition inflow, and clear toxins from the neurons. Calcium is required to generate neurotransmitter release and also to release signals when something is not in balance for neural operation. The high voltage calcium channels signal to pain sensing nerves; and we feel a migraine. Magnesium helps in the opening of the voltage gated pumps as it attaches to ATPase, which is the energy providing molecule for pump opening.

These biochemical fundamentals are the key for understanding the basis of migraine-free life.

Biochemical Imbalance Caused by Hypersensitivity

I am offering a cursory, mostly hypothetical, explanation here intending to highlight some new angles for answering the question that fMRI scanning investigations have found and have no explanation for their findings[296]: why migraineurs' sensory sensitivities lead to the signs that appear hours or minutes before a migraine hits. Recall that a migraine-brain is a special brain that is always on alert to notice what is different from the norm. Recall also the hypersensitivity survey I asked migraineurs to fill out. Most migraine sufferers reported having heightened sensory sensitivities years before their migraines appeared. The following basic characteristics are present in all migraineurs:

1) Low threshold levels in sensing external stimuli
2) Stress hormone release in response to sensed external stimuli
3) Biochemical imbalance results

Migraineurs have general hypersensitivity to external stimuli such as smells, sounds, light, etc. These stimuli are inputs to brain processes that utilize the multiple sensory connections among specific neurons responsible for sensory stimulus[7]. Thus, migraineurs sensory organs are more sensitive and are highly integrated[3] to alert better and faster in case of danger.

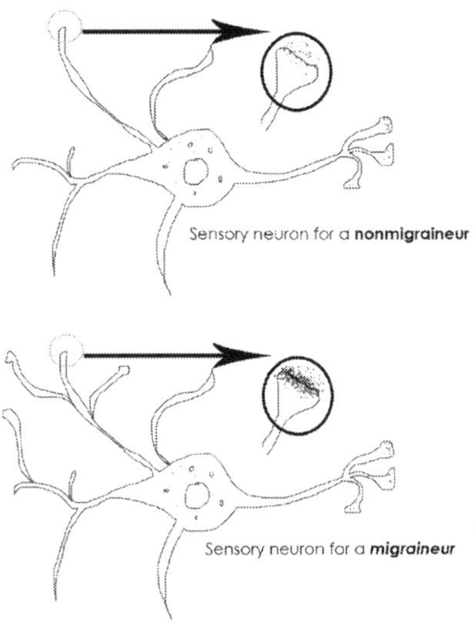

Figure 8. Hyper sensory neuron sensitivity; multiple receptor connections

The top image represents a sensory neuron (hypothetical cartoon) in the brain of a non-migraineur. Note that the dendrites (encircled) have several little black dots, representing neurotransmitters that can exit into the synapse (space between neurons). Another neuron on the other side of the synapse picks up the neurotransmitters. If you look at the bottom sketch, you can see the same in the brain of a migraineur. Much more neurotransmitters are in the synapse so more (or louder) signal is sent.

The consequences of the above depicted anatomical difference are:

1. In case of migraine-brains, more neurotransmitters are created – this is a voltage expensive process that requires more energy

2. If a non-migraineur has (illustrative and simplified assumption) 10 neurotransmitter vesicles, while a migraineur has 100, the migraineur will transmit more neurotransmitters and at a higher intensity
3. The increased output of neurotransmitters in the synapse is more excitatory for the receptors of the nearby neuron in the relevant brain region, resulting in an earlier and/or higher level of alertness to stimulation

Such hypersensitivity, because of more sensory connections, may provide an evolutionary advantage by initiating the fight-or-flight response for an early escape from danger, releasing adrenaline and cortisol for fast action. Today's migraineurs do not live in the savanna where they would fear a lion behind the bush; nonetheless they still possess this ability and they react to a stimulus that is not the norm in their environment. The heightened sensory abilities come with many disadvantages in our modern lives. In addition to being more sensitive in general, when the brain has used up all its available nourishment and energy dealing with the effects of this extra sensory overload[4,6], a biochemical imbalance emerges. The brain over-reacts to the external signals and prompts the release of stress hormones to the perceived threat. Adrenaline stops the work of all non-essential organs and functions (like digestion) to make energy available for the increased muscle and brain power needed for the fight-or-flight. In the brain, the sudden heightened energy requirement of the fight-or-flight response creates a greater level of energy demand, necessitating an increased need for those nutritional elements that are vital for satisfying this demand. If this increased need is unmet, an electrolyte imbalance in the affected brain region will follow. To avoid the above scenario, a migraineur needs to supply more of the vital electrolyte elements, in harmony with the special attributes of her migraine-brain.

It is also likely that many migraineurs have extra adrenaline floating in their bodies between migraine episodes as a result of the frequent fight-or-flight reactions, explaining the prevalence of anxiety and restless leg syndrome among migraineurs, even without a migraine pain episode. Migraineurs are also genetically predisposed to having more dopamine in their brains, which – among its many other roles – also helps with a fast reaction to danger[298,299].

There are many visible and invisible signs that – if correctly interpreted – inform the migraineur that a migraine is about to be triggered. These signs let her know that her brain has crossed a threshold in its ability to deal with external stimuli, and that a migraine is imminent unless energy is provided for the extra workload, the brain must perform to counter the misapplied evolutionary reflex to the stress. To rehash what may prompt a heightened response of a migraine-brain, here is a typical list:

- Sudden scent change (perfume, deodorant, fresh laundry, cigarette smoke, hair spray, lotions, smells of infections).
- Sudden change in the level of sound, or sudden awareness of ongoing sounds like crowds, clock ticking, fireworks,

airplane/helicopter overflights, noisy muffler, music, drums, fallen large objects, ice cubes falling in the freezer's automated ice cube maker, sound of transmission line electricity (Yeah! Migraineurs hear the sound of electricity), forceful chomping/chewing, cars backing up using a beeper, dogs barking, etc.

- Live concerts may be a problem also because of their noise level!
- Sudden light change – what seems like normal light in one minute may appear to be too bright; flickering light (like fluorescent), greenish hue light, sudden appearance of street lights or car headlights at night.
- Full moon – evoking the ancient fear of predators hunting humans at night under the bright light of a full moon
- Taste busters – many migraineurs are super tasters, so what may taste great for others may be terribly bitter to a migraineur. If your child refuses Brussels sprouts, you may have a migraineur (or at least a super taster) on your hand! Spices that are hot or overpoweringly flavorful may not go over well with migraineurs.
- Sudden barometric pressure changes cause ionic balance shifts in the body. Such ionic shifts cause pain to migraineurs. This also includes driving to high altitudes (low pressure), to low altitude like Death Valley salt flats (high pressure), scuba diving (very high pressure), and airplane flights (low pressure). Changes in pressure due to changing weather conditions can be excruciating for a migraineur.

- Very dry air with its increased potential for static electrical charge generation is not a friend of migraineurs.
- Hormonal fluctuations – particularly those hormones that use insulin

I want to take a moment to expand a bit on one of the points I mentioned above that no one has yet studied and thus I am not able to provide a citation for. The hyper sensitivity of the visual sensory organs manifests itself in many ways. Migraineurs are more on alert during the night and sleep with a "cat's eye" (not fully closed). Consequently, many migraineurs wear an eye mask in order to reduce unwanted light during sleep. However, a migraineur can navigate quite well in what to others seems like pitch dark. As noted earlier, bright light appears really bright to migraineurs; dark sunglasses are a must. And here is perhaps the most bizarre example:

An eye exam for a migraineur where the pupils must be dilated ends in 5 days of torture if the standard solution is used for pupil dilation. Luckily, a child-solution with a lower concentration is available if one asks for it. The explanation is quite simple: the migraineur's pupils are never at full closure, so they are in a somewhat dilated state to start with. In addition, the light shined into the eye during the exam can cause an instant migraine.

We are not getting our ulcers being chased by Saber-tooth tigers, we're inventing our social stressors — and if some baboons are good at dealing with this, we should be able to as well. Insofar as we're smart enough to have invented this stuff and stupid enough to fall for it, we have the potential to be wise enough to keep the stuff in perspective.

--ROBERT SAPOLSKY

Stress in Biology

Stress is probably one of the most common words in our everyday use. By stress we normally mean something that makes us busy or angry or simply not feeling right for the moment. Here is a well-accepted definition of stress in biology:

> *"...a person's response to a stressor such as an environmental condition or a stimulus. Stress is a body's method of reacting to a challenge... Stress typically describes a negative condition or a positive condition that can have an impact on a person's mental and physical well-being"*[300].

The body's reaction to the negative or positive environmental stimulus takes place by the activation of the sympathetic and the parasympathetic (unconscious) nervous system via biochemical processes. This was a mouthful so let's take it apart: environmental stress on the body initiates undesirable internal chemical processes that activate those systems in our body that are not under conscious control, such as anxiety, fight-or-flight, IBS, RLS, heartbeat, breathing, nausea, vomiting, diarrhea, dizziness, etc. Stress need not be negative. Positive environmental influences can just as much affect our well-being. For example, extreme happiness about getting an A on a test in a hard subject, ending up with a sunny warm day when the forecast predicted cold and gloomy weather, getting a new job, getting engaged or married, all can bring on a euphoric high, causing a hormonal imbalance that results in a migraine. Such a stressor is also one of the reasons why by being extremely happy or laughing strongly we may find ourselves crying. Thus, a stressor can come from both positive and negative stimulus, and it can cause stress on the body that can disrupt the biochemical processes.

Many people respond to stressors by eating sweets. Eating a piece of cake at a wedding makes one feel good because it releases dopamine in the brain[301,302] but this can cause many undesirable effects such as hunger, shakiness (sugar crash), as well as a migraine. Thus, while eating sweets is a customary celebration of life events and a happy end to dining out or watching a favorite movie, for migraineurs it is a major stressor. Add to this that migraineurs are also glucose sensitive[13,14,220,303,304], and you can see how by eating a piece of cake a major electrolyte imbalance will follow.

For a very long time I've heard people say that stress brings on headaches, but not migraines. This – now we know – is incorrect; once the electrolyte is out of balance the potential for a migraine is real. Our nervous system translates external stress and transmits it to relevant hormonal variations. In response to this change, the affected cells adjust or change their biochemistry. This internal biochemical change is the *stress response* to the external stress events and conditions. Just as there are internal stressors, such as the menstrual cycle, that can change the body's chemistry, so can external stressors create biochemical imbalances or disturb hormonal processes. To help you distinguish very clearly between external and internal stressors, here are three short examples, and note the connection to a chain reaction of effects:

External stressor: a migraineur driver gets stressed out about the traffic jam on the freeway. This causes her adrenaline, steroid, cortisol, and other stress hormones to increase, blood pressure to rise, and heart to pump faster and stronger, creating a potential for heart attack or stroke. In this case, an external factor directly caused the internal stress on the vascular system.

Internal stressor: the increase in our driver's blood pressure causes extra stress on her arteries. This causes trouble for the vascular system but let's continue to the brain. The extra stress causes the brain and its neurotransmitter activities to create and use energy for the higher demands of certain brain regions that are either recognizing and acknowledging the external stimulus or are preparing for a possible response to it. This unplanned, extra physiological activity may force the neurons in the driver's brain to work at a pace that is above her threshold at that moment. Increased energy levels are needed, but as she is fuming over the traffic jam, she is not providing any extra energy to address the deficit. During this unexpected energy expenditure – this internal stress – the body must suddenly work harder without any increase in nutrition and hydration. If not mitigated, this will lead to a biochemical imbalance, causing a migraine. So even if the external conditions have not directly caused a life threatening, vascular reaction, that is, she was not hit by a stroke or a heart attack, the stress may still end up giving our driver a migraine.

Stress on the Brain: a neuron is stimulated by the unpleasantness of the traffic. The neuron's message is transferred to another neuron by the neurotransmitters it passes into the synapse. Since the migraine-brain is endowed with more sensory receptor connections, whatever neurotransmitters a sensory neuron releases, more receptors will pick them up, which has the effect of amplifying the signal[305]. This is why migraineurs are "hyper sensitive" to odors, sounds, etc. The migraineurs' hyper sensitive brain amplifies everything sensory.

How does this become a migraine? The answer is quite simple. If we stimulate a single neuron and no other neuron pays attention (as in a non-migraine-brain), all the effort of that neuron is *inhibited*, the fire is put out, and not much extra energy is used. When a migraine-brain is stimulated, the activation of the neurons with many more receptor connections pass the signals to a multitude of neurons—the signal will be *amplified.* More stimulation results in intensified, sometimes alarm level, reactions. The release of the extra neurotransmitters uses more energy; a migraine-brain uses a ton more brain energy than the brain of a non-migraineur. Using more energy means the brain needs more energy. Unfortunately, if the migraineur doesn't recognize the need for more energy, does not know how to properly make up the deficit, or is not in the position of doing something about it, sugar cravings will follow! The more sweets are eaten, the more trouble the migraineur gets into. Glucose needs sodium to be carried into the cells and sodium is also used to provide voltage energy. Without quickly re-establishing an electrolyte balance by eating salt, the region deficient in energy will stop producing action potential and will go off-line. Migraine pain is on the way!

Stressors as Triggers

A stressor is a biological response to an internal or an external stress. However, while there are plenty of real stressors, there are many false ones as well. They are named as possible stressors because of a lack of clear understanding of what they really are. We call those stressors that are proven to have the ability to initiate the cascading events that lead to migraines, triggers.

False Triggers

There are many "triggers" that don't disrupt electrolyte homeostasis but may end up giving you a headache. Often these give headaches to everyone or many people, migraineur or not. Some of these triggers belong to a category that I label "false triggers" simply because they are not cause for a migraine.

Plastics

I have heard many times that migraines are caused by the use of plastics. Migraines existed way before water and food came in plastic containers, and before the microwave oven was invented—people had migraines thousands of years ago. The recent scare of plastics as migraine-cause due to the use of bisphenol A (BPA) in plastic is one of these fake triggers. I know plenty of people who never use plastics for anything yet are migraine sufferers. I also know many people who often drink out of plastic bottles and eat out of plastic microwave food trays and who have never had a single migraine. As a scientist, I am skeptical of findings that associate the cause of migraines with something that a large population of migraine sufferers never ever uses. BPA might cause other problems for people but not migraines. Migraine is only possible for the population with a special ancient brain. Can it make it worse? I suppose if someone has a special sensitivity to BPA, it can. But this would not be a primary cause of a migraine since there is nothing in plastic that will disrupt electrolyte homeostasis.

Nitrates & Nitrites

Many people believe that nitrates are migraine triggers. You may be surprised to learn that your saliva naturally contains variable amounts of nitrate at all times[306]. Since your own saliva does not trigger your migraine, it is safe to assume that nitrates in general don't trigger migraine either. Some people have commented that the nitrates in the saliva are "natural" and as food additives they are not. To me this sounds similar to saying that nitrate as a chemical in the mouth is somehow different from nitrate as a chemical added to foods. Chemically we only have one nitrate. Many people opt for nitrate free foods, in which celery juice is used instead of nitrates. Now if you open up a chemistry book and look at what celery juice is, you will find it is full of nitrates. This is a trick of the trade that allows food makers to advertise no added nitrates, while adding them in a different form! Nitrates are part of you; adding more or less will not harm you, and they definitely cannot cause a migraine—nitrate is not a migraine trigger. Nitrites have also been brought up in many conversations as migraine triggers—nitrites are used as food coloring and have many useful functions in our body—including signaling about pathogens. Our body naturally contains both nitrates and nitrites and so our sensitivity is limited to our infant period but young children already have increased amounts of both. If nitrate is a problem for migraineurs in any shape or form, it can be for one reason only and that is actually considered to be a benefit for people in general: it lowers blood pressure[307,308]. Nevertheless, lowering blood pressure can cause a problem for migraineurs, who already have low blood pressure. This may cause a headache though, not a migraine.

MSG

MSG (monosodium glutamate) is commonly held hostage as a migraine cause. MSG is a chemical that is found in nature. MSG *"is the sodium salt of the common amino acid glutamic acid. Glutamic acid is naturally present in our bodies, and in many foods and food additives. MSG occurs naturally in many foods, such as tomatoes and cheeses. People around the world have eaten glutamate-rich foods throughout history."*

(https://www.fda.gov/Food/IngredientsPackagingLabeling/FoodAdditivesIngredients/ucm328728.htm)

A banana is 19% glutamic acid so if you are sensitive to MSG, have no banana, tomatoes, cheeses, and many more foods like these—and avoid any stock or broth since bones cooked in soups release glutamate. Glutamate is an amino acid (protein). Many migraineurs enjoy drinking bone broth full of glutamate without getting a migraine. The longer we cook broth the more glutamate leaches out of the bones. While MSG can certainly cause headaches for many people but it is not a migraine trigger.

Histamine Intolerance

Histamine is a natural and vital element in our bodies. For example, when there is too much pollen in the air and they stick to the mucus in our nasal passages we may get runny nose, teary eyes, cough, etc. Our own histamines activate the immune system when alien elements enter the body. Histamines collect water from every source possible (this can disrupt electrolyte) and wash out the invading organism, be it pollen, dust, mold, or perfume. Histamine intolerance refers to a problem in histamine management within the body. Diamine Oxidase (DAO) is the enzyme for the metabolism of histamine and its activity can sometimes result in histamine oversupply. This can cause headaches (not migraine), asthma, cough, and a host of other symptoms. Note, however, that it is not the histamine that is causing the trouble, but a misfiring DAO system. Histamine intolerance is an unwelcome malady but is not a trigger for migraines. The function of histamine itself however is another matter. In a well-functioning body, histamine collects water to help the immune system wash out the invaders. This capacity of histamine can cause migraines, since the water that is collected reduces available water elsewhere, electrolyte imbalance may follow.

Tyramine

Tyramine is another chemical that is often blamed as being a migraine trigger but in truth foods rich in tyramine are preferred foods for migraineurs. Tyramine is naturally found in some foods and is induced in those that are fermented or marinated. Pickles, for example, or sauerkraut, are often filled with tyramine, and not only do they not cause migraine, they can help relieve them because of their saltiness. Unfortunately, tyramine is also found in meat that is spoiled, which can cause major intestinal problems and headaches; combined these symptoms may mimic a migraine prodrome and migraine pain. But, Tyramine is not a migraine trigger.

Adrenal Fatigue

Many migraineurs explain to me that they have adrenal fatigue and therefore migraine. There are two issues here: does adrenal fatigue exist and if it does, can it trigger a migraine?

Adrenal fatigue is a misused term. The official term is *adrenal insufficiency*, a condition of having not enough steroid hormones. Adrenal insufficiency (Addison's Disease) is a serious health condition that is fully testable by a blood test (usually taking two hours). The test can then show if one has adrenal insufficiency or not. This condition is really not a guessing game and so concoctions provided for adrenal fatigue are somewhat of a scam. Lots of money can be made by selling supplements that don't address the underlying concern. If you find you have adrenal insufficiency, you will be placed on life-long medicines. Adrenal insufficiency doesn't disrupt electrolyte but the medicine (corticosteroids) used to treat it can cause migraines.

Iron deficiency

Some migraineurs believe that iron deficiency contributes to migraines. Iron deficiency is a symptom of many possible health conditions. A symptom doesn't cause migraines. If you have iron deficiency, please consult your doctor.

Real Triggers

Whatever disrupts electrolyte homeostasis in any way is a real migraine trigger. Many things that are completely unrelated to foods can also upset electrolyte homeostasis: hormonal changes, travel, pressure changes, exercise, full moon, a bug your immune system is fighting, skipping meals or hydration, and preparation for surgery, to name a few. There are literally hundreds of triggers and it is impossible to list them all, and there may even be some triggers that are specific to only you. It is not possible to eliminate triggers from our life since we are not in control of many things around us. However, we are in full control of our body and how it reacts to triggers. Once the mechanism of triggers is understood, all triggers can be neutralized. Being a migraineur is a prerequisite of the possibility for a stressor to become a trigger.

Common Real Triggers

Full Moon

Many doctors and scientists dismiss the full moon as an influence for migraine as nonsense. They refer to the impossibly small amount of gravitational change (as in tides) that cannot have any effect on the "enclosed water" in the brain, and they may be right. The relative amount of gravitational pull is likely to be miniscule and even less than the average daily variations caused by blood pressure changes or the amount of water in the body at any given time. So let's look past this theory to see what's really going on.

The reason for the moon as a migraine stressor is hidden in our evolutionary history. For this I have to link a few seemingly independent points together:

Full moon has bright light ➔ man-eating predators can hunt easier in the bright light of a night with full moon, therefore danger is associated with the full moon ➔ the possibility of danger initiates a stress response and the body releases adrenaline ➔ migraineurs are very alert a few days prior to and during a full moon ➔ in ancient times this was an evolutionary advantage (watching out for predators) ➔ a higher level of adrenaline ties up insulin, preventing glucose from reaching the brain. While alert needs more voltage energy ➔ more voltage energy needs more sodium and nutrition ➔ without extra sodium and nutrition migraine is imminent during full moon.

Sitting in our modern apartment or house, with lights on 24/7, TV and the Internet on demand, and food available from our grocery store ready to be cooked or is even precooked, means that most people will find it difficult to identify with what I wrote above.

It is very true that migraineurs have no need to use any of their sensory organs to protect their tribe from the man-eaters that may hunt in the bright night of a full moon in Manhattan. However, not every brain is adapted to living in a big city. Migraineurs still possess an ancient brain form and simply have not adapted through genetic variations to modern life. In ancient times when all humans still lived in the wild, having a brain like the brain of today's migraineur would have been a highly-desired advantage. Read this article for more on this:

https://www.hormonesmatter.com/migraine-all-wrong/

Weather

Weather changes are serious stressors. It would be nice if our skull had the ability to change its size and shape to accommodate pressure and temperature changes that our flexible internal cells go through. The explanation of why weather changes affect our cells is somewhat difficult to understand for people without a background in physics but an example or two may help you relate to it better.

There are four interrelated parts to weather as triggers: altitude change, barometric pressure change, temperature change, and humidity change. However, for a living organism that is as sensitive to external factors as a migraine sufferer is, temperature changes, pressure changes, and temperatures themselves have completely different "feel" responses given a particular altitude. Exceedingly hot or low temperatures, increasing or decreasing barometric pressure (even if we sit in a climate controlled room), and temperature changes in any direction that are sudden and exceed the threshold of our body's ability to cope, have all been proven to be migraine triggers. The body's average normal temperature is what the body wants to maintain. An external temperature significantly over or below that is a challenge, and it can evoke a stress response. For instance, there are many people who are not sensitive to heat; they just sweat but otherwise carry on with their lives. The sensitives, on the other hand, may or may not sweat enough but – at a minimum – feel physically beat up.

Our body always wants to remain in homeostasis, so our brain works harder to orchestrate a cooling response to heat, a heating response to cold, or for countering the effects of the pressure change. Working harder means that the regions of the brain that control your body temperature or your blood pressure are electrically more active at this time than they normally would be. Those who are sensitive to this, feel a kind of vibration in the air that I call "buzzing". It is not a comfortable feeling—it doesn't hurt—but it can make one feel restless and beat up. One may also hear crackling sounds as if things were popping in the head. For us "sensitives", weather change related stressors can easily cause a biochemical imbalance which leads to an electrolyte disturbance as a result of the increased brain activity. This is why it is even more important for migraine sufferers to follow the advice we learned in kindergarten: "hydrate more when it is hot" or "hydrate more at high elevation." That is, drink more water AND eat extra salt! When pressure increases though, do the opposite: rather than increasing salt and water, increase potassium by eating potassium-rich foods.

Pressure change is very complex and requires some more explanation. My first chemistry class in college demonstrated what pressure change does to liquids in closed spaces. We placed room temperature water in a very thick glass jar halfway filling it and sealed it. Next, we used an apparatus that could depressurize the bottle to near vacuum. The more air we removed, the hotter the water got, and at one point the water started to boil from the pressure decrease. This is a good example how changes in pressure affect water temperature if air and water are enclosed together, as they are in your body. Our skull's contents are not immune from the effects of pressure changes, and pressure changes also come with changes in the amount of oxygen available—one need only to look at mountain climbers and their struggle for oxygen. So any change in pressure can play games with our head; the larger the experienced pressure difference, the more severe the consequences may be.

Obviously, barometric pressure changes beyond a certain level are a perfect example of stress. Migraine sufferers with their higher level of sensitivity are prime candidates for experiencing difficulties with barometric pressure changes. Generally speaking, weather related pressure changes are usually small, but can be significant for our unique physiology. Migraineurs can be sensitive to an increase in pressure as small as 0.01 inHg, like an increase from 29.99 in Hg to 30.00 inHg. I spent some time calculating what such a pressure change would be equivalent to in elevation change, and how that translates to the weight of the column of air over our heads. I have posted a detailed calculation of this into the Facebook migraine group "Migraine Sufferers Who Want to be Cured." Join us there to see various pressure levels and how they affect the brain.

Migraineurs are sensitive enough to experience ear popping from an altitude change of as little as 150 feet up or down the hill. And it makes sense once you see the calculations and realize that 150 feet change equals to a 0.156 in Hg change in pressure, which is more than what I noted earlier that migraineurs are sensitive to. It is important to note that pressure changes differ between altitudes since the weight of the atmosphere changes proportionately to its density as well. Going from sea level to 1000 feet, the pressure decreases more than going from 5000 to 6000 feet.

Pressure change can also be demonstrated easily when you take a flight. During flight planes are depressurized to a level corresponding to a 3,000 - 5,000 feet altitude. We can see how the pressure change affects a bottle of water both as the plane gets depressurized during takeoff and also upon landing as it gets re-pressurized. You can try this.

Buy a plastic bottle of water at the airport. On the plane, before the doors close, place the bottle into the seat-back pocket in front of you. Wait until the plane has reached its cruising altitude, at which point the plane is fully depressurized. Pull the bottle of water out and examine it. It will look fat! Then open it while holding it close to your ears so you can hear the psssssssssss coming from it as the pressure equalizes between the inside and the outside of the bottle—it will regain its normal shape. The opposite will happen when the airplane returns to an airport (assuming your flight takes you from and to approximately the same elevation). Close the bottle back tightly again and place it back at the back of the seat in front of you again. After the plane landed and the doors open, take the bottle out and you will see it is sucked in and twisted. Open it and watch it regain its normal shape.

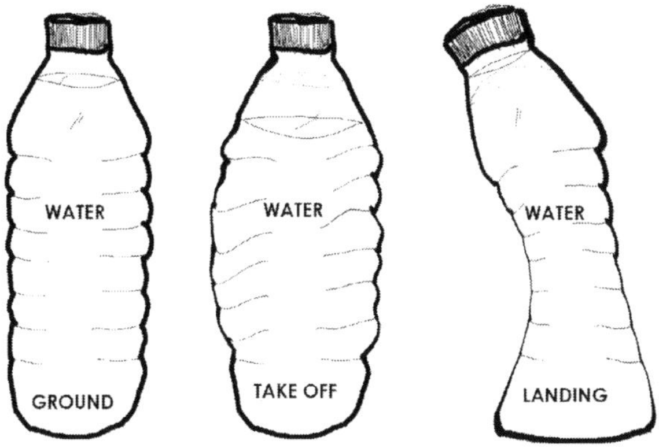

Figure 9. Pressure change effects

Keep in mind that what you see happening with the bottle is what is also happening in your brain and the rest of your body to your organs and your cells, most of which are chockfull of water. A migraineur commented online in response to the above example by saying she wished she could have a needle to let the air out of her head; that is exactly how the pressure decrease feels. What I found is that by keeping my body fully hydrated and properly supplied with all the important nutrients, I have been able to avoid migraines even in challenging and stressful situations like sudden or significant barometric pressure changes. These are precisely the situations when your neurons need all the help they can get. In principle, this is consistent with the commonly held wisdom of increasing hydration at a higher altitude—this increases blood volume which in turn allows for better oxygenation in the thinner air of higher altitude and increases blood volume. Altitude sickness (moderate altitude sickness of just headaches or migraines) can be averted by the extra hydration.

An increase in barometric pressure is harder on our body—we need to reduce blood volume and that is not instantaneous. As the pressure increases, the weight of the atmosphere increases over our head and body, pressing from the outside in all directions, trying to squeeze us into a smaller shape. This increased pressure causes narrowing of the arteries and blood vessels, creating an internal stressor for our body when suddenly there is too much blood volume relative to the available space in the veins. So a migraineur, when the pressure increases, needs to shed some water from the blood, and also from within the cells. To do so, potassium is needed. Seek a source of fast absorbing potassium from food (never supplement): avocado, nuts, and milk are the fastest absorbing potassium sources.

Foods

Most migraineurs tell me they have their trigger lists and they accept what's on them as unavoidable facts. Few care to investigate or are even curious about *why* some food items may trigger migraines. Just about anywhere I look today I see advertisements for migraine prevention methods with catch phrases like "migraine diet" or "eliminate your migraine triggers" or "3-day migraine cure". Some of these list hundreds of foods a migraineur should avoid, which leaves some migraineurs with nearly nothing to eat. Yet, I see comments from migraine sufferers who have followed such trigger elimination diets and they still have migraines.

There is no such thing as a migraine-trigger food (with the exception of sugar); only certain chemicals in food may act as triggers, depending on the mixture of other foods they are consumed with. If a food eaten provides the brain with all the minerals it needs to stay in balance, assuming it doesn't set off an allergic reaction, it is fine to eat. Some foods, if eaten without consideration for what chemicals they contain and what chemicals the brain may already have too much or too little of, may trigger migraines because having too much or too little of some chemicals poses a challenge for electrolyte homeostasis and thereby creates the potential for a stress response.

This is very important to understand so I repeat: it is not the particular food that triggers the migraine. Rather, it is some element of that food that contributes to a chemical imbalance that influences the likelihood of having a migraine. In other words, you can eat anything and everything (except sweetened things) that you are not allergic to, but you have to eat things in the proper combination and quantity to ensure biochemical balance is maintained in the environment of your neurons. This is reinforced by frequent comments made in pretty much every migraine group—that foods are triggers sometimes, but not always—this simply means that when they are not triggers, they are eaten in the right amount, and they are paired with a food companion that balances the nutrients in a way that prevents the initiation of stress.

How does this work? Let me explain it with a specific example. If you eat a particular food, say an ice cream, to you it looks like cold, sweet, good tasting stuff. For your stomach it looks like this: milk (fat, potassium, salt, lactose, protein, calcium, etc.,), sugar (glucose, fructose), water, and flavoring (say chocolate, which is cacao, fiber, caffeine, sugar, and potassium). For your cells the full nutritional value of a single serving of chocolate flavored ice cream appears as: 127 Calories, 41.77 gr water, 3.4 gr protein, 4.89 gr fat, 17.48 gr carbohydrate, 0.5 gr fiber, 16.80 gr total sugars, 108 mg calcium, 0.47 mg Iron, 14 mg magnesium, 56 mg phosphorus, 116 mg potassium, 48 mg sodium, 0.29 mg zinc, 1 mg caffeine, etc. While the ice cream may taste good, if you have chosen the ice cream because it is hot outside, the caffeine and sugars will get you! Caffeine increases blood pressure reducing potassium[309] and sodium[310] as well as water (it is diuretic), while sugar removes water and sodium from your cells. Not only will these upset your brain's ability to meet its voltage requirement but your hydration will be halted as a result of the constricted blood vessels. As you see, what you eat is not what your body eats because everything you eat breaks down into its chemical elements and they affect your body in unexpected ways. Chemical components do matter!

For instance, I read in migraine forums that bananas are migraine triggers for many people. It is not the bananas that trigger the migraine but the nutrients and other elements that the bananas contain. Let's say you have very little time for lunch and you eat a banana. A medium banana has approximately 400 mg potassium and approximately 6 teaspoons of sugar equivalent (more if the banana is fully ripened). There is not much else in a banana. So, what will 6 teaspoons of potassium enriched sugar do to your body? As we learned: sugar will remove water and sodium from your cells. Potassium also has a vasodilating effect of your blood vessels and will remove additional water. By eating that banana you will have created a major electrolyte disruption by dehydrating yourself. You will immediately be thirsty after eating the banana, and if you drink you will become even more dehydrated by diluting your electrolytes further, since sodium was also removed by the sugar and there is nothing to hold water for your cells. Now you are on the verge of a migraine. How can you cancel the banana's migraine trigger effect? You have to balance the just consumed potassium with sodium. Take a 1/8th of a teaspoon of salt after the banana instead of drinking water; just salt, no water, no matter how thirsty you are.

Why salt? You are thirsty as a result of water and sodium leaving your cells—it is not that you have no water only it was removed from the cells and you need to pull it back. The only way you can bring water back is by adding salt, which will attract water back. As the water that was removed by the glucose returns inside the cell, your thirst will disappear. This way you can have your banana – if you must. To be honest, a banana is never a recommended food item for a migraineur. It is not nutrition dense enough and has way too much sugar.

Another frequently mentioned food trigger for many migraine sensitive people is peanuts. I used to love peanuts before I became allergic to them. Spanish Peanuts (red skin) were my favorites; they contain a lot of salt and oil, and for me they never triggered a single migraine. I switched to raw Spanish peanuts thinking it was a healthier choice with less processing but I ended up triggering migraines. What was going on? Same food prepared differently; one a migraine trigger and the other not? A serving size of the Spanish roasted salted peanuts is about 100 grams so based on that: potassium 776 mg and sodium 433 mg, a 2:1.5 ratio of potassium to sodium in oil roasted Spanish peanuts—perfect potassium to sodium ratio. Consequently I never got a migraine from them. But look what I found when I looked at a 100-gram serving of the raw Spanish peanuts: potassium 744 mg and sodium 22 mg! Major trouble! Now the ratio of potassium to sodium is way off! A ratio of 33-parts potassium to 1-part sodium. No wonder raw Spanish peanuts without added salt became a migraine trigger for me—and they may be for you too! Now, if you still want to eat raw peanuts for the taste but don't want a migraine, you either need to salt them well or eat them alongside something quite salty that has no potassium in it. Even a pinch of loose salt will do the trick or stuff olives with peanuts or just take a salt pill.

I have mentioned earlier repeatedly that this book was helped tremendously by migraine sufferers of various forums with whom I have had a productive information exchange. This paragraph is specifically for the few who brought up cashew nuts, which in some cases had been recommended to them by doctors. I always asked these migraineurs if the doctor had suggested raw or roasted and salted cashew nuts. The reason for my question should be obvious by now but let me go ahead and give you the exact numbers so you can see why salt makes a huge difference. A serving size of cashew nuts is not given in the USDA database, so again let's use 100 grams (3.5 oz). In 100 gr of raw cashew nuts the amount of potassium is 660 mg and sodium is 12 mg. There is 55 times as much potassium in 100 gr raw cashew nuts as sodium. Raw cashew nuts would seem to be a great way to balance the high sodium diet that doctors believe their patients eat—I understand why a doctor would suggest it. But note that not everyone has high sodium in their diets and cashew nuts are also heavier in carbohydrate than other types of nuts. Raw cashew nuts will throw your balance of electrolytes out of homeostasis and trigger a migraine!

I got a bad migraine that lasted 3 years, and the pills I took made my fingers disappear.

David Bowie

Migraines, Hormones, Genders, & Age

In this subsection I would like to discuss the role of hormones in relation to migraines as possible stressors. The understanding of this subject is obscured by myths and misinformation. Let's see if I can make things clearer.

Female Hormonal Changes

Much blame has been placed on the influence of female hormonal variations as the cause of migraines. But interestingly, the metabolic pressure that acts as a stressor: hormones occupying insulin receptors backing glucose up (explained in a moment), has been excluded as a possible cause[13,220,311-313]. If migraines have a direct correlation with the presence and fluctuation of female hormones alone, one would assume that anyone who lacks such hormonal changes—say men, or very small children, or women who are in their menopause—would not have migraines. The truth is that there are children migraineurs, men with migraines, and menopause or post menopause provide no migraine relief either. These facts eliminate the female hormonal theory as the cause of migraines.

The connection to hormonal variations is indirect and is explained by, in the case of females, how monthly hormonal cycles create stress on the body, transforming the preparation for the cycles into stressors. The monthly menstrual cycle works with hormonal changes from estrogen dominance to progesterone dominance (often referred to as PMS). This trigger can lead to migraine if steps aren't taken to counteract the cause. Hormones, or their variations, do not cause migraines directly but they can cause glucose backup as noted earlier, which in turn starves the brain. Let's take this further apart.

Both progesterone and estrogen use insulin receptors in the blood for getting picked up and carried away[314-317]. Glucose must also be taken up by insulin receptors. So there is a problem of priority: what will insulin pick up from the blood first, hormones or glucose? Because insulin's primary role is hormonal signaling, the priority job is to take care of hormones. As a result, insulin gets tied down by hormones, while whatever glucose is in the blood sits pretty, waiting for unoccupied insulin. This is a problem for organs that need insulin to deliver glucose to them—such as the brain. The brain communicates with other organs and requests more glucose for energy, so several things happen to the unsuspecting female migraineur:

1. She will start craving sweets.
2. Her liver will release glycogen—stored glucose.
3. Her brain will still not get glucose until insulin is free so she continues to crave sweets and the liver continues to release glycogen.

4. Once the hormones release insulin to it can deliver glucose to the brain and other organs, the sudden entry of a lot of glucose will cause an electrolyte imbalance which leads to a migraine.

Regardless whether she will eat sweets or the liver "dumps" glucose (glycogen) into her blood, the consequence will only be an increase of glucose in the blood, as insulin is tied down with hormones until the job is finished. The backed-up glucose will thus cause a biochemical imbalance, causing migraines. Unfortunately this is a vicious cycle that can place women at a greater risk for insulin resistance[318-320]. Rather than eating sweets when the brain demands it during PMS, the healthiest thing for migraineurs (and all women actually) is to cut back on carbs and increase hydration to provide more voltage power for the necessary action potential. Knowing that the liver will provide the required glucose backup from its reserves, migraineurs not giving in to their sugar cravings can be migraine-free during this time of the month.

The Female brain uses more voltage to organize a menstrual cycle.
Each month a fertile female goes through two key changes: half the month her body prepares for an egg to be fertilized and the other half it destroys the unfertilized layer and cleans it out from the uterus. These changes come with important visible (changes in how women look) and invisible (preparation for pregnancy or for menstrual cycle) consequences. When she is most fertile, her face becomes more beautiful, more symmetrical, cheeks a bit more pink,

lips a bit more full, and her body odor becomes more attractive to males[321]. A woman's sexual preference for higher testosterone males increases and peaks at the time of the most fertile phase of her cycle[41,42,322-324]. Imagine how much stress this puts on the female body. Now go a step further and envision what happens at menstruation time: everything in the female body that has become so beautified gets reversed. Her sexual preference now turns toward low testosterone males. She has also switched off estrogen and turned on progesterone to remove the fertile lining of the uterus with the help of some blood. The hormone-driven changes require more cellular communication; more cellular communication requires more voltage energy, and her brain needs more sodium-enriched electrolyte in order to meet this greater energy need. Migraines are more prominent before the cycle, or in other words they are clustered around pre-menses rather than ovulation, corresponding to the fluctuating energy requirements. How much stress does all this mean to her? The brain that orchestrates all this, of course, must have extra energy, and if it is not provided migraine can result. Most doctors refer to this as a "hormonal migraine" and will hand you a pill. Medicines are not needed for this natural cycle, proper nutrition and hydration will eliminate the occurrence of migraine.

Insulin and glucose connection associated with progesterone and estrogen changes

The monthly cycles are driven by many hormones but two of them are critical: estrogen and progesterone (female steroid). Both estrogen and steroid hormones use insulin for their proper uptake[312,313,325].

Steroid is a major anti-inflammatory hormone of the body. I would like to give you a personal example of its connection to insulin. I discovered totally by accident (taking a dose of corticosteroids for an infection) that steroids can increase blood sugar to diabetic level; this connection is confirmed by academic literature, stating that Prednisone can cause type 2 diabetes[311].

My experience was a scary one. I was prescribed Prednisone for bronchitis while I was on a very low carbohydrate diet (a ketogenic diet, discussed under "Real Migraine Diet" later), and so I measured my blood sugar regularly several times a day. My normal fasting blood sugar is around 80 mg/dL, and after a meal or at any other time I rarely, if ever, exceed 99 mg/dL. A healthy blood sugar level is between 70-99 mg/dL (3.9-5.5 mmol/L) during fasting and a random healthy blood sugar reading is less than 140 mg/gL (7.8 mmol/L). Prediabetic fasting blood sugar levels are between 100 – 126 mg/dL and random readings are between 140 – 200 mg/dL. Diabetic fasting blood glucose is over 126 mg/dL and random is over 200 mg/dL.

Given how normal my blood glucose had been for a very long time, I just about fainted when I found my blood sugar jumping over 180 mg/dL after the first Prednisone (50 mg) pill. That one pill pushed my blood sugar to a level associated with near diabetes! I had eaten absolutely no food before I took the Prednisone (blood sugar reading of 80 mg/dL), and 30 minutes after taking the first pill (still no food) the reading was 180 mg/dL—a 100-point increase. What happened? What happened to me is what happens to a female body from a hormonal perspective—only perhaps not this extreme.

Based on what I explained about glucose backup before, as insulin is used by the steroids, this is like people (glucose) waiting in line for taxi cabs (insulin) in the rain and all the cabs are taken. As more people arrive and begin looking for taxi cabs the backup simply grows! Having this much glucose in the blood from Prednisone is what is responsible for steroid induced insulin resistance[326-328]. Prednisone is also often used as a medicine for patients with adrenal insufficiency—a condition when not enough steroid is produced by the body[329]. Many women are placed on corticosteroids for a variety of reasons; please be careful. Now you know, Prednisone may cause insulin resistance and type 2 diabetes[330].

Perimenopause

Women are often told that when they enter menopause their migraines will stop—this is not true. There is an interval between the time when a woman is fertile and has standard menstrual cycles and the time when she is fully free from normal female-hormone fluctuations. This is known as perimenopause. During perimenopause, the female hormones that orchestrate all the reproductive processes in the body slowly change. This change is caused by a decrease in hormone levels that occurs in variable and uneven increments. While a woman is fertile, her cycles are fairly regular, and so she can easily tell when her next menses will arrive and prepare accordingly to prevent her migraine. During perimenopause, the cycles become irregular and she may have no idea in the morning that her period will arrive at 2 pm in the middle of a meeting.

However, this is not nearly as difficult a problem to tackle as it appears; it requires the same preparation as for women who are still fully fertile—as discussed earlier. Use your favorite search engine with key term "Hormone levels predict attractiveness of women" (with the quotation marks included) and look at the images that come up. You may be shocked! You can find a very good picture here:

https://d1o50x50snmhul.cloudfront.net/wp-content/uploads/2005/11/dn8251-1_650.jpg

What this suggests is that, although female sexuality is no longer tied to regular monthly cycles, the female facial and body changes continue to follow the same pattern as in a fully fertile woman, since the body is going through the same routine, only in a less predictable way. Thus, taking selfies every day for a month and comparing them, will help you identify the time your body is switching into PMS mode based on how your face changes. Once you have taken selfies and can see the changes, you will be able to recognize them by simply looking into the mirror.

Menopause

You may be dismayed to learn that reaching menopause will not stop your migraines. There are no more monthly changes in body and face, no more changes from estrogen to progesterone and back, and all that brain energy that used to be lost is now saved. However, with menopause may come many other changes in life: retirement, travel, grandchildren, an increased probability of illnesses, and a decline in general health and strength. All of these can put internal stress (stressors) on the body. Stressors are alive and well during the rest of a woman's life. A reduction in migraines can be expected as the brain starts its ageing related natural atrophy and the neurons start to trim off excess connections. Since migraines develop as a result of the extra energy required for creation and maintenance of the extra receptor connections, as those connections are trimmed off, less and less energy is needed. There is a lesser chance for electrolyte disruption once the brain is in atrophy stage[331].

In menopause one eventually does reach a migraine free status—the question is: when. Luckily (so to speak), I know several migraineurs who still have their migraine-brain at age 80+. This suggests that there is no mandatory natural ageing schedule for the brain and synaptic pruning need not occur with menopause.

Post-Menopausal Migraines

Recently I heard a migraine friend telling me that someone she knows had a hysterectomy (removal of the uterus but not the ovaries) for migraine prevention! The fascinating thing is that all researchers and doctors would have to do is ask post-menopausal women (better yet, ask one with a complete hysterectomy) if their migraines have lessened. Doctors would then learn that a hysterectomy not only will not help, but may even make things worse. The uterus doesn't have hormonal connections of importance since the most important hormonal changes are driven by the ovaries. So, despite having no uterus, the woman still cycles, only she has no idea when she does (no periods), yet the migraines remain!

There are several women in my migraine group who needed to have their uterus removed for whatever reason (not for migraine prevention) and retained their ovaries still producing eggs. These women – not having any menses – can only tell that they are in the middle of a cycle by recognizing breast tenderness, if any, and that happens when it is too late to prepare for the possibility of a migraine.

However, it really doesn't make any difference to migraines whether the sufferer has or does not have any of her female organs. While the menstrual cycle does contribute to electrolyte imbalance, this is a once-a-month event. More significant is the fact that migraine is related to the quantity of sensory neuron receptor connections. If the numbers increase with age – at any age, so will migraines, and that is independent of any hormonal variations or age.

Male Cycles

It is not widely known that males also "cycle," likely in synchrony with female cycles. Males in relationships change their looks similarly to how females move into estrus: they become more masculine, more muscular, and a bit more aggressive. During the female menstrual time, and also at the time their baby is born, their testosterone levels drop and they become more "homey" looking and less aggressive[332].

It is said than men outgrow the migraines after puberty[125]. It has also been suggested that men usually get cluster headaches rather than migraines, whereas women usually get migraines rather than cluster headaches[124]. While all this may be true, I find a great number of misdiagnoses in the migraine group both in males and females. Indeed, the number of men joining the group is insignificant in numbers compared with women. However, I find boys at age 8 or even younger, way before puberty, having migraines, and many men with migraines way past puberty. I therefore am filled with skepticism of the available statistics, though I understand that one migraine group may not be representative of the whole world's migraine population

Kids and Migraine

I receive many calls from parents with respect to their children having migraines. Why and how do kids get migraines? Girls prior to puberty have no menstrual cycles. Menstrual cycle is a sexual hormonal cycle that happens to represent reproduction but there are other hormonal cycles. For example, both boys and girls, between the ages of 2 and 4, go through the "terrible twos". This period represents hormonal changes occurring within the brain. The hormonal changes in a child need not be precisely timed to a specific age—hormonal changes depend on the developmental stage of the child—so don't expect your child to suddenly come down with a migraine on her 2nd birthday and then stop all migraines at age 4 any more than you should expect the terrible 2's to start precisely at age 2!

What happens is that the brain develops a huge number of connections at approximately between 2 and 4 years of age, but this spurt may start earlier or later. Some connections are created in overdrive, while others develop more slowly, and so kids at this stage are uncomfortable. The "terrible two's" have a definite meaning but for a different reason from what we believe to be "kids behaving terrible for no reason". If you ever had to cram for an exam in school and felt what I call a "brain ache" from studying very hard, that is similar to what a child is experiencing during this period! While you are studying, and you know why you have a brain ache, and can take a break by taking a nap to refresh, a 2-year old has no clue what is happening, and, as I see it, their parents are often quite unaware and helpless in their ability to respond. Kids go through such fast and irregular brain connection development that they can indeed end up with a migraine simply because their brain runs out of voltage. It is important for you to help your child by providing voltage enhancing nutrients, and by not providing sugary foods, which is trouble for electrolyte homeostasis! The type of nutrients they need are the same nutrients you need as an adult. The key to a happy and balanced child is keeping their electrolytes in homeostasis at all times. And, by far, the best hydrating electrolyte solution for the body is whole fat milk.

Since the brain keeps growing and new connections and receptors are developing all through life, getting out of electrolyte balance because of irregular brain energy use is common. Particularly in boys, migraines are very common in puberty when their hormonal variations are high. Testosterone increases, occupying insulin receptors, backing glucose up, and preventing nutrients from reaching brain areas that develop fast. Once puberty is over, many boys stop having migraines, though a few continue into adulthood and some to old age.

Metabolic Disorders & Health

Many triggers and prodromes are connected to migraineurs' metabolic challenges. In almost all academic literature about migraines, the connection of migraine to metabolic disorder is noted but not explained[8-12,140]. I propose the following explanation. We already know that the migraine-brain has trouble metabolizing glucose efficiently. Migraineurs have heightened responses to the electrolyte imbalance caused by the consumption of even a small amount of glucose. Migraineurs are genetically predisposed to having issues with glucose transport and management[208]. Listing the oral glucose tolerance test (when the body's reaction to a sudden surge of glucose is measured) would not have appeared appropriate in the earlier section about triggers but it would have been correct. That is because migraineurs have such a huge response to glucose that the response itself becomes a trigger. Understanding how to prevent glucose from becoming a trigger requires grasping what glucose does, how it does it, how to measure it, and how to control it. One can always get a glucose tolerance test in a laboratory setting but such a huge amount of glucose (50gr or 75 gr and for geriatric patients 100 gr) is sure to give a 3-5-day long migraine. A less aggressive approach can approximate the results of a lab test, using standard blood glucose measuring kits.

The speed with which the body responds to glucose consumed and the magnitude of the reaction provides a clear sign for determining how advanced the glucose intolerance and potential insulin resistance has become. A healthy response with the desired level of insulin sensitivity is nearly immediate and returns to normal rapidly.

A healthy glucose response is a glucose-peak 30 minutes after a meal, after which the blood sugar reduces within an hour to a similar level of what it was before the meal. To make sense of at-home blood glucose testing, you need to develop a test schedule. Please make sure you do the testing safely by investing in sanitizing foam, gel, or tissues that you use both before and after each test. This avoids any possible infection. Don't reuse the lancet (the needle); trash it after it is used and use a fresh one every time.

Start checking your glucose as soon as possible. The schedule for testing: morning fasting before you take your salt pill and water (this is optional and I explain in a moment why), right before a meal (any of your meals), 30 minutes after you *finished* that meal, and for every

30 minutes thereafter until your next meal or 5 hours, whichever comes first. Jot down the date, the time, what you ate—including if you had nothing to eat—and continue until you have obtained at least a week's worth of data. The American Diabetic Association suggests a fasted (12-hour fast) blood glucose level of between 70 and 99 mg/dL, an after-meal level of between 70 and 140 mg/dL, and a random any time level of also between 70 and 140 mg/dL. This means that if before the meal your blood sugar is 70 mg/dl and 30 minutes after the meal it is 141 mg/dL, you've just found out that you are a tad into the danger zone of insulin resistance. This is suggestive of something important: the increase of your blood sugar after a meal should be limited and the more it goes beyond the healthy range, the more it represents a potential problem. It is also a problem if your highest reading is delayed past the 30-minute after-meal reading; the further out the worse it is.

If your random reading any time between meals or your fasting glucose is lower than 70, or if after eating your blood sugar drops below what it was before you ate, you have a reactive hypoglycemic response—a cause for concern. I wrote above to keep records for every 30 minutes for 5 hours. Can you go for 5 hours without eating and not getting a headache or a stomach ache? Do you get dizzy or ravenously hungry? If so, these also signal trouble.

The speed with which your blood glucose increases and decreases matters the most, magnitude is important but secondary. For better visualization, I created a hypothetical graph of four different blood glucose responses to two meals on the same day. The blood sugar measures are taken 30 minutes apart.

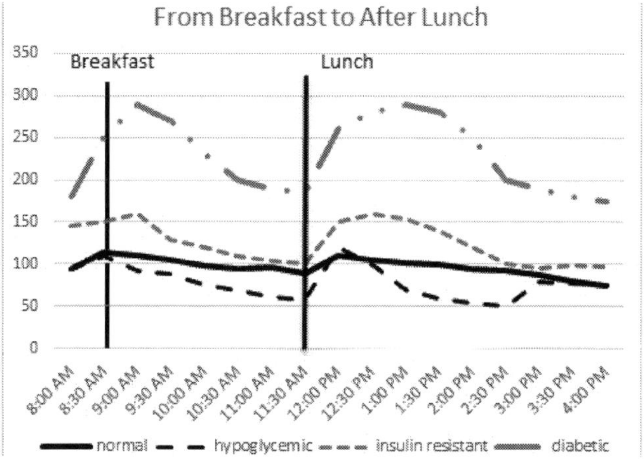

Figure 10. Blood glucose measure before and after 2 meals

The solid black line is the healthy ideal blood glucose response: sharp but not significant increase 30 minutes after the meal, a fast return to baseline after the meal, and staying stable. The black dashed line is a reactive hypoglycemic response. Reactive hypoglycemia is very common for migraineurs—it is an early stage of insulin resistance, and if part of the day the glucose is very high, it may be representative of more serious insulin resistance. The increase after a meal is similar to normal but the drop after the meal is significantly deeper than normal, ending in a lower blood glucose reading than before meal, with a possible sugar crash: feeling jittery, cold sweat, shaky, panicky, may faint, could be a medical emergency. The gray dashed line is a hypothetical insulin resistant response with hyperinsulinemia. It starts with high blood glucose, increases for longer than

30 minutes after the meal is over and decreases only marginally. The gray dash and dots line is a hypothetical type 2 diabetic response.

Reactive hypoglycemia (postprandial hypoglycemia)[333] seems to be frequent among migraineurs and though distinct from diabetes as shown on the graph above, it is representative of the beginning stages of diabetes[334]. Unfortunately, it is my experience that most migraineurs either have undiagnosed insulin resistance, diabetes, or reactive hypoglycemia[304]. This can be corrected by diet—perhaps not cured but placed into remission. Although there are many theories about what causes insulin resistance, its connection to carbohydrates is clear. Migraineurs in particular, with their glucose intolerance, really should reduce their carbohydrate consumption to the bare minimum. Consuming carbs is not essential because our body can make its own glucose—discussed earlier. If you feel uncomfortable with poking your fingers constantly for blood sugar readings, you should schedule an appointment with your doctor for an oral glucose tolerance test and a serum insulin test—or better yet, the Kraft insulin in-situ test[335]. There is only a very slim chance that your doctor will know (or can order even if she knows) a Kraft insulin in-situ test. In that case just progress with the oral glucose tolerance test.

Note: in the US the oral glucose tolerance test is only 2 hours with only 2 measures, so highly insufficient. If you decide to get the oral glucose test, please request additional blood tests every 30 minutes and also proceed to ask for longer than 2 hours. You may have to pay out of pocket for such a test—this is why a home glucose testing kit is much more convenient.

I deliberately excluded the fasting glucose from testing. The morning Dawn Effect interferes with fasting glucose levels and since the Dawn Effect is all about steroid release that uses insulin backing glucose up, migraineurs' morning fasting glucose test result is often higher than it should be leading to meaningless conclusions. In addition, for each person, the length of fasting turns the production of glycogen on at different times by the liver. It is understood that glycogen production usually starts after 8 hours of not eating. This is certainly true for some people; for others the time may differ—this is greatly dependent upon insulin sensitivity[336-339]. While most doctors often request a fasting glucose test, in reality it provides misleading results. When blood test is done in a fasted state, the liver generates glucose from its glycogen reserves, invalidating the result[340-344]. Another often requested test is the hemoglobin A1c (HbA1c) test. The HbA1c[345,346] test (based on 6-12 weeks glucose average) is not very useful. There is no linear relationship between glucose consumption and insulin[340,347-349]. Kraft explains well how full-blown diabetics and also prediabetics can go through the HbA1c test with flying colors[335] but a non-diabetic who sometimes eats sugar may get trapped. Also, because the HbA1c is an average of blood glucose levels over a period of time, those with hypoglycemia with big swings from very low blood sugar to very high, usually show a completely normal HbA1c, failing to signal the presence of hypoglycemia.

After having been at baseline for many months on the low carbohydrate diet, migraineurs notice an increase in sensitivity to glucose. They show edema, thirst, and other signs of glucose consumption faster than what they are used to (faster reduction of glucose from the blood and entry into the interstitial fluid) and this makes them nervous! Many comment that they don't want to be more sensitive to glucose because that means they can only eat less of it! They believe that responding faster to eating carbohydrates is a sign of heading in the wrong direction. In fact, they are recovering from their insulin resistance. The more sugar sensitive (the faster the reaction) a person is, the easier it is to prevent a migraine, and the less likely it is that the person is insulin resistant. A quick reaction implies that insulin picked up all the consumed glucose from the blood and delivered it fast to the cells.

Section 5

Migraine Prevention & Treatment

The purpose of science in understanding who we are as humans is not to rob us of our sense of mystery, not to cure us of our sense of mystery. The purpose of science is to constantly reinvent and reinvigorate that mystery. To always use it in a context where we are helping people in trying to resist the forces of ideology that we are all familiar with.

--*Robert Sapolsky*

In Part II of the book, I covered what to do in the quick when you get a migraine, but I didn't provide explanation as to why you needed to take those steps. In this section, you will find a more detailed version of what you read in Part II. This is the heart of the explanation behind the steps of the Stanton Migraine Protocol®. It is expected that you are by now familiar with the cause of migraine and you also know that water and salt (hydration) are very important in migraine prevention.

Step by Step You Will Get There

Learn to feel what your body needs. To be able to feel your body's plea, you need to reach a healthy baseline from which you can judge how far you have derailed. In this section, you learn what the healthy baseline means, how to get to that healthy baseline, and how you can tell which direction to head if you have strayed away from it. To start with, you first need to drink enough water.

How much water do you need?

Many "experts" suggest that 8 glasses of water per day is all you need, and other liquids, such as juices, sodas, teas, soups, etc., count toward that water intake. Scientific studies researching water-need provide mixed solutions[350]. The Institute of Medicine recommends as "adequate intake" 125 fl oz (3.7 L or 15.6 glasses, 8 oz per glass) daily for men and 91 fl oz (2.7 L or 11.375 glasses) for women including all beverages and liquid foods, such as soups[351] without distinction for age, activity level, and weight[352-356]. In truth, everyone needs an amount of water that is proportional to their gender, size, level of activity, altitude, and climate. I somehow can't see that the same amount of water a day equally meets the need of a 5-year old, a little old lady aged 90 weighing 100 lbs, a 40-year old overweight woman of 200 lbs, or in case of men a little boy, a teenager, an athlete, or a 350 lbs giant. Sorry. It just doesn't work like that. Since migraineurs need more water and more minerals in their electrolyte to keep their hyper active brain going, I like a different approach based on a widely used formula. The minimum daily water a woman needs is equivalent to the amount of water her body contains in ounces. An adult woman's body is about 55% water[354], so take your weight in lbs. and multiply that by 55% or 0.55. The number you get is the minimum amount of water you need in ounces[357]. A glass of water is 8 oz. and it is easy to relate to. A women's minimum daily water need in number of 8 oz. glasses is 55 % of her weight divided by 8. Example: assume you weigh 132 lbs. Take 55% of that, so 132 x 0.55 = 73 oz. is your daily minimum water intake. Divide this by 8: 73/8=9 glasses of water. If you are a male, over 70% of your body is water so instead of 0.55, multiply by 0.70. As a male with the above weight of 132 lbs., you need 92.4 oz. water or 11.6 glasses of water, minimum. You can trigger a migraine if you don't drink enough water[358].

Experts also suggest drinking water when you are thirsty. This is also incorrect—particularly for migraineurs and type 2 diabetics, since thirst can represent a loss of electrolyte minerals and not just water—and diabetics are always thirsty. You have already read, and will read in future sections as well, about the benefits of increased dietary sodium for reducing edema, bringing water back into the interstitial fluid, and removing glucose. It thus makes common sense to increase sodium instead of drinking water, particularly if you are also short of minerals. While there are hundreds of papers about the benefits of cutting sodium for diabetics, most discussions center on the benefits for reducing hunger[359]. Whether cutting dietary sodium really cuts hunger has come under fire from several scientists and two showed that increased sodium reduces thirst and increases the number of calories burned—hence reduces weight[360,361]. The assumption is that all diabetics are obese and hunger control is what is needed, and that reduced salt in the diet controls both—neither of which is true[362]. Migraineurs are not typically obese but are often thirsty—for a very similar reason to diabetics, which is connected to electrolyte disturbance by glucose. Thus, when you feel thirsty, assuming you have been drinking enough water, instead of drinking more water, take a bit of salt—1/8th teaspoon or 1 salt pill—without water (just a sip). Wait 5-10 minutes and watch your thirst vanish. This works both for migraineurs and diabetics (type 2).

It is easy to judge if you are drinking enough water by looking at your urine color. To ensure urine color stability, I do three very important things. These steps help to keep proper hydration levels and electrolyte homeostasis during the night and prepare for the day ahead (These instructions are intentionally repeated in this book, they are important, you should memorize them):

1. About an hour before bed time I drink a glass of whole milk. This provides the energy for the body and brain as my active over-sensitized brain tries to sleep. If you cannot tolerate milk, eat its equivalent in protein, carbs, and fat.

2. About 30 minutes after the milk, I drink a glass of water (at least 15-30 minutes before lying down) with a salt pill or 1/8th teaspoon of salt. I personally use the Health by Principle electrolyte capsules (www.healthbyprinciple.com), which I designed with iodine (I receive no financial gains from any purchase; I have no conflict of interest). This is the only salt supplement (capsule) with iodine in the market at the time I write this book. If you have Hashimoto's or Grave's disease, please pick a different brand of salt supplement that does not contain iodine. Hydrating this way before sleep also helps you avoid getting up at night to visit the bathroom, helps you sleep better[363], reducing nightmares!
3. In the morning, before I even get out of bed, I drink a glass of water and take a salt pill. This replenishes my body and rehydrates it after a night of sleep.

Most people have a change of urine color from a more concentrated darker one in the morning to clear water color as the day progresses. While this is considered to be normal by many doctors, it is not normal for a migraineur. A migraineur cannot afford to see large changes in her urine color. Changes represent hydration, and thus electrolyte, changes: too dark is dehydrated and too light is over hydrated (not enough minerals in the electrolyte). Your urine should be light yellow—like mild lemonade—but never like water.

Baseline

Baseline is the foundation from which you can build up your health using the Stanton Migraine Protocol®. Without reaching baseline, nothing will work with certainty and your migraines will still be unpredictable, even if you learn to manage them to some degree.

It is where you need to be with your food and drink choices at all times. This is the base against which you adjust on a moment's notice should you feel that the light is getting brighter, the noise is getting noisier, your kids seem suddenly too wild, though they are doing exactly the same thing they were doing 5 minutes ago, etc. The reason why baseline is a must is because it brings your body to an optimal and predictable state, and allows your body to clear out leftover edema that you never knew you had. It also allows you to identify and remove interference caused by incompatible foods. From baseline you can assess the true impact of a particular food. For example, most migraineurs, when I get to know them, tell me that they have no edema. Of course, they don't see that they do. Their edema exists in a permanently low-level state. At baseline, no one has edema. Thus you can notice the slightest water retention once you reached baseline.

Baseline is where your electrolytes are in perfect homeostasis, your body is fully hydrated, and your brain cells are energized. You are not thirsty, not tired, and no longer crave sweets, or salt, or water. So how do you get to baseline? Here are several rules for you to follow:

1. You must completely give up all added sweeteners—cold turkey is the easiest way to quit since sweeteners are highly addictive. This means that all sweetener types (all sugars no matter what type: brown, white, raw, natural, fruit sugar, honey, maple syrup, etc.), all sugar substitutes and so-called naturals (like stevia) need to be stopped. Sugar substitutes are not sugar and cause a ton of problems for the body. For some people they are also irritants. In general, sugar substitutes spike insulin, cause obesity, and contribute to metabolic syndrome[364-367]. Furthermore, some sugar substitutes, such as Stevia, are the plant's natural insecticide for protection against insects that intend to destroy the plant. Thus, when eating Stevia, as natural of a substance it is, one is actually consuming a mild nerve toxin. Not sure about you but a nerve toxin is definitely not my idea of an enjoyable indulgence!
2. You cannot have any smoothies, shakes, sauces, juices, gels, or any fruits, vegetables, grains, or higher-carb nuts and seeds, in any shape or form, where they are separated from their fiber. Most fruits, vegetables, nuts, seeds, and grains are very high in carbs, with fructose, glucose, and starches. Much of the fructose is chemically bonded to insoluble fibers and glucose to soluble fibers. Removing the fiber or breaking the chemical bonds between the fibers and the sugars by blending, shaking, grinding, or squeezing the fruits, vegetables, nuts, seeds, or grains turns them into sugar water, or sugary spreads in the case of nuts or seeds or flour. Artificial milk

made from nuts or soy or similar also falls into this category. Once the chemical bond of the fiber is broken, the carbohydrate portion in the food readily converts to glucose during digestion, spiking insulin and, in the case of fructose, heading to the liver to transform into triglycerides.

3. You need to stop alcohol—while a glass of wine or another alcoholic beverage every now and then is healthy for you, until you learn to prevent all migraines, I ask you to quit all alcohol. Alcohol that is fermented fruit or grain, without its fiber, is all sugar even if it does not taste sweet. Distilled spirits such as vodka have no carbs in them. No matter the type of alcohol, they are all diuretic (dehydrates you), and thereby work counter to our efforts to remain hydrated. Alcohol crosses the blood brain barrier, something that can give you a headache, though not a migraine. It is not advisable to drink any alcohol before you have fully mastered the protocol.
4. Avoid prepared foods because they all, without exception, contain sugar, preservatives, and additives that may lead to migraine, and nearly zero fiber. This also applies to canned soups, canned vegetables, those little fruit or fruit sauce cups, and prepared meals. You can use frozen whole raw vegetables that have no seasoning on them—let it be you who seasons them to taste. We have a motto for migraineurs: "If you are not the one who prepared it, don't eat it."
5. You can consume water, whole cow or goat milk (only whole fat please), cream, butter, sour cream, crème fraiche,

mascarpone, yogurt (unsweetened and live cultured, avoid Greek-style strained yogurt because it contains too much protein and less nutrients than unstrained yogurt), kefir, and enjoy maximum 1 small cup of coffee per day. Yep, that's it. No soda pops, no teas, not even herbal tea, and no Kombucha either.

6. You need to devote time learning how to read food labels, ingredient lists, and using the USDA Foods Database or any alternate available in your country. As crazy as it sounds, most labels contain words you've never heard of, including many names for sugars and sugar substitutes that resemble nothing you would have ever imagined! Although there is a list of current names of sugars and sugar substitutes in a later section, the list changes regularly so continue to update your knowledge.
7. Calculate your minimum and maximum water need based on the previous sub-section. Never drink less than your minimum and never exceed your maximum. Make sure that you "hydrate", meaning water with salt every now and then (not every glass) to produce electrolyte, versus simply drinking water. Let your urine color be your guide.
8. Reduce all complex carbs in your diet to 50 - 70 net carbs grams for women and 65 - 85 for men. Below 50 carb grams you are at risk for experiencing headaches caused by too little carbohydrates—this refers to the standard baseline diet only. The term "complex carbs" refers to all fruits, vegetables, nuts, and seeds with their natural fiber attached. Minimize

and eliminate grains as much as you can. Avoid starches, such as tapioca, rice, potato, corn, cereals, breads, pastas, and avoid all forms of flours, including so-called gluten-free flours which often are nothing more than starch. The complex carbs that you should consider adding to your diet should only be dark green leafy lettuces, spinach, broccoli, cauliflower, tomatoes, zucchini, cucumbers and alike, and for fruits mostly only blackberries, strawberries, raspberries, apricots, and maximum 10 ball (100 gr) cantaloupe. If you must have some starches, chose wild rice or quinoa (neither is a real grain).

9. When extra water is in the extracellular space in the interstitial fluid (edema, generated after eating carbs), it causes pressure on the cells from the outside. It will also be visible in the areas where it has collected in the form of swelling. You can test for edema by pressing a finger deeply into the fleshy part just above your ankle, and then pull it back right away. If your skin takes more than a count of 2 or to come back to normal, you have edema. Skin popping right back is the sign of no edema.
10. You will also become thirsty after eating carbs because salt and water will have left the cells. It makes sense that your cells signal for the need of more water. However, since sodium is needed to retain water in the cells, there is no chance for any water to remain no matter how much you drink, unless salt is also consumed. You will likely have to urinate within 20-30 minutes after eating carbs. This urine is water

that was removed from your cells and managed to find its way to your kidneys. The more you drink the more edema you will end-up with and the thirstier you will get. This is the same mechanism by which type 2 diabetics are also thirsty all the time. Drinking water at this time is the worst thing you can do. Instead, take 1/8th teaspoon of salt with just a sip of water when you feel thirsty after eating carbs. This will pull the water back inside where it needs to be and your thirst will magically vanish.

11. A very important function of baseline hydration is that is prepares you for peaceful sleep at night and ensures that the 3:30 am migraines don't happen. Here I repeat again the importance of the evening glass of whole milk followed by a glass of water and a salt pill. The purpose of the whole milk is to provide protein, fat, and some glucose for your brain while you sleep. Migraineurs have very busy brains, nightmares, and restless sleep. Waking up for a wee-hour migraine is caused by running out of nutrition and voltage in the middle of the night.
12. The final important step for migraine prevention in baseline is the morning salt and water. Keep salt by your bedside and a glass of water too. When you awaken in the morning, and before you even get out of bed, take 1/8th teaspoon of salt or a salt pill and a glass of water. Wait at least 30 minutes before you eat breakfast. The role of the morning treatment is to rehydrate you. As you sleep, your body enters fasting mode (breakfast stands for "break[ing] fast") and so hydration is

critically important. If you are properly hydrated, your urine color will always be the same.

Salt versus Sodium & Sodium versus Potassium

I often refer to salt and sodium interchangeably since we eat salt but salt label contains sodium. To remind you, salt is 40% sodium and 60% chloride. Thus 1-gram (1000 mg) salt has 400 mg sodium. The USDA recommends between 1500 and 2300 mg sodium per day for the general population—2300 mg sodium is 1 teaspoon of salt. There is no scientific evidence suggesting where this number came from (history of research shows mixed results)[368]. The latest study shows that the low sodium range recommended by the USDA is unhealthy for the general population[242]. Since migraineurs need more sodium than non-migraineurs by about 50% - 70%, you should try to maintain your ideal ratio, which is somewhere between 2:1.5 and 1:1 potassium to sodium. The USDA recommends eating between 3500 mg to 4700 mg potassium a day. When people try to eat 4700 mg potassium to meet this guideline, most find it an impossible task—4700 mg potassium is approximately 5 medium sized baked russet potatoes a day, which is 166 net carb grams. This is about 100 carb grams more than what, on average, a migraineur can consume a day with average migraine preventive control. If you ate these many potatoes, you would consume 839 calories with little protein, almost zero fat and other than a small amount of vitamin C, not much else but starch. Alternatively, you could eat 4.5 avocados or several pounds of fish or steak a day to consume that much in potassium. It requires a lot of food to eat 4700 mg potassium a day and most people don't need and don't want that many Calories. 3000 – 3500 mg potassium seems more achievable. The ratio of potassium to sodium is not only more important for migraineurs, it is also more important than actual quantity in maintaining optimal cardiovascular health[256,369,370].

Where do you find the potassium information per food item? Use the database:

https://ndb.nal.usda.gov/ndb/search/list for information of all the foods you eat! Don't leave home without this database.

When You Feel The Pain Already

If you missed all the signs and you feel the pain already, you must act immediately. At the start of a migraine, first you have to remember what you have eaten within the past 24 hours—keeping a diary helps. Possible problem areas: too much or too little carbs, too much or too little salt, too much or too little potassium, too much or too little water. If you are still eating sweets, your carbs are too high so don't be surprised to have a migraine. You may find that you need to quit all grains—most migraineurs need to. If you are drinking too little water and slowly increasing it but aren't quite at the level you need to be, that can also be a cause. Don't drink up all the water you need at once—have a glass of whole milk instead.

If you can recall or look up what you ate, check to see if your meals were balanced. In the Facebook migraine group, Kristin, one of our admins, created an Excel database that allows you to enter what you eat and all the data will automatically populate and sum for you: total carbs, fiber, net carbs, fat, protein, calories, potassium, sodium, magnesium, calcium, and nearly all vitamins of importance. If net carbs exceed 5 gr, the carbs Excel cell will pop a yellow warning up, indicating that you need to pay attention to your carbs. If your meal exceeded 12 net carb grams, a red warning will pop up to remind you that you must take salt after the meal, and no water with or immediately following the meal. To get a hold of this awesome resource, you need to become a participating member in the migraine group:

https://www.facebook.com/groups/219182458276615/

When & How to Make A Full Electrolyte

There are many options out there to provide proper nutrition for the body in order to reach the ideal biochemical balance, but what if you are in another country and the food or drink you need is not available? Or what if you have a tummy bug and spent the past day next to your toilet. In such cases you need to create a fully hydrating liquid, which includes the full spectrum of electrolyte: sodium, potassium, magnesium, calcium, phosphate, and glucose. You can hydrate to perfection by creating electrolyte yourself. You have two options: make the hydrating fluid yourself from scratch or purchase and modify a sport drink. Let me detail each.

Homemade full electrolyte: in a 16 oz glass of water add 1/8th of a teaspoon of salt and one teaspoon unsweetened and undiluted frozen orange juice concentrate (or 2-3 tablespoons of fresh orange juice). Mix it well, and take it a spoonful at a time 10 minutes apart, little by little as discussed in Part II, reducing the time between spoonful as you are able to hold more and more the fluid down. Repeat with several glasses that day—the more the better. If you are at home or have access to milk and your stomach is no longer upset, drink whole milk. Once you can hold fluids down steady, you can return to standard hydration; start by eating soups.

If you would rather use a sport drink: purchase a bottle of high potassium, low sugar, (no sugar substitutes or naturals like Stevia please, only sugar) sport drink. Pour an 8-oz glass only a quarter full of the sport drink. Fill the rest with water and add 1/16th teaspoon of salt. A sport drink doesn't have the full spectrum of electrolyte minerals so the moment you can switch to whole milk or homemade electrolyte, do so.

If your vomiting for over 4 hours or diarrhea doesn't stop within 8 hours and you cannot hold any fluids down, please head to the ER to receive electrolyte solution via IV.

Word of caution:

This method of hydration is not for everyday use. It should be reserved for those emergency times when you are dehydrated due to illness, cannot keep anything down, and/or have diarrhea. Soft-drinks and store-bought electrolyte drinks appear to hydrate but dehydrate instead, because they have sugar in them—and as we have learned earlier, sugar removes water and salt from the cells. Avoid drinking store-brought prepared sport or electrolyte drinks as much as possible. For the best hydration with full electrolyte, drink whole milk.

Worthless people live only to eat and drink;
people of worth eat and drink only to live.

SOCRATES

Essential Minerals for Migraineurs

Go ahead; ask your acquaintances, friends, and relatives to explain what being hydrated means. I guarantee that almost all of them will say that it is drinking water and maybe a few might mention a sport drink or coconut water or something similar. None of that is correct. Hydration does not mean drinking water (with or without flavoring). Hydration implies that water goes into your body and then stays there to hydrate. How do you keep water in your body? You will be amazed at how many people drink very little water because if they drink more, they spend the day running to urinate. A new branch of the medical industry was born for women drinking water rather than hydrating, creating what is called "urinary incontinence" or "urinary frequency" or "urinary inefficiency" or "bladder is too small" or "overactive bladder" treatments. Humbug. I am not saying that some women do not have these kinds of problems as a result of giving birth or some infection or a surgery gone wrong. But yes: HUMBUG! And I say this because a very large percentage of women shows the *symptoms* (not illness) of one or more of the above-mentioned conditions as a result of drinking only water or some sweet drinks, rather than a hydrating fluid (salt and water).

The functionality of the water that we drink is to get inside our cells carrying nutrients, then wash waste products and toxins out[134,354,371-379]. Our urine color is "transparent yellow" which is distinctly yellow but not neon yellow (like after taking vitamin B), not dark (like honey), and not clear (like water). The color of the urine represents what it carries out of your system and it better be carrying toxins! Urine also should have a smell. Clear color urine has no smell—it is simply wasted water that has just run through you. Urine that is too dark and has a strong odor represents too much toxin in the little water you drink. Neither represents proper hydration.

For hydration, meaning to get water inside your cells, you need to make sure you have proper amounts of salt and potassium in your body! Sodium and chloride make sure that water can enter the cells, as we described it in detail before. Potassium is required to remove the water from the cell. Hydration is a process by which your cells take water in and send waste and toxins out. If water remains inside your cells long enough to do its job, you are hydrated. You will know because you will not need to urinate every hour.

Minerals and the Nervous System

I could write a whole book on the importance of salt to just the heart alone; salt is the most important essential mineral for the whole body. Salt is one of the most essential minerals for the brain as well. Salt, or the lack of enough salt to be precise, is very strongly connected to migraines. However, this doesn't mean that you need to put the book down and dump a bunch of salt in your mouth right now. There is much more to proper salt consumption than meets the eye. Here we shall set the record straight: without salt there is no heartbeat, no brain function, and no blood.

Given how many minerals need to be in perfect balance for electrolyte homeostasis, where does one start the search for the missing mineral? I started by analyzing how a cell lives, what it does and how, and which important element in electrolyte is most likely to be low and why. The technical background is somewhat complex so most of the details are left for Part IV. The challenge is to find out the relationship between what migraineurs eat and their ionic homeostasis failure. This failure can be caused by the inappropriate amount of any of the following elements: sodium, potassium, chloride, magnesium, calcium, phosphate, glucose, and water. Are there any food groups that can cause electrolyte disruption in a way that would bring about a lack of any of these elements? Indeed, there are.

That Evil salt

We have been and are still being told that salt is bad for us, but there is big confusion about why that would be so or how much is too much. Scare stories with findings that salt is harmful are abound by medical practitioners who claim that salt and its effects have been "well understood" and "properly researched". None of that is correct, as noted earlier.

Fetuses in amniotic fluid are in salt water at nearly the same level of saltiness as seawater (we are descendants of predecessors from the sea after all). We all start (and have always started) our lives in salt water. Our vital body fluids are made of salt and water plus other important minerals. If we sweat from heat, exercise, have fever, or are nervous, what we sweat is a mixture of salt and water. Our tears are salt water and our breath evaporates salt water. Our blood tastes salty as well. So then, a body that spent 9 months in salt water before being born, a body that requires salt and water in every one of its cells to survive, is somehow better off without salt? How is that?

Salt is an essential mineral, meaning we cannot make it ourselves, and so we must eat it. Our bodies contain a lot of salt; 0.4% or so[380]. So, a skinny 110-pound female has nearly a half a pound of salt in her body; a 200-pound average male 0.8 (almost 1) pound. It takes quite a stretch of logic to say that "salt is bad," particularly coupled with the lack of any well-conducted or well-analyzed research that can explain how an increase of a single teaspoon of salt would negatively affect the body and justify a recommendation for reduced level of daily salt intake. Most typically, fasting urine samples are collected from people and their blood pressure is then measured. Researchers look for the correlation of higher blood pressure among those subjects who had more than the reference level of sodium in their urine. Frequently correlations are drawn based upon a higher than expected sodium amount and higher than normal blood pressure[226,242,258]. There are several problems with this approach and they are nearly always glossed over by reduced salt advocates. Let's review the many problems with the tests that measure urine samples for sodium and then correlate the results with blood pressure.

a) The kidneys regulate what leaves the body, as well as what stays in the body and for how long. The actual regulation of how much salt will end up in the kidneys to create electrolyte is performed by the Renin-Angiotensin-Aldosterone System (RAAS). Any defect to either the RAAS or the kidneys, or any medicines taken that affect the operation of either of them, will affect how much sodium will be in the urine, independent from how much salt has been consumed by the person. There are also heart medicines that cause the retention of potassium, which in turn changes the amount of sodium excreted. Diabetics excrete different amounts of urinary sodium as well because of glycosuria, a well-understood process of too much glucose of the urine. We also know that glucose removes sodium and water from cells, thereby increasing urinary sodium without an increase in dietary sodium.
b) Migraineurs use more voltage energy in their brain, and more voltage generation uses more salt. In the 20th Century researchers have already found that the urine of migraineurs contained 50% more sodium than non-migraineurs and that they were "busy brain" people[144]. Almost no one paid attention to the findings that migraineurs have very low blood pressure[19,238,381,382]. Very few studies inquire about blood pressure of migraineurs when they are not in the middle of a migraine pain attack. Of course, during an intense pain

episode blood pressure increases. There are a few studies that verified the low blood pressure of migraineurs when not in a state of pain[18,383,384]. The low blood pressure of migraineurs helps some medicines, such as triptans, succeed simply by increasing the migraineurs' blood pressure due to their vasoconstriction effects[385-387]; albeit they leave the migraineur with major side effects[388,389]. A cup of coffee can bring about the same result in a much safer manner.

c) When carbohydrates are eaten (any type: complex, simple, refined) glucose removes sodium from cells[39]. No study has ever inquired if the subject consumed any sweets in the 24 hours prior to the experiment, or if they drank a lot of water when they became thirsty after eating sweets. Patients who eat a lot of sweets the day before sample collection will have variable sodium levels in their urine depending on their insulin sensitivity status.
d) General health and mood affect blood pressure as does the traffic, how much one slept, what she had for dinner. None of these had ever been considered in the measurement of blood pressure
e) We also now understand that people who eat a lot of simple carbohydrates and drink sweetened beverages end up with higher blood pressure[235,254]. No study has ever controlled for this.

Increased salt is not only not harmful, but beneficial. A most recent study showed that increased dietary salt helped the subjects feel better, they had more energy, and even lost weight[360]. This study also showed that subjects excreted more sodium in their urine. That is because salt induced the burning of fat in the body—something normally does not happen with carbohydrate metabolism easily! If increased dietary sodium reduces weight and water, it cannot possibly increase blood pressure, which is associated with increased weight and increase blood volume.

As you can see, urinary sodium level's reported connection to blood pressure is misleading by faulty research that neither asked enough questions nor set meaningful health condition boundaries[390]. The confusion generated by imperfect science can actually hurt people[242,391]. We obviously are getting misleading recommendations by which to live a healthy life. Much newer research tells us that *too little* salt is bad for us[226,242,245,246,251,253,255,390,392] and salt does not cause high blood pressure[393-401]. Whom do we believe? While there is considerable debate on how much salt humans need, recent research shows that the more the better and healthier[242,243]. A study also showed the inverse relationship between the amount of dietary salt (measured as urinary sodium) and the frequency of migraines[226]. Admittedly, these studies were published after the 1st edition of this book had come out, so I understand that at the time my concept of extra salt must have sounded strange and was received with much skepticism.

Consider this quote:

> *"The metabolic syndrome (MetS), defined as a cluster of disorders including obesity and diabetes, is reaching epidemic levels*

in the American population, and the prospect that it can reduce neurological function is alarming. The weaknesses imposed by the MetS are particularly alarming if we consider that the pathology of most brain disorders has some failure in the capacity of neurons to metabolize energy. Dietary factors such as increasing consumption of fructose is considered as an important contributor to the MetS in humans, and rodents treated with high fructose diet display signs of MetS such as increased hepatic lipid and triglyceride level, and peripheral insulin resistance. Fructose-induced MetS reduces synaptic plasticity and learning and memory performance in animals, and alter molecules which play important roles in mitochondrial bioenergetics. MetS disrupts signaling through insulin receptors which are strategically localized to brain areas involved in cognitive processing such as the hippocampus."[402]

It is clear that it is sugar that affects the entire metabolic system in a very negative way rather than salt. In the past, we have heard very little to warn us about sugar's effects upon our health. Now though, in 2017, this seems to have taken a marked turn and I cannot have a day without bumping into an anti-sugar article. As of this writing, "my plate", the official US food pyramid, considers cereals and breads (all refined and highly processed carbs and most filled with sugar) to be among the healthiest food items for your diet. Salt is not even on the plate! Yet research from all over the world shows a direct relationship between carbohydrate consumption, high blood pressure, metabolic syndrome, and a connection to cardiac events.

Unfortunately, many research results have been ignored because of commercial interests[235,279,281].

Furthermore, the findings on the connection of salt and blood pressure are comical even in terms of the percentages and numbers. Based on salt-reduced diets, researchers found that healthy adult males achieved a 2.4 mm Hg fall in systolic blood pressure[392]. The systolic blood pressure is assumed to be normal between 100 and 139 mm Hg any time during the day. That is, a range of 39 mm Hg systolic change all through the day is considered normal. One cannot have two identical blood pressure (BP) readings one after the other within the same minute because every time we breathe or our heart beats, our blood pressure changes (try it at home). Since a 39 mm Hg daytime variation is normal for a person, what makes us think that a 2.4 mm Hg (less than 10% of normal variability) increase in BP is such a large increase that it requires a reduction in sodium[390]? In hypertensive individuals, the change in BP from the reduced sodium diet was 5.8 mm Hg, which also falls within the 39 mm Hg variation of normal. Are we alarmed by toothpicks in the forest? Were the 2.4 or 5.8 mm Hg changes larger in importance than the 39 mm Hg variation during the day? And if so, why?

I can see absolutely no reason for the reduction of sodium in heart-healthy or even hypertensive individuals given the relatively small amount of change sodium reduction is capable of producing[242]. Patients with serious heart disease still need to eat salt just to keep their heart beating! So how can we provide the salt necessary to have a functioning heart if, at the same time, we remove the salt from the diet? A recent study shows that there is such a thing as "too low" salt level, below which the heart can no longer function[242]. This study found that the daily sodium intake for a hypertensive individual has a low end of 1200 mg (early death increases by reducing it further) and an upper end of 5000 mg sodium (slightly over 2 teaspoons of salt) a day. By comparison, current USDA recommendations are 2300 mg sodium for healthy adults and 1500 mg sodium or less for elderly or hypertensive adults, both of which are close to dangerously low levels. Healthy individuals suffered a much higher rate of cardiovascular death when their sodium was reduced to 1200 mg or less a day[242].

To close the discussion on the salt debate, consider the generalization of sodium requirement for a person who weighs 100 lb versus one who weighs 300 lb, or a person who lives in a cold climate versus one living in a hot and dry desert, or a person who sits by her computer all day long versus one who runs Marathons. The amount of sodium required for all these people will be completely different because salt evaporates and is used up faster in the larger, heavier, younger, and more active persons versus the little old lady sitting in her rocking chair all day. Generalizations always fail. People are simply too different to state that all people need to eat the same amount of sodium. USDA or AHA guidelines should have a *range* that encapsulates all possibilities, even leaving room for exceptions, such as the different sodium needs of migraineurs.

Consider the following testimonial I received from a migraineur in my Facebook group who had very high blood pressure when she had joined:

> *"Wanted to share something. I've had medication induced hypertension for many years. I was put on a [Lopressor] (can't remember the name) at age 18, propranolol around age 30, for my migraines. Started off innocently enough, 10 mg daily. My last increase was 80 mg, four times daily. I have been on more bp meds than my dad, who has had 5 heart attacks, quadruple bypass, and too many stents to count, even in his legs. I've been in this [migraine] group less than a week, trying to push fluids, and keep my electrolytes balanced. I'm doing my best. As of yesterday, I've not had a full-blown migraine in almost a week, I've lost 10 pounds, and my blood pressure went from an average 174/132, down to 122/62. I'd not had meds in 11 hours, in case my doc wanted blood work. After telling [the doctor] about Dr. Stanton's protocol, she became very interested.... Yeehaw!! Thanks Angela!!*

As you can see, blood pressure can easily be controlled by a medicine-free lifestyle, simply by controlling what and how one eats and drinks. Artificial sodium control is not necessary—the body knows what it needs.

Instead, I recommend we focus on what really causes high blood pressure, insulin resistance, metabolic syndrome, and cardiovascular disease: sugar and carbohydrates, in general. I find tons of articles about sugar causing high blood pressure and cardiovascular disease[224,225,235,254,275-279,403-411]. Even in medical manuals sugar is labeled as the cause; yet interestingly when it comes to controlling blood pressure, suddenly it is salt that is reduced and not sugar[39]. Why? If sugar caused it, shouldn't it be sugar that is removed? I have no explanation for such a twist of logic and cannot help but assume ulterior motives. The take home message is this: There are plenty of reasons to fear carbohydrates rich in easy glucose, sugars, and sugar substitutes, and none for fearing salt!

Too Little Salt vs Too Much Salt

Many times, when I had a migraine, I could not control it with medications, and so after the third day of terror I would end up in the ER. The nurses immediately started treatment by pumping saline solution—electrolyte—into my veins. The nurses would always tell me that I was dehydrated. According to the prevailing American diet recommendations, I ate a very healthy diet full of vegetables, fruits and healthy grains. I also drank plenty of water (8-10 glasses a day, which for my weight and activity level was ideal). So what was in my diet that made me dehydrated? In retrospect it is clear: lack of enough salt.

The vascular constrictors often prescribed, such as triptans or medicines with caffeine in them, appear to do wonders for people with low blood pressure because the constriction of the blood vessels reestablishes the blood pressure necessary for proper blood flow (120/80). Notice, however that, while we have made the veins tighter so blood can flow through them with higher pressure, we have also modified something that was not sick on its own. To make up for the inadequate cell hydration we have artificially increased blood pressure! It would have been better to simply rehydrate the cells! Low blood pressure can hurt the brain; less blood may not carry enough oxygen for the neurons' requirements.

An important and welcome finding happened in my life after I had discovered the secret of biochemical balance and started to thrive for a proper ratio of sodium, potassium and water. My blood pressure did not change over the years but my blood volume did. This is counter to scientific findings[412]. Blood pressure does not change from increased salt consumption over the long run, provided that potassium and water are increased simultaneously in a healthy ratio with salt. Salt management alone, ignoring potassium, does not suffice.

It is very hard to tell if someone has too much or too little salt in her body. Fortunately, we have learned a few "tricks of the trade" through the years that help. Many migraineurs have signs on their faces, fingers, toes, ankles, etc., that lets them evaluate what they need. As you have read it earlier, I found in the migraine group years ago that nearly all migraineurs (probably all, only some may not have noticed it) have one eye becoming smaller than the other prior to a migraine. My personal experience is this: when my right eye gets smaller than the left I need salt, but if it gets bigger, I have too much salt in me and need potassium. This valuable observation relates to neuronal activity specific to managing the muscles of that eye. When the right eye gets smaller, I am running low on voltage in a specific brain area and the affected neurons cannot open the eye properly or hold the muscle of the eye firmly. Taking salt at this point changes my eye back to its normal size within 10 minutes. If the eye is larger than normal and I feel a tad off, my brain is likely receiving too much stimulus. In this case I have too much salt in me and I need to increase potassium.

Salt, be it in pill, powder, or rock form, reduces swelling and edema in the body and transports glucose into the cells[39]. You should talk to your doctor before taking extra salt but not because of any concern about your blood pressure. There are certain rare health conditions to consider, or you may be taking medicines that do not permit the intake of extra salt. For example, if you have damaged kidneys, only one kidney, or have had a urostomy, your body may not convert salt into electrolyte as intended. Some people have salt sensitivity, thus for them taking extra salt can cause injury[413].

If you are a vegetarian or vegan you will need to supplement your daily salt intake more than those eating a broader variety of foods; fruits and vegetables are very poor in salt content and also high in carbohydrates. Salt is an essential mineral for all mammals. Apes have been seen dipping their fruits in the ocean for the salty taste as well as for washing parasites off the food (salt may kill parasites)[414]. Many bird types regularly eat salt and mammals seek out salt patches[415-417]. Farmers provide "salt licks" to their farm animals[418]. We are creatures of salt and whatever salt we lose as part of our daily activities, we must replace. We lose most of our salt in our urine and some as perspiration and even breathing.

Which Salt?

There are a number of salt products available on the market today, many of them cleverly marketed on the internet. I know several members in my migraine group, for example, who tried the "Himalayan salt lemon juice" treatment, only to vomit it up on the spot. Plus, unbeknown to them, Himalayan salt—also highly advocated by many as healthy due to the many "minerals" in it—is fossilized salt that ascended to the mountains via tectonic forces from under the sea in Pakistan. Under the mountain's immense weight the salt-deposits had been compressed by the pressure and its high heat, forming fossilized rock salt. The colors represent the many metals that were seeping through the salt as it had been under enormous heat and pressure, forming "minerals", some of which are made of radioactive isotopes, such as mercury, and lead. I wrote an article about Himalayan salt and its harmful ingredients:

https://www.hormonesmatter.com/himalayan-salt-lead-poisoning-global-scale/.

If you really want to dig into the full spectrum of potentially harmful ingredients, check this out:

http://themeadow.com/pages/minerals-in-himalayan-pink-salt-spectral-analysis (the larger the atomic number, the heavier and more dangerous the metal).

It is interesting to note that while arsenic, mercury and lead are too toxic to be near us in the same room (we removed lead paints from our walls and mercury fillings from our cavities), yet when they are ingredients in Himalayan salt many people drop their guard and go after the "pink fad" because of its romantic name. They believe it is better for them to eat this than purified table salt because, as they say, "purified table salt is stripped off its nutrients." True. Purified table salt is "pure" and contains nothing else but salt—precisely what our body needs. Salt has 2 elements: sodium and chloride. The rest are not part of salt so they are instantly removed and cleared from our bodies by our built-in detox machines: kidneys and liver (except for heavy metals and radioactive elements, which remain in our bones). Salt itself breaks up into ions of sodium (Na+) and chloride (Cl-) that are indispensable for the neurons' voltage generation. Some believe that the anticaking material used in table salt is a poison—of course the same anticaking in sugar, flour, and various supplements are ignored. An interesting anecdote: there is a Dr. M whose website is very popular with many people in the US. He has some interesting and useful articles on human health. He also sells many (unhealthy) nutritional bars, supplements and, among other things, advocates Himalayan salt. I sent him an email asking if he knew that Himalayan salt is full of toxic elements. His response was (sent to me by his staff):

> *"He [Dr. M] feels the crystalline structure of crystal salt is balanced and not isolated from the 84 inherent mineral elements.* ***They are connected in a harmonious state****. He agrees with the composition of the minerals but* ***does not find anything harmful about the amounts of mercury or lead.****"* (emphasis added by me)

I responded with the following:

> *"This would be a true statement if the salt did not break into ions in our bodies such as sodium (Na+) and chloride (Cl-) to form part of the cellular mechanism. In the process of becoming ions they release mercury, lead and other chemicals. Thus, mercury is released without any crystals to protect us from it. The same is true with lead and all radioactive isotopes in Himalayan salt. Perhaps Dr. M forgot that in the body everything becomes ions and what was a crystal at one point will not stay a crystal--unless it is silica a.k.a. sand."*

I received no response to this one.

There was a time when most people knew that originally all salt came from the sea. Today we pay a premium for the packages that have "sea salt" printed on them, even though the cheapest table salt is also sea salt. One should always make an educated decision regarding what one eats. Unpurified sea salt is impure, meaning that organic materials (such as fish poop, other debris, and even bacterial spores) build up on it and thus delivers impurities to our diet that may cause illness.

Calcium & Magnesium

Two other minerals important to discuss that need to enter the body together are calcium and magnesium. Many women take calcium supplements, thinking they will help improve the strength of their bones. The truth, unfortunately, is that they will not. Calcium is a fat-soluble mineral, which means that one must take calcium with some good fat—for example milk or cheese. Calcium taken as a supplement can end up as calcium deposit in arteries instead of strengthening the bones. Calcium supplements can bring with them stroke danger as well[419]. To optimize your calcium intake for your bones, drink whole milk and eat plenty of dairy. Meats and eggs are also great calcium sources, as are sardines that have the bones in them—and eat the bones. If you must take calcium for thyroid or other conditions, please be sure to take the minimum dose you need and always consume it with natural animal fats or fatty foods.

Magnesium supplementation is recommended for all migraineurs and should be taken with calcium containing food—such as milk. The type and amount is discussed under the section of vitamins. Here I would only like to remind you that the highest magnesium containing foods are dark green leafy salads and vegetables. Since most high magnesium containing salads and vegetables are low in carbohydrate and also high in potassium, they are highly beneficial for migraineurs. Examples are romaine or cos lettuces, spinach, broccoli, zucchini, avocados, and similar greens.

Potassium

Potassium is an essential nutrient that has been given little consideration in the past—except in the case of heart patients. While foods rich in salt are pretty obviously identifiable (one can taste salt), we have no idea what foods have potassium in them and how much. It does not help that potassium does not have a specific taste. And what exactly does potassium look like?

I often receive the question if potassium should/could be supplemented in a pill form. The answer is no, you should not. Potassium is a dangerous mineral if too much is consumed (hyperkalemia) and if too little is consumed (hypokalemia). In both cases, if dietary changes don't improve the condition, hospitalization is necessary[420]. The harm in taking potassium as a supplement comes from the fact that it all absorbs at once. Recall that potassium initiates the resting potential of neurons (you learned this several sections back). If you take potassium supplement, it will do just that: cause neural resting potential, and take water out of your blood reducing blood volume, which leads to reduced blood pressure[421-423]. Taken as a supplement by a migraineur, who normally has low blood pressure, it can cause fainting, palpitations, and potential heart damage, and may cause seizures[132,424-427]. You are also likely to end up with a migraine.

It is highly recommended that you consume your potassium in foods. All migraineurs should eat high potassium foods and balance the potassium load with salt. In general, most foods that nature created and which have not been tinkered with by humans (unprocessed) are full of potassium. Most people think of bananas when potassium is discussed but in reality, bananas are a poor choice of potassium: they have less potassium than many other foods, and contribute way too much sugar. A medium size banana has approximately half as much potassium as a medium size avocado but it contains a ton of sugar, whereas there is not much sugar in an avocado. Or consider a slice of salmon or steak, each of which has more potassium than a banana and no sugar at all. Consuming foods rich in potassium allows for a slow entry of potassium into our blood, assuring toxin removal. Many electrolyte salt supplements have 20mg or so potassium added. That amount of potassium simply helps the sodium get to the right place. That amount does not count as potassium supplementation so it is perfectly fine.

No one actually has defined an ideal potassium or sodium amount for the general population. I found with the assistance and experience of the migraine group that the majority of migraineurs do best with a potassium to sodium ratio of 2:1.5 to 1:1. Individual requirements can vary, so a trial and error period is highly recommended. To calculate the ratio one must use the correct, full nutritional information as provided by the USDA.

People are fed by the food industry, which pays no attention to health; and are treated by the health industry, which pays no attention to food.

--Wendell Berry

Non-Essential Minerals

Carbohydrate, Glucose, and the Nervous System

Would figuring out the relationship between carbohydrates consumption and insulin be helpful in understanding why migraineurs run out of important minerals, and if so, what can we do about it? Harrison's Medical Manual comes to the rescue, clearly summarizing in one sentence what happens:

> *"...serum Na^+ falls by 1.4 mM for every 100-mg/dL increase in glucose, due to glucose-induced H_2O efflux from cells" (page 4)*[39]

It is important to understand what the above quote really means. As mentioned before already, it is unexpected from a healthy (insulin sensitive) individual to have a 100 mg/dL blood sugar increase after consuming foods containing glucose. The normal fasting range tops out at 99 mg/dL, and the normal maximum high after eating or at any random time is supposed to be less than 140 mg/dL. A normal reaction to food of any kind is not supposed to be as large as 100 mg/dL, unless the person is diabetic. However, this doesn't consider migraineurs and other groups who are genetically glucose sensitive or intolerant! One need not be diabetic to have a huge reaction to glucose if one is intolerant of glucose. To give you an example from my personal experience, after a baseline of 95 mg/dL random blood sugar reading (I am not diabetic), I ate 10 small white-flesh Ranier cherries, 10 cherries and nothing else. My 30-minute-after-cherries reading was 175—not quite an increase of 100 mg/dL but pretty close and this is only after 10 cherries. Now imagine if I eat a large slice of cake! As a migraineur, I am glucose intolerant and my reaction will be diabetic in magnitude without being a diabetic. Eating watermelon gave an even bigger glucose spike. Starting blood sugar was 88 (this was my fasting blood sugar) and I ate 414 gr—a 3-inch slice of a large watermelon. 30 minutes after my last bite, my blood sugar was 167 mg/dL, an 85-point jump. And while this is not an accepted "normal" range for a healthy individual, it is normal for a migraineur whose body doesn't use glucose properly.

Another concern is medicines. Many medicines increase blood glucose concentration as they tie down insulin receptors. Remember my experience with Prednisone mentioned earlier in relations to hormones? Prednisone tied up all my insulin and "backed up" my glucose to a very high level, waiting to be picked up by insulin. It took several hours for my blood sugar to return to normal because Prednisone is a hormone and not food.

It is also important to note that every single person reacts to every food item differently. For example, milk is known as a highly insulinogenic food—meaning that it spikes insulin. Milk is said to have sugar—at least that is what it says on the label. In reality, milk has no sugar. It has lactose that needs to be broken up by the lactase enzymes in the intestines to become sugar. So milk doesn't spike glucose or insulin prior to the lactose being broken up into glucose and galactose. This delay does not play out the same way for everyone. For some people milk spikes to the extreme and for others almost none. For me it is almost none. Check your glucose spike reaction to food items you consume regularly.

The speed with which insulin can remove glucose from the blood and pass it onto cells is crucial. Simply put: every time a migraineur eats carbohydrates (be it sugar, fruit, vegetable, nuts and seeds, a slice of bread or cake, soft drink, candy, or a glass of orange juice) it converts to glucose and in the case of fruits, to fructose as well. Glucose from carbs enters the neurons and kicks both water and sodium out, leaving the neurons void of two key elements of electrolyte. In other words, causing a "*dramatic failure of brain ion homeostasis*". You may ask at this point: well what about those who have no migraines? Since their brain is more adapted to modern nutrition, and their voltage gated ionic channels are different from the ones in the brain of migraineurs, they will not suffer the same consequences as migraineurs do. There are many genetic variance connections to migraineurs having different pumps and channels of importance for electrolyte homeostasis[113,114,428]; this is discussed in greater detail in Part IV. Of course, even though they don't get migraines, plenty of non-migraineurs end up with type 2 diabetes and so they are not immune from getting into trouble. Only it takes a longer time for type 2 diabetes to show its ugly head to which migraineurs are genetically predisposed[79].

Having read the book this far, I trust you have got the message: you must stop eating sugar and sweetened things in general, and reduce your carbohydrates, including fruits, high glucose vegetables, and starch as much as possible.

Understanding Nutrients

"Last night I had an awesome breakthrough in my nutritional paradigm. I was hungry and wanted something good to eat. My first thought was "what would taste good right now?" Then I thought, "what does my body NEED right now?" Huge, right? So, I looked at my food journal and noted that I was a little low on protein and fat, so I made myself a nice 150 g salmon steak with a cream and butter sauce. So, delicious, more importantly, it was just what my body needed. Why was this such a breakthrough?

Because Angela's protocol [the Stanton Migraine Protocol®] is (or should be) so easy to implement. I find the hardest part, for me, is overcoming the mental conditioning of the last 30+ years. "Fat is bad, fat makes you fatter, sicker, slower. Animal fat and protein will damage your heart, your kidneys, your liver, and your brain. If you want to live become a vegetarian." And, of course, calories are king. "Every calorie counts. Limit calories to lose weight. If calories eaten exceed calories burned you will get fatter." It goes on and on.

All my life I have heard (and still hear) this on the TV, read in the newspaper, and in magazines. Not to mention that I hear from my friends, my family, medical professionals, and even complete strangers.

Because of all of that, when preparing a good [Stanton Migraine Protocol®] friendly meal, my brain looks at my daily food log and begins to panic. "Good God" it cries "look at all that fat, look at all those calories, are you trying to kill yourself?" Before the initial panic can set in to a full-blown anxiety I must stop, take a deep breath, and remind myself that all that propaganda is messing with my mind. Calories only matter as a guide to how much fat, protein, and carbs you should be eating. Other than that, they are completely meaningless. Fat is not going to make me fat; quite the opposite, in fact. Fat is good for the brain, the heart, and the rest of the internal organs.

It will take more time, overcoming 30+ years of brainwashing will not happen overnight, but I will eventually overcome. And so will anyone who is willing to ignore "conventional wisdom" and eat healthy animal fats and proteins." --SG

The above is a quote from one of the migraine group members, as posted in the group one day. Her message brings home something very important: we tend to pick what we eat based on what we feel like eating rather than what our body needs as nutrition. This is a very important revelation about how we, particularly migraineurs, should focus on what our body needs, rather than what our taste buds desire.

Assume for an instant that you watched a TV commercial stating that too much salt is bad for you, so you should lower your salt intake. You are shown some great tasting low-salt foods or salt-substituted foods. The message also includes that eating lots of fruits, veggies, whole grains, and nuts are healthy for you and fat is bad so stick with low fat. You opt for eating lots of fruits, vegetables, grains, and nuts and convert to low fat everything from that point on (this is not farfetched since this is what has happened from the middle of the 20th Century to the present day to an awful lot of people in the developed world). In other words, you follow what is now called "my plate" by the USDA in their nutritional recommendations, referred to as SAD (Standard American Diet). However, science advances inexorably and we have learned new things, reached new conclusions about our health and nutrition.

Most foods consumed today as part of the SAD formulation contain nearly zero essential nutrients. Recall I noted that nutrients that are essential are so because our body cannot make them and thus we must consume them. Let's understand what macronutrients are, which ones are essential and why, and how they fit into the biochemical balancing challenge of a migraineur.

Macronutrients

There are three macronutrients and two of the three have vital (essential) role in our body. The macronutrients are:

- carbohydrates (not essential)
- fats (essential and non-essential fatty acids)
- protein (essential and non-essential amino acids)

Note that of the three macronutrients, carbohydrates are not essential—meaning the human body can make all the nutrients they provide from other sources. We need not consume an ounce of carbohydrates to remain perfectly healthy. Fats (fatty acids) and protein (amino acids) contain essential nutrients and so we must eat both. Most foods are of mixed macronutrients. For example, we consider an apple as carbohydrate but it also has small amounts of protein and fat. Over 50% of proteins also convert to glucose during digestion. This is based on the protein's amino acid composition. All non-essential amino acids convert to glucose, some essential amino acids can convert to both glucose and ketones (ketones are discussed under the ketogenic diet section later), and two essential amino acids convert only to ketones. Thus protein has variable conversion rate to glucose. The only macronutrient that contains nothing but its principle element is fat; fats only contain fat and nothing else. Fats typically remain fats though under some uncommon conditions can convert to glucose[429-434].

Macronutrients come in a variety of shapes and forms. I found that many people are not familiar with the basics of macronutrients and are not sure what is what. For example, I often hear vegans or vegetarians claim they eat no carbohydrates. I used to laugh at that since everything vegans eat and most of what vegetarians eat is carbs. I no longer laugh because I have heard it so often that it is becoming clear they have been misled and have no idea that fruits, vegetables, grains, nuts, and seeds are all carbohydrates. Many vegans have gotten angry with me when I told them that their diet was all carbs! Let's examine each macronutrient for what it is and what it does.

Carbohydrates

It is worth repeating, carbohydrates aren't essential for us at all; they represent a macronutrient group that we can live without—read the evolution of the human diet in two excellent open access articles[230,435]. While this may come as a surprise to you, humans have lived for eons without eating a single piece of fruit or vegetable[230]. The definition of carbohydrates: "any of various neutral compounds of carbon, hydrogen, and oxygen (such as sugars, starches, and celluloses) most of which are formed by green plants" (Meriam Webster Dictionary). Thus carbohydrates, as a macronutrient group, contain sugars (glucose, fructose, lactose, galactose), starches, and cellulose (fibers). It should be noted that some carbs are pure sugar without any other nutrients, such as glucose, whereas other carbs contain both protein and fat only usually in very small amounts—such as lettuce. On the other hand, nuts, seeds, and grains that you would think are not carbohydrates, actually are. A piece of lettuce is just as much a carbohydrate as is an apple, or a piece of candy, a drop of honey, a slice of bread, a bowl of cereal, almonds, soy, or a baked potato. What differs is how fast the carbs within them convert to glucose in the body.

Carbohydrates contain only small amounts of fatty acids (fats) and small amounts of amino acids (proteins). Since both fatty acids and amino acids have essential forms, eating a strict carbohydrate diet can leave a person deficient in essential elements unless they are supplemented.

I believe what confuses many people about carbohydrates is that they have not learned to differentiate between "refined" and "unrefined" (often referred to as "simple" and "complex" or "processed" and "unprocessed") carbohydrates. Refined carbohydrates are the ones in which glucose exists in its most ingestible and simple form: monosaccharide (one glucose molecule). This isn't just candy, as most people would think. When the fiber is separated from fruits, vegetables, nuts, seeds, or grains, what is left behind in terms of carbohydrates are monosaccharides (glucose and fructose), which are the simplest of sugars. For example, assume you pick a few fresh apples off your own tree. If you eat one of those apples whole with skin, you are eating a "whole food" that contains unrefined complex carbohydrates. These have longer sugar chains and take longer to convert into glucose in your body. When you eat the fruit whole, the fibers (soluble and insoluble) are bound to glucose and fructose in the fruit and some digestion of separating fibers from the sugars must occur before the sugars can be absorbed. This digestion period ensures that some of the sugars, the ones bound to fiber, end up in your gut as food for a healthy gut biome.

If you, instead, put that same apple into a juicer or a blender and create an apple juice or a smoothie or a shake, you will have transformed the complex carbohydrates into refined carbohydrates by separating the sugars from the fibers. Now the same apple no longer provides nutrition to your gut microbes since the sugar is absorbed earlier in the digestive process and heads to your liver, where some of it will enter your blood circulation as glucose to feed cells while the rest will become triglycerides (fat), which insulin packs away for storage. Thus, it takes very little effort to transform unrefined carbohydrates into refined carbohydrates, but for your body, the difference is significant. Every time we eat or drink something, we need to consider and understand the metabolic consequences.

How about milk imitations? Those who cannot drink animal milk for whatever reason often drink soy or almond or similar milk instead. Such milk substitutes represent refined carbohydrates and are not much different from eating pure table sugar.

There are other refined carbohydrates of concern as well. For example, anything highly processed turns into glucose quickly in our body after initiating an insulin spike. An example is corn flour, wheat flour, or any flour. While eating corn whole on the cob is wholesome (although with a high sugar content), after it is dried it becomes a grain (popcorn is a grain). Its glycemic index (the amount of insulin it will spike in percentage to what the pancreas is capable of producing in response to pure glucose) is 100%. So, whether someone eats a slice of gluten free corn flour baked muffin, corn tortilla, or popcorn, for the body (in terms of insulin) it is the same thing as eating pure glucose. The glycemic index, while not a reliable tool for all things, can at least be used to identify those carbohydrates migraineurs want to avoid. Wheat flour has the exact same problem; it makes very little difference if you eat whole wheat or white wheat. Both are ground and convert to glucose immediately. A single flour tortilla has 23 gr of net carbs, which is equal to almost 6 teaspoons of sugar. One medium corn muffin has 54 net carb gr, which is equal to 13.5 teaspoons of sugar. An avocado has so much fiber that once you subtract the fiber from the total carbohydrates, the net carbs (the amount that will become sugar in your body) is minimal. By contrast, a banana typically contains the equivalent of 6-10 teaspoons of sugar.

All sugar types are carbohydrates. This means that it doesn't matter if you select table sugar, raw sugar, coconut sugar, date sugar, etc., they are all the same: glucose and fructose. They all get absorbed by our digestive system in identical ways.

Here are the methods of sugar absorption:

Glucose (dextrose): is a monosaccharide (simple sugar of one molecule) causing an instant spike of insulin which is required for the transport of glucose into the cells. Glucose can provide energy to our body while the unused part converts to triglycerides and is deposited as fat[436]. Eating glucose is not essential since the body can create glucose (via gluconeogenesis) from proteins and sometimes from fats[437].

Fructose (levulose): is a monosaccharide that does not spike insulin according to accepted scientific knowledge but this is debatable[438]. Fructose (without attached fiber) goes through the liver, where it gets converted to ethanol first[439] and then to triglycerides to be deposited as fat[440]. Approximately 41% of fructose converts to glucose as well[441]. Fructose causes non-alcoholic fatty liver disease, gout[276,442], heart disease, and obesity[443-445]. Fructose ends up as triglycerides (3 fat molecules connected with a glycerol), they form the small particles of sticky plaques that block arteries[411].

Galactose: is a monosaccharide that is less sweet than glucose or fructose. Galactose converts quickly to glucose[446,447].

Lactose: is a disaccharide, meaning two types of sugar molecules bonded. The two sugars are glucose and galactose. Lactose, found in milk, is therefore not recognized by insulin as sugar until the bond between glucose and galactose is broken, which is done by lactase enzymes in the intestines. Since lactose converts to sugar deep in the intestines, where hungry bacteria also live, not all of its glucose is returned to the blood. Nonetheless, milk is believed to be insulinogenic, meaning it spikes insulin but it appears to do so only in some people and not all. Perhaps this has something to do with life-long adaptation versus restarting milk consumption at a later time.

Starch: is polysaccharide (made from more than one molecule of glucose). I am sure you have often heard that starches are healthy and good for us. Nothing could be further from the truth, particularly for migraineurs. Starches are long chain (polymeric) glucose molecules that are connected together by bonds forming a polysaccharide. Starch is converted into sugar, for example by malting, or fermented to produce ethanol in the manufacture of beer, whisky and biofuel. It is processed to produce many of the sugars used in processed foods. Tapioca starch is commonly used as a replacement for wheat in gluten free foods. Starchy foods, such as potatoes or rice, turn into glucose by enzymes before you even swallow them.

Fibers (cellulose): If you look in the USDA database, you will find that fibers, both soluble and insoluble, are grouped with other forms of carbohydrates. In many other countries this is not the case, so if you are reading this book in another country, please check to be sure you understand how your foods are labeled. Fibers are not digestible by the human body and so they don't ever become sugars. As a result, while they are listed with carbohydrates, they don't count as such. There are officially two types of fibers listed, though in reality there are three. I detail all three below.

Insoluble fiber: doesn't dissolve in water, remains metabolically stable (will not metabolize); it is a bulking agent. With sufficient fructose attached, it is a prebiotic (food for gut bacteria) that is fermented by the microbiota (probiotics) in the large intestine.

Soluble fiber: dissolves in water, and ferments in the colon into gases and prebiotics. Soluble fiber is an aid to loosen up feces. It increases the time of digestion and reduces the rate at which glucose is metabolized. It can also reduce hunger because it takes up stomach space but is indigestible.

Resistant starch: as the name suggests, it is a special starch that behaves like fiber. Some types of resistant starch are fermented by the microbiota in the large intestine, conferring benefits to human health through the production of short-chain fatty acids, increased bacterial mass, and the promotion of butyrate-producing bacteria[3] [448].

3 butyrate-producing bacteria produce short chain fatty acid. Butyrates are important for cells lining the colon. Without butyrates for energy, colon cells undergo autophagy and apoptosis (programmed cell death).

So now we know that carbohydrates are a macronutrient that we don't have to consume to survive. Migraineurs have a genetic variance in glucose metabolism, they are glucose and fructose intolerant[449]. The majority of them cannot consume sugar, refined carbohydrates (bread, cereals, etc.,), high sugar fruits (apple, grapes, tropical fruits, dates, etc.,), and high starch foods (potatoes, rice, etc.,), without increasing their risk for a migraine! Whatever glucose the human body needs it can perfectly create from protein by gluconeogenesis in the liver[437,450].

Sugar is extremely addictive[403,451] and unfortunately it is added to everything that is commercially prepared! This is a serious problem. Migraineurs who join my migraine group learn from veteran members about the importance of quitting all forms of sugar. Simple sugar is unhealthy for all people[406,410,439,452,453] not just migraineurs but for migraineurs it is toxic.

Fructose is sold in stores on its own as though it was a sugar substitute that is healthier, but we now know that is not true[223,438,441,454]. Fructose without insoluble fiber (as in agave, honey, high fructose corn syrup, or juices) is particularly unhealthy. As discussed earlier, fruit juices turn into ethanol and then to triglycerides. Think about this next time when you hand apple or orange juice to your child; you are feeding your child something that transforms into ethanol alcohol and then to unhealthy triglycerides[406,409,410,439,452,455-457]. This has already caused a childhood non-alcoholic fatty disease epidemic[458-460]. And the next time you reach for a soft drink (or give one to your child), loaded with fructose, consider what is happening inside your own (and your child's) body[409,410].

When liver inflammation is not connected to alcohol addiction it is called non-alcoholic fatty liver disease. It is a metabolic disease that is fully reversible if one stops eating/drinking fructose. Since the liver is not an endless alcohol storage unit, it must convert it to something else it can store: fat. It would be great for you to watch these two videos:

https://www.youtube.com/watch?v=dBnniua6-oM

https://www.youtube.com/watch?v=sJGS3jdjJGE

Sugar substitutes must also be stopped---they cause obesity and type 2 diabetes[367]. Most sugar substitutes spike insulin, and with a gene variance common to migraineurs that predisposes them to insulin resistance, it is very important to avoid insulin spike as much as possible[364-366,461,462]. Sugar substitutes don't provide any nutrition to the body but since they spike insulin, and since insulin makes you hungry, the more substitutes you consume, the hungrier you will get[463]. This may lead to eating more than you would have eaten had you chosen regular sugar instead. Eating more than you need, particularly if that spikes your insulin, can lead to insulin resistance, obesity, and other metabolic disorders. Here is a great review by sugar substitute type[366], one studying it from a different perspective[464], and several connecting them to obesity and other metabolic disorders[365,463,465]. I'm sure I have given you plenty to digest in this section but there is more!

Glycemic Index & Glycemic Load

The Glycemic Index (GI) was created to describe the degree to which insulin is spiked by carbohydrates, independent of the amount consumed. Glycemic Load (GL) describes the amount of insulin that is released based on the amount of carbs consumed. There is an excellent table in a historical write-up of human food[230] in which you can find GI and GL of many foods:

http://ajcn.nutrition.org/content/81/2/341/T2.expansion.html

In case the link changes, you will find it in the middle of this article[230]. A smaller version that is more user-friendly can be found here:

http://www.madaboutberries.com/articles/glycemic-index-and-glycemic-load.html. While I won't copy and paste the table here, I will give you a few examples and explain their significance.

Most everyone loves Cheerios Cereal and we are told it is "heart healthy", "lowers cholesterol", and "helps control type 2 diabetes". But is any of this true? The GI of plain Cheerios is 74 and the GL is 54. What do these numbers mean? GI is independent of quantity, so whether you eat a single Cheerio or a whole box in one sitting, the GI remains the same. It represents how much your glucose will spike as a percentage of the maximum glucose spike a food item is capable of inducing. Glucose spike is independent from the amount of glucose ingested but the accompanying insulin spike will be very much dependent upon glucose amount consumption[335,466]. The general wisdom is that if the GI is over 50, you should avoid eating that food. GL is quantity dependent; the more Cheerios you eat, the greater the insulin amount needed to pack away all that glucose. A standard recommended serving of Cheerios is 54 on the GL index. This is over 10 times as high as the maximum recommended GL of 5. Could this food then really be healthy for your heart and lower your cholesterol? The answer is an unequivocal *no* in regard to heart health[452,467,468]. In terms of type 2 diabetes, the news is not any better. Type 2 diabetics should not be eating anything that spikes their insulin, since their insulin has a very hard time picking glucose up (this is insulin resistance in a very simplified form). Anything spiking insulin will cause further insulin resistance ➔ deeper type 2 diabetes ➔ obesity.

A bit more on why GL is important. As noted, GL refers to how much a particular food spikes your insulin. Insulin is a priceless commodity! It is manufactured by the pancreas, which has a finite capacity and an upper limit for insulin production. Insulin is primarily a growth hormone[469]. Once we are fully grown, particularly as we age, insulin is in decline[470,471]. Insulin's other jobs are hormone signaling[472] and fat storage management[473]. Insulin as a signaling hormone has many duties in our body: hormone management, hunger management, satiety management, fat storage, and conversion. In other words, one of insulin's functions is to increase our fat reserves for leaner months! So those with insulin resistance are storing the fat away as per nature intended it. Packing fat away for leaner months is nature's protection to allow the species to survive and to procreate later, when more food is available. In fact, insulin, as a fat storage mechanism, is a prehistoric adaptation. In ancient times, the ones who survived were those who were able to become insulin resistant in order to store fat for leaner months[474]. Those with compromised insulin, such as type 1 diabetics, are not able to store fat without insulin[475]. Bears and other hibernating animals become insulin resistant in order to store more fat in the summer and then use that fat during their hibernation, thereby reversing their insulin resistance every winter[476].

Thus being insulin resistant is not the problem. The problem comes from not having lean months in which insulin's role reverses from packing fat away to taking the stored fat and having the body convert it back to fuel. We don't reverse insulin resistance with annual regularity. Hibernating animals do and for them insulin resistance is a necessary survival skill and advantage, and seasonal[477,478]. For humans of today (in most places of the world) food is not only plentiful but seasonal availability is round the clock all year long as if seasons didn't exist. Most carbohydrates (that ancient humans may have consumed only a little when available) are now bred for sweetness (higher sugar content than ever before), and are available in abundance. Reversing insulin resistance in modern humans is not dictated by our environmental circumstances since we have artificially modified them for our convenience. This then leads to the permanence of insulin resistance, which causes major health concerns—including obesity[479]. It is particularly true for migraineurs with their ancient and glucose intolerant brain.

To give you an example of how easy it is to get insulin resistance: the human body contains 1.2-1.5 gallons of blood, in which you will find approximately 1 teaspoon of glucose[480]. That's all. Imagine what a can of soft drink will do to your blood glucose? A typical can of soda contains 45 carb grams, or slightly over 11 teaspoons of sugar.

But let's eat something "healthy" that is "good" for us, like an apple—make it Granny Smith since we think of it as sour and assume it must have very little glucose. The GI of a Granny Smith apple is not high: 37 (50 is considered to be high) but its GL is 70 (very high). Let's eat a small one. A small Granny Smith apple contains 15.6 grams of net carbs, which is about 4 teaspoons of sugar. Sugar is a mix of glucose and fructose so as per the USDA database, our apple has 1 teaspoon of glucose, 2 teaspoons of fructose, and 3/4 teaspoon of sucrose (half of sucrose is glucose and the other half is fructose). So in sum, we eat 1.5 teaspoons of glucose total in that apple—not counting that some of the fructose also converts to glucose[441] (~54% of fructose is converted in the liver to glucose, and about quarter of fructose is converted to lactate.

15% - 18% is converted to glycogen, the from in which the liver stores glucose[481]). Our entire blood glucose prior to this apple was only one teaspoon and with eating a small sour apple we have more than doubled that! Suddenly our blood is so full of glucose that insulin must drop whatever it is doing to start removing the glucose from the blood. Glucose that stays in the blood in excess of 1 teaspoon for an extended time is toxic, causes insulin resistance, type 2 diabetes, stroke, and cardiovascular diseases, so the job is urgent[225,482-485]. As you see, while the GI of an apple is not overly high, it creates quite a chaos for our insulin—and an apple a day is supposed to be good for us; right? Maybe not…

Now let's pick a food that we have been told to avoid because it is unhealthy for us, like whole fat milk, and compare it to skim milk, which we have been told is healthier. The GI of whole fat milk is 27 and of skim milk is 32. A serving of whole fat milk has a GL of 3 and skim milk has 4. Why did I pick milk specifically for comparison? Because many migraineurs drink milk as it is a perfect electrolyte. I find that most of them prefer to drink skim or low-fat milk because they have been told that fat was unhealthy. Once they join our migraine group they quickly learn about the fallacy of this accepted wisdom. Because it is a perfect electrolyte, you can always drink whole milk to prevent a migraine or to help you recover from one. I would also like to point out that the word "sugar" on milk labels is misleading. Milk has no sugar only lactose, which converts to sugar in the intestines as described earlier. Because it converts in the intestines, its sugar load on the blood is significantly less than that of a Granny Smith apple, which becomes glucose in the mouth with the help of certain saliva enzymes, though their GI is similar! That is why the glycemic load for whole milk is 3 whereas for a Granny Smith apple it is around 6 (this is for a typical apple)! The GL of one spoon of pure lactose is 2, whereas for the same amount of sugar it is 4. For this reason, we calculate the carbohydrate content in regular lactose milk only at 50% of the label amount. Not so in lactose free milk, in which lactose is broken up before you drink it. Whatever carbs are listed on lactose free milk, we count them fully.

How about another food we have always been told is beneficial to our health: whole wheat bread? I show its relevant indexes in comparison to white bread, which we are told is the worst form of bread (1 slice each):

White bread:	GI: 75	GL: 12 (twice that of the apple)
Whole wheat bread:	GI: 69	GL: 9

Thus whole wheat bread is marginally better than white bread and much worse than a cup of whole milk and even worse than an apple. This should make you pause for a moment.

GI and GL values are taken from http://www.sugar-and-sweetener-guide.com/glycemic-load-list.html

or

https://www.health.harvard.edu/diseases-and-conditions/glycemic-index-and-glycemic-load-for-100-foods

or

http://www.madaboutberries.com/articles/glycemic-index-and-glycemic-load.html

(whichever had the particular information I was looking for).

Electrolytes and Carbohydrates

The connection of carbohydrates and electrolyte disruption to migraines has eluded scientists. Electrolyte is a basic, vital substance in the human body but no one seems to have considered how its variability may affect migraineurs or others afflicted with metabolic diseases such as type 2 diabetes[117]. What happens when electrolyte concentration changes inside the human body? What causes the concentration variation in the first place?

As noted earlier, as glucose increases in the blood, it expels water and sodium from of cells[39]. This is a critical electrolyte disruption. While this is written in every medical manual, many doctors and neuroscientists I have talked to either forgot about this or actually held erroneous ideas about the process. When it comes to migraineurs, electrolyte homeostasis and glucose don't mix well! Because glucose-rich carbohydrates so severely affect the electrolyte of migraineurs, they are harshly disadvantaged when it comes to their migraine management and nutritional choices.

Perhaps my most important contribution to the science of understanding migraines is this realization of the connection between electrolyte variations and migraines, and that the cause of the electrolyte variations is glucose.

Sugar Substitutes & Naturals

So-called "Naturals" like Stevia, are not sugars at all. Indeed, they are natural, but so too are heroin, psychedelic mushrooms, and rattlesnakes. "Natural" doesn't automatically mean the stuff is good for you! Stevia is the most commonly used sugar substitute because it is natural. However, it is used as an anti-pathogenic agent to fight later stage Lyme disease[486]. If something kills pathogens in the body, chances are it is not something you should consume as an everyday sweetener. Stevia is up to 350 times as sweet as sugar, so it is often mixed with erythritol to be able to give it some volume and mask the bitter aftertaste. New formulations have also been developed that don't leave a bitter taste behind—one of these is called Rebaudioside M[487]. Erythritol is a sugar alcohol and is the main ingredient of Truvia®, along with Stevia. Erythritol is regarded as a "palatable insecticide"[488]. Stevia is a glycoside. Glycosides are often found in nature, and are used to store elements that are toxic.

Insecticides (be it Erythritol, or man-made others) are for the purpose of deterring and/or killing invading insects. Fruit flies are killed by Erythritol[488] and, in fact, talk has started as to whether or not orchards should use this sweetener as an insecticide to deter insects from our fruits and vegetables! What an interesting turn of events if, what we call a sugar substitute, is in reality a nerve toxin. While our innate taste prefers sweet and considers it nontoxic, not everything that tastes sweet is harmless.

To see that some scientists are considering using Erythritol as a real insecticide that we spray on our crops for insect protection, read:

http://www.naturalnews.com/045450_Truvia_erythritol_natural_pesticide.html

or here:

http://www.seeker.com/sugar-substitute-turns-out-to-be-potent-insecticide-1768623162.html[488].

As early as 1942 a patent was filed by the Shell Corp to use Erythritol as a crop insecticide. Patent no: US 2369429 A and in 2014[489] under patent number: WO 2015153957 A1 by Drexel university.

Proteins

Protein with some of its amino acids is one of the essential macronutrients. Without proper amino acids, your muscles will waste away—and this includes one of your most important muscles: your heart. Therefore, eating protein is essential. We also want to know which kind we want to eat: animal or plant based. Importantly, regardless which kind we pick, some amount of the protein we eat converts to glucose in the body, at a slower pace than carbs. Those who elect not to eat carbs (zero carbs diets) can still get glucose to their brain and other vital organs from protein. Furthermore, some proteins, such as organ meats, are sources of ready-to-use glucose. The liver is a giant glycogen (glucose) storage. So, by eating liver, one is also eating glucose. Eating much protein may or may not be hard on the liver and kidneys, hard to tell since research shows contradictory results[490-493].

Because most amino acids are found in inadequate quantities in plants, vegans often supplement their diet with soy protein. Soy beans are meant to substitute meats in a vegan diet. Unfortunately, soy proteins do not fully address dietary amino acid needs, and on top of that too much soy can be harmful for the thyroid[494]. Vegetarians can consume some of the missing essential amino acids by consuming fish, eggs, and dairy.

Essential Amino Acids	Infant RDA	Adult RDA	1 Cup Soybean
Tryptophan	17	3.5	0.42
Threonine	87	7	1.321
Isoleucine	70	10	1.459
Lysine	103	12	1.984
Methionine+Cystine	58	12	1.98
Phenylalanoine+Tyrosine	125	114	1.500
Valine	93	10	1.475
Histidine	28	8-12	0.891
Leucine	161	14	2.371

Table 1. RDA of essential amino acid need vs soy bean

As you can see in Table 1, meeting the daily *essential* amino acid needs eating a vegan diet is not possible. This is troublesome and is one of the explanations why a vegan diet is not nearly as healthy as proponents believe.

Insulinogenic Index

An interesting factor of importance mentioned earlier is that over 50% of protein converts to glucose. While eating a steak may not appear to have much to do with spiking insulin, it may surprise you. Here I list all amino acids and categorize according to whether they are essential or not and if they convert to glucose or not:

	Glucogenic	Ketogenic	Both
Nonessential	Alanine Arginine Asparagine Aspartate Cysteine Glutamate Glutamine Glycine Proline Serine		Tyrosine
Essential	Histidine Methionine Valine	Leucine Lycine	Isoleucine Phenylalanine Tryptophan Threonine

Table 2. All amino acids per type

Most every animal protein contains all of these amino acids in variable amounts. The USDA database often details these (not always) if you click on "full nutrition" information. When choosing food, pick those with the most essential amino acids relative to nonessential ones. For example, beef liver has 15.653 gr nonessential amino acids per

100 gr serving and 28.409 gr essential amino acids. To find the ratio of essential to nonessential amino acids, divide essential by nonessential ➔ 28.409/15.653=1.82 which means that 1.82 times as much of the amino acids are essential as the non-essentials; this would mean it is a good choice of a meal. Almonds are amazingly good in essential amino acids, considering that it is a nut: 72.15% of the amino acids in almonds are essential and in near comparable amount to meats, although 100 gr of almonds is nearly a quarter pound so not likely that you eat that much. In general red meat, lamb, pork, salmon, and the dark meat of turkey appear to contain the most essential amino acids.

Since over 50% of protein converts to glucose, we need to evaluate also to what degree it is insulinogenic, meaning how much insulin will be needed to metabolize that protein. Unlike carbs, insulin merely increases rather than spikes from protein. There are studies that have generated these insulin scores (similar to glycemic index) using the following formula[495,496]:

$$\% \, ins \, cal = \frac{(0.54 * \text{protein}) * \frac{4 \, cal}{gr}}{\text{total cal}}$$

(https://optimisingnutrition.com/tag/insulinogenic-calories/).

To find an online calculator that can help you calculate the insulinogenic index of any food, look here:

https://jscalc.io/calc/QaltoCGzlT7FTf3j

Note that the above formula works perfectly well for butter, fish, or meat, but there is a tad of a problem. The insulinogenic index is not precise as each protein has different glucogenic amino acids in them and all the protein foods you eat together will modify the total insulinogenic index. So use the insulinogenic index with a grain of salt, as a rough guide and not as a gold standard.

Fats

Fats comprise the third essential macronutrient group—they contain neither protein nor carbohydrate at all.

As noted earlier, there are two essential fatty acids: omega 3 and omega 6. Omega 3 fatty acids are difficult to incorporate into your diet. There are three forms available, but the human body can only use two of the three. DHA and EPA are the types the human body can use—these are only available from animal sources. Alpha-linolenic acid, ALA, is the vegetable form of omega 3 fatty acid but the human body cannot synthesize it efficiently. Vegans who eat omega 3 only in ALA form from vegetable sources are very low in this essential fatty acid. Omega 6 is linoleic acid. Most animal products, vegetables, fruits, nuts, seeds, and grains contain omega 6 fatty acids, readily absorbable by humans. The many other types of fats are not essential fatty acids, meaning the human body can create them. The USDA RDA of omega 3 fatty acids for adults is 2 gr and of omega 6 fatty acids is 10 gr.

Fats can be categorized into three types according to their molecular composition:

1. Saturated fat
2. Monounsaturated fat
3. Polyunsaturated fat

Most animal foods contain approximately equal percentages of saturated and monounsaturated fat (approximately 49% each), and much smaller amount of polyunsaturated fat (usually around 2%). Plants vary considerably. For example, olive oil is very high in monounsaturated fat and low in the other two. Coconut oil is very high in saturated fat (in fact higher than any other fat, including lard) and low in mono and polyunsaturated fats. Bone marrow (beef in particular) is very rich in monounsaturated fat (similar to olive oil) and less in the other two. Seed and vegetable oils are high in polyunsaturated fats and low in the other two types.

Through the eons of human evolution, human diet mostly consisted of meat and fat from animals and sea creatures. Based on highly questionable studies in the middle to late 20th Century, animal fats were equated with saturated fat, even though they contain less saturated fat than coconut oil[497] and demonized as responsible for cardiovascular disease for no reason[498-500]. Some animal meat, pork for example, contains more monounsaturated fat than saturated fat. And since all three fat types are in all foods, we cannot demonize saturated fat alone. Courageous and diligent work by a group of scientists and journalists at the start of the 21st Century opened the door to understanding what this amazing macronutrient really is and how important it is for humans[211,212,232,233]. The nutritional paradigm is slowly changing and we are no longer discouraged from eating foods with saturated fats in them, such as red meat, butter, whole fat milk, eggs, etc. Returning to consuming animal fats is not only beneficial for us, but as many of you will agree, it also makes the food taste better.

There is a 4th fat type I didn't mention above: the group of hydrogenated fats and oils. Hydrogenated fats and oils are created in laboratories in a process of modifying fat molecules by chemically adding hydrogen to them. Hydrogenated fats are polyunsaturated fats made into saturated fats artificially, creating what is known by all as "trans-fats". This way the structure is so changed that, to the body, this fat doesn't act as fat and it causes great damage. Items made from hydrogenated fats are margarines, "Can't believe it's not butter", and similar concoctions, in addition to all oils that have their label contain the words hydrogenated fat, partially hydrogenated fat, or trans-fat. The reason for the creation of trans-fats is that saturated fat (hydrogenation creates saturated fat) is stable, can be reused, and doesn't become rancid—however, it becomes a goo that combusts spontaneously (even when used as fuel for engines[501]). Vegetable oils, heated on high temperature also turn into goo and can burst into flames spontaneously[502].

Polyunsaturated and monounsaturated fats are unstable because they are not fully bonded molecules like saturated fats are. Therefore, it is important for you to stop cooking with oils of all kinds, including olive oil. For high heat cooking use only animal fat and medium smoke point coconut oil. Olive oil is so sensitive that it is best consumed only cold on salads or condiments for taste. For cooking return to the days of your grandmother and use bacon dripping, butter, ghee (clarified butter), beef tallow, pork lard (not the hydrogenated grocery store brand!), chicken, or duck fat. Use anything but oil! Coconut oil has some benefits when used as cooking oil or eaten in general. It is available in capsules, powder, and regular liquid oil and has the ability to boost energy for athletes and improve cognitive functions for those with cognitive decline, such as people with Alzheimer's disease[503-506]. However, it can also help in packing on the pounds. So unless you know you will be working the extra energy off, I don't recommend you use much of it. It is essential that you replace margarine and all fake butters with true animal-fat made butter.

Why We Need Fats and Cholesterol

We had been told since the 1960s that fat (particularly saturated fat) was bad for us[507-513]. They said that it causes metabolic disorders, obesity, and cardiac disease, so most prepared foods were changed to reduce fat content, fake fats like margarine became prevalent (see "Women's Health Initiative, Diet Modification Trial", which was a very badly designed study lasting 80 years). While the study showed that a low-fat diet actually harmed women—breast cancer increased in the group with reduced fat—the conclusion in all of the research papers that analyzed the study was that "breast cancer was not significantly reduced by the low-fat diet"—of course not; it actually increased. The story goes that if we eat fat (including dairy and fatty meats such as red meat), it makes us fat and causes coronary heart disease because the fat goes straight into our arteries, clogging them up and then, before we know it, we have a huge cholesterol plug and we die from cardiac failure[514-517]. Since then, many studies have published showing the problems and errors of this theory but even to this day, publishing a paper that opposes that camp is still extremely difficult[233]. As a result, most works revealing new, verifiable, contrarian findings are published in books[211,212,232,234,518-520]. A major breakthrough in this regard is a recent publication in the highly esteemed scientific journal The Lancet[233].

There are several problems with reduced fats, particularly reduced saturated fats[521]. Fat reduction can make huge difference in how our brain works and also how healthy and migraine-free we are:

- Our brain is over 60% fat and 25% of our body's cholesterol is in the brain forming the white matter[522]; the brain makes its own cholesterol[260,263,264,267]. Fat is necessary for proper electronic signaling in both brain and heart.
- Every cell in our body has its membrane made from a lipid bilayer (lipid = fat).

- Every cell in our body uses fat and cholesterol. Humans need to consume animal fats if they are to utilize essential fatty acids and most vitamins and minerals—including calcium, vitamin A and D.
- A gram of carbohydrate or protein provides only 4 Calories whereas a gram of fat provides 9 Calories of energy. We need to eat 2.25 times as much in carbohydrates or proteins as we do in fats—that much more in time and in amount! This would indicate that if you are a vegan or a vegetarian, you must eat over twice as much as your fat-eating brethren for equal Calorie intake, and still will be deficient in most fatty and amino acids!
- The metabolic paths of glucose and protein from fat are so different that they are not interchangeable! Much of the metabolic diseases we see today result directly from the belief that it doesn't matter what our calories are made of: a calorie is a calorie argument, which is incorrect[523].
- Our cells are built from fat and prefer it for obtaining energy[522]. Fat is so important that the body keeps it on reserve. The liver converts sugar into triglycerides[409,411]—the fat we store. Fat's metabolic pathway is significantly shorter than that of carbohydrates or protein, excluding the pyruvate process, hence fat burning is much more efficient[524].
- Cholesterol has earned a very bad name, courtesy of the fraudulent research performed by Ancel Keys and his followers[507,508,525-527]. Without cholesterol our body and brain

> cannot function and we die. Cholesterol reducing drugs have caused more trouble than provided benefits[528].

Because we have been told to cut down on eating egg yolks and animal fats, we replaced them with "heart healthy" grains, cereals, a ton of carbohydrates, and vegetable based oils. I did a little comparison of the oils using the USDA database, so here are samples of all fat and oil types that are available to us. At the end I also included "unhealthy red meat": porterhouse steak, a "healthy meat": wild caught Coho salmon, and a so-called "extremely healthy" avocado to compare their fat content. I bolded the fat type that is most dominant:

Fat, 1 Tblsp	**Saturated gr**	**Monounsaturated gr**	**Polyunsaturated gr**
Olive oil	1.864	**9.850**	1.421
Lard (pork or beef tallow)	5.018	**5.773**	1.434
Butter	**7.169**	3.327	0.427
Duck fat	4.250	**6.310**	1.651
Chicken fat	3.814	**5.722**	2.675
Mutton fat	**6.054**	5.197	0.998
Bacon dripping	6.709	**7.718**	1.917
Coconut oil	**11.217**	0.861	3.710
Grapeseed oil	1.306	2.190	**9.506**
Canola oil	1.031	**8.859**	3.094
Porterhouse steak 100 gr	4.026	**4.516**	0.513
Avocado 100 gr	2.125	**9.799**	1.816
Coho salmon 100 gr	1.595	**2.702**	2.521

Table 3. Fat comparison chart[4]

We have always been told to avoid red meat because of its "high saturated fat content". As you can see, coconut oil has much more saturated fat than red meat or any other oil or meat on the list. Yet it

4 Data taken from the USDA database

is a health food that is used now to help reverse or cure various diseases[503,529-531]. You can also see that pork lard, and porterhouse steak have more monounsaturated fats than saturated. The exception are butter, mutton fat, and coconut oil. So why exactly were red meat chosen as the evil saturated fats is unknown to me.

In case you are wondering how "human" fat may compare, in terms of fatty acid composition, to animal fats, the data is elusive. There is a study dating back to 1960 that analyzed human fats and their constituents but they only looked at fat beneath the skin (subcutaneous fat), which is brown fat full of mitochondria—and thus can produce energy (ATP)—the "good fat". It has different properties from visceral white fat (around the organs), which is the "bad fat," or beige fat in between the other two types (the most active endocrine (hormone regulating) organ)[532]. What kind of dietary fats contribute to the creation of the different types of fats in humans? And how are our bodies using fat in order to survive and live a healthy life? It is very hard to find an answer to these simple sounding questions—though how we use fat is now starting to be understood and discussed among academicians and practitioners of the ketogenic and the LCHF (Low Carbs High Fat) diets[533,534]. Given that we are mammals and not vegetables, our fat composition is likely much more similar to the fat composition of cows or pigs and other mammals than to carrots, not to mention canola or corn oil.

The only thing I have been able to find about human fat is that females on average have about 5 times as much fat in their bodies

(10-12%) as males do (2-3%), and body mass index (BMI) difference, which is quite useless for our purpose here. It is now understood that fats are endocrine (hormonal) organs[535]. They contain nerve tissues, blood connections, and immune cells that communicate with the brain[536,537]. The adipose (fat) tissue responds to signals from hormone systems, the central nervous system, and expresses important endocrine factors such as leptin (controls hunger), proteins of the renin-angiotensin system (sodium, chloride, and potassium management to create electrolytes), and many others. It is also a major signaling agent for sex steroids and the metabolism of glucocorticoids. The importance of its endocrine function is shown by the adverse metabolic consequences of the excess or the deficiency of fat. While there is no doubt that having too much adipose tissue is unhealthy and is connected to various diseases[538], including insulin resistance, it is somewhat contradictory what builds up the adipose tissue and how. The "heart healthy" diet proponents force the theory that eating food high in saturated fat causes high levels of adipose tissue but many studies show that since stored fat is made from carbohydrates by the liver, and not from eating fat, dietary fat's role is misidentified[512,539-542]. Research about the ketogenic diet in the general population and about the tribes that eat a ketogenic equivalent diet of saturated fats and no carbs or grains demonstrate that eating fat doesn't create fat people with high cholesterol[211,212,232,543-547].

The role of insulin in depositing fat into adipose tissue that the liver creates from carbohydrates has much more to do with obesity, type 2 diabetes, and cardiac diseases than eating fat on its own[224,452,467,548-553].

The more insulin floods the system in response to carbohydrates consumed, the more triglycerides are generated by the liver to be stored in the adipose tissue. It is this the feedback mechanism between glucose transport and insulin that deposits more adipose tissue, and since fat does not spike insulin[282,404,405,552,554], there is really no reason for us to fear fat. Though the lack of connection has been well muddied in the past 60+ years by proponents of the low-fat movement, the real culprit of obesity and cardiac disease is glucose and fructose[225,280,555-557].

I suspect you didn't expect to read a lecture on the history of fat research and I will not give you more but I wanted you to know that all of the bad things you have been told about fat and cholesterol are based on misinformation. Having a low-fat diet is certainly totally wrong for migraine prevention, so forget all you have ever heard about "fat is bad", and instead open your mind to updated facts.

Astrocytes, a form of glial cells that perform a variety of support roles in the brain, manufacture cholesterol for the brain. Some amount of cholesterol from the body also cross the blood brain barrier[261-264,266,267]. It is clear then that rather than cutting back on cholesterol, we need to eat more foods of the type that can be converted to cholesterol or is cholesterol rich itself. It is rarely mentioned but the body has a "cholesterol clock" so to speak. What I mean is that if we eat all the cholesterol our body needs, our body will not make more. If we don't eat enough, the body will make as much as it needs. Therefore, everyone seems to have an ideal cholesterol level and that may not be what the guidelines suggest[558]. Fat and cholesterol are also critical for the transport and absorption of fat soluble vitamins and minerals and for vitamin D synthesis through the skin. Most people on low fat diets have to supplement vitamin D.

What I am about to say should give you pause before trusting most medical professionals on the subject of fat's and cholesterol's role for the human body—especially when it comes to migraineurs. I am certain every single reader of this book has had a blood test for "lipid panel" that gives information about cholesterol level in the body in the form of LDL (the bad cholesterol), HDL (the good cholesterol), triglycerides (who knows what that means cholesterol), some random ratio that no one seems to understand, and a "total cholesterol" value which seems to be the only number most (not all) doctors consider important and understand. The current common lipid panel tests – including total cholesterol results – are quite meaningless. The paradigm shift that is taking place is so new that most doctors have never heard of it, let alone appreciate its significance. It is important for you to understand what cholesterol really is, why it is so vitally important to brain health, and what type of cholesterol you should and shouldn't have. In Part IV I give a thorough explanation of the current cholesterol test, why it fails, and also discuss a newer, more promising cholesterol test. For now, I would like you to relax about your cholesterol test results.

With so much concern about cholesterol being too high, note a few important things:

1. No one has ever established the ideal cholesterol levels—it is different for everyone
2. The liver controls the body's cholesterol need and the brain controls the brain's cholesterol need. Therefore, the ideal cholesterol level is based on how cholesterol is used by each person's particular body and brain[267], and there is no magic number that is right for everyone
3. Cholesterol is so vital for the brain that each cholesterol molecule is used for a very long time in the brain[267,559]
4. Increased triglycerides (they are not cholesterol but fats) are more associated with coronary artery disease than LDL, HDL, or total cholesterol[560].
5. Total cholesterol in the standard lipid test results is a sum of the bad cholesterol (calculated), the good cholesterol (HDL), and triglycerides (assumed). The importance of this is that total cholesterol increases if your good cholesterol increases. Therefore, having a high total cholesterol result may mean you are very healthy! Amazingly, some physicians fail to grasp this fact.

Cholesterol & Migraines

How does all this talk about cholesterol connect to your migraines and why should you care? Cholesterol and fat form the white matter, a most important brain layer for migraineurs[561,562]. People with seizures, migraines, Multiple Sclerosis, Parkinson's disease, and many other conditions seem to have one thing in common: myelin damage[563-565]. White matter is the layer that is made of myelin and one of myelin's jobs is to coat each axon. Since the brain is full of fat and cholesterol, it is a crucial reality that migraineurs need lots of cholesterol and fats. It is important that migraineurs have adequate amount of fats and cholesterol in their brain to successfully insulate the axons through myelination. Glucose damages myelin, and insulin resistance compounds the problem as glucose stays longer in the blood and has thus more time to cause damage[285,566,567].

Migraineurs should eat more fat and more cholesterol to ensure proper reserves of myelin. The simplest and easiest way to eat your cholesterol is by eating egg yolks and high cholesterol containing meats. Migraineurs also have difficulty absorbing certain vitamins and minerals, all of which are found in the nutrient rich eggs, organ meats, and meats. Here are important mineral and vitamins in egg yolks, in addition to cholesterol: B6, B12, B9, B5, B1, A, E, K, and D. Egg whites contribute B2 and B3[568-573]. Omega 3 eggs are now also available. Omega 3 fat (particularly DHA) is vital for a healthy brain.

I know all this information about fats and cholesterol appears heresy for many of you. I've been relaying the results of my many years of investigation and I believe I would be dishonest if I compromised on this issue. I hope you read all this with an open mind.

Milk and Milk Types: The Truth

Cow's Milk

Milk does a body good is what the slogan says, and indeed, for once, this slogan is right on for migraineurs! In addition to sodium and potassium, milk is a rich source of calcium, fat, as well as protein, and has just the right amount of carbohydrates. Because of its balance of nutrients, milk is the perfect electrolyte. If you are not lactose intolerant, whole milk is your best friend; if you cannot have lactose, try lactose free whole milk. I recommend that every migraineur who has recognized a migraine prodrome immediately drink a glass of milk! According to the NIH (National Institute of Health), if you cannot drink milk, you can still meet your daily calcium need by eating salmon or sardines that are canned with soft bones (yep, you need to eat the bones!), or eat almonds, Brazil nuts, sunflowers seeds, tahini, and dried beans. To learn more about calcium and the food sources, check out the NIH website[574].

There are two casein (protein) types in cows' milk: A1 and A2. The ancient casein is A2. A1 is a mutated form that didn't exist in the olden times. Most people who are sensitive to milk are sensitive to the A1 casein type milk, which is believed to have inflamatory properties. A2 casein type milk is not inflamatory. Unfortunately, most high-milk yielding cows produce a combination of A1/A2 types and thus their milk, to various degrees, is inflamatory. In some states A2 casein milk is available. Look in your store for A2 brand milk (Australian) that is pure A2 casein milk or visit local dairy farms and inquire. Gurnstein cows are all A2 casein milk producing cows and many Jersey cows are as well. If you are lactose intolerant, you may actually be A1 casein intolerant. So try A2 milk before lactose free milk—all lactose free milk brands in stores are A1/A2.

Warning: Soy Milk

Soy contains a very high amount of estrogen! Particularly if you take birth control pills or estrogen replacement medicines, watch how much soy you eat! One cup of soy milk contains 330 mg potassium, 100 mg sodium, and about 100 mg calcium. However, soy milk is not nutritionally equivalent to milk (less essential fatty and amino acids), and most often contains added sugar to make it palatable. It is not good substitute milk for migraineurs. Eating too much soy can also harm your thyroid[575].

Warning: Almond Milk

Almond milk is not useful for migraineurs, and is not that great for the average non-migraineur either. The ratio of potassium to sodium is way off—160mg sodium to 35 mg potassium. It can also contain a lot of sugar, depending on the brand you buy. While it provides 45% of your daily requirement for calcium, it seriously lacks protein and fat; and you will likely be hit with a migraine. I recommend you enjoy some fresh almonds instead!

Warning: Coconut Water and Coconut Milk

Many people believe that coconut water or coconut milk, sold in cans or bottles, serves as "electrolyte." First of all, I have not found coconut water or milk without added sugar or sugar substitutes—even those products that don't list any added sweeteners contain significantly higher carbohydrate content than natural coconut water does out of a fresh coconut. In the bottling process the carbs get to be concentrated. There are a few other things to consider as well. When you visit a grocery store, how many bottles of coconut water and coconut milk do you see? Multiply that by the number of stores that sell the same in every store in the US. Now envision how much coconut water is in a coconut. Have you ever opened a coconut? I have. One large coconut usually contains about half a glass to 2 glasses max (size dependent) of coconut water. Can you envision the number of coconuts needed to be grown and processed to get "real" coconut water into every single can or bottle? We would need another planet earth just for growing coconuts. Don't trust what you get from that bottle or can, even if it says 100% coconut water. It is not. It is water mixed with coconut water, coconut juice concentrate, or coconut flavors added to water and supplemented with potassium—they can legally ignore the added ingredients as long as some part of the drink is real coconut water. I recommend you buy a fresh coconut instead, chop its top off, and drink the coconut water inside—you will taste the difference (it has very little taste).

Coconut milk is a fruit juice (or nut juice). It is coconut water squeezed from the flesh of the coconut. It is, therefore, by definition, a juice and has nothing to do with milk—other than that it is white.

Additionally, it is not proper electrolyte at all. Real coconut juice is very high in potassium; it does not have the desired potassium to sodium ratio. Also, coconut water can serve as a diuretic for a hypertensive heart patient. It is definitely not a healthy drink after exercise either since the heart needs time to reduce its activity and oxygen use—the high potassium content of coconuts reduces the heart's ability to do so effectively. Avoid coconut water, coconut milk, or coconut juice.

Grains

You believe you know what your ideal nutrition is but you may be surprised to find out you are wrong in some of your choices. If you look at our current food pyramid[576], the biggest section (the most recommended foods) is that of grains—6-11 servings of grains per day due to their supposed benefit of high fiber and their purported type 2 diabetes reducing effect[577]. One of the biggest problems with grains is that they intrinsically lack nutrition! Because of this, they are often fortified to become more nutritious but grains also block the absorption of the added nutrition-- no real benefit[578]. The human body cannot absorb any of grains' nutrients, no matter what it contains[578]; grains cause inflammation and disease[579]. As a result, eating grains is eating bulk, glucose, and nothing else.

Grains are high glycemic index foods[580]. Research articles, such as the one I am quoting below—and there are thousands like it—send a confused message, some recommending them and suggest that they reduce type 2 diabetes, others suggest the exact opposite.

> *"Eating many high-glycemic-index foods – which cause powerful spikes in blood sugar – can lead to an increased risk for type 2 diabetes, heart disease, and overweight. There is also preliminary work linking high-glycemic diets to age-related macular degeneration, ovulatory infertility, and colorectal cancer"*[581].

> *"It's the germ and bran of the whole grain you're after. It contains all the nutrients a grain product has to offer. When you purchase processed grains like bread made from enriched wheat flour, you don't get these. A few more of the nutrients these foods offer are magnesium, chromium, omega 3 fatty acids and folate"*[582]

I checked on the validity of this last quote from the American Diabetes Association on the nutrients in grains. Again, I found conflicting evidence, since as noted before, while grains surely are full of nutrients, they are not available for the human body. I also found that a slice of whole-grain multigrain bread contains a ton of carbs that convert to glucose and no other nutrients. In comparison, I also looked up a slice of oat bran bread, supposedly very high in nutrition. One slice contains 10.5 net carb grams (approximately 2.5 teaspoons of sugar). To get a daily nutrition equivalent of a single serving slice of red meat, you would need to eat over 3 pounds of oat bran breads, which contains approximately 100 teaspoons of sugar and more sodium than what you should have in a day.

The very fact that grains add bulk, and – as a result – are recommended for healthy bowel movement, reduces your body's ability to remain properly hydrated and absorb nutrients. Grains must suck moisture out of your body in order for you to be able to pass the bulk. The bulk formation of grain causes terrible constipation to millions of people who don't drink enough water. Many grain-eaters regularly take laxatives—an entire industry was founded specifically for this purpose.

Grains may play a lot of unexpected tricks with our body as well. Here is a message I received from one of the migraineurs who used to be extremely sick all the time but has been with the group for over three years now without migraines. She initially quit grains (because we recommend to everyone to quit, not because she was sensitive to it) and here is what happened when she returned eating bread, thinking she had no issues with grain:

> *"... I got Ezekiel bread in for my physical assistant to try help her transition off white bread. As an experiment I ended up, on two separate occasions, having a slice. The 2nd time, to make sure the first was the actual reaction. I really am allergic, I'd come out in hives / skin rash I'd swollen up in places and skin was extremely itchy and burning, oh and stomach cramps. I know I have carb intolerance and now I realised wheat was the problem not milk, which kept me from trying to become vegan lol. Says me, who happily eats beef, bacon, and avocado now 😄. But wow it was an amazing response, and I remember going through this* ***daily*** *living like this. It's so weird. Just added*

it to all my other systems. Ezekiel bread had been a great transition to come off a bread diet, but that's all it was." AD

Grains can cover up many health conditions that you may attribute to something else. Grains modify your intestines' ability to absorb nutrients (this is true for everyone, even if you are not a celiac). Grains, particularly those with gluten and gliadin, are very sticky. The sticky stuff adheres to the intestines, preventing nutrition absorption and protein synthesis. Since we consume so much grain, we end up deficient in vitamins and minerals. This is one of the major contributors on the demand side of the market for vitamins and supplements. And finally, grains are not beneficial for type 2 diabetics either. Grains are high glycemic index foods and increase blood sugar, spiking insulin very high[583,584]. The fact that grains contain nearly zero potassium is downright insulting given how grains are pushed for heart health, which requires lots of potassium. Unfortunately one cannot find out what health conditions grains interfere with until grains are stopped for at least 2-6 months. It takes that long for the body to wash all that stuck-on gliadin and gluten from the intestines so healing can start.

I started my grain removal journey by reading two books: Grain Brain by Dr. David Perlmutter[259] and Wheat Belly Total Health by William Davis, MD[578]. Grain Brain discusses some of the bad things about grains but its main focus is the ketogenic diet. The Wheat Belly Total Health book made a lot more sense in terms of the problems grains cause in general. I finally understood that it is not *just* gluten we need to be concerned about but the entire spectrum of grains! Gluten is just one of many proteins in grains that our body cannot utilize. Gliadin is another one and it is potentially even worse[585,586]. These proteins turn against our own protein synthesis, mineral and nutrient absorption, and cause inflammation in the intestines and the gut, and in the case of gliadin, they are toxic. The protein gliadin combines with gluten in grains to create a glue-like substance that deposits on your intestinal walls and blocks all absorption[587-589]. Lectin, another substance, is even stickier and greatly contributes to inflammation[579]. Intrigued, I decided to quit eating grains to see what would happen. This was by far the best decision I have ever made, although it was also one of the hardest in terms of mastering the discipline to push forward. To better understand what you will need to dot when you want to go grain free, read my article here:

https://www.hormonesmatter.com/evil-grains-gluten-free-grain-free/

Grains are more addictive than sugar—this is not talked about in polite circles, and so most people have no idea how addictive grains are. Grains release a morphine-like substance that keeps us very happy when we eat them[578]. As it happens, I now have what I call a "grain cough." Foods that you would never ever suspect in a million years to have any association with grains, have grain in them, only hidden. It can be extremely dangerous for a Celiac, for example, to eat some French fries! As per the following link:

http://food.ndtv.com/food-drinks/there-are-19-ingredients-in-your-mcdonalds-french-fries-736343

McDonald's French fries contain both flour and sugar:

> *"Potatoes, Vegetable Oil (Canola Oil, Soybean Oil, Hydrogenated Soybean Oil), Natural Beef Flavor [**Wheat** and Milk Derivatives], Citric Acid [Preservative], Dextrose [**glucose**], Sodium Acid Pyrophosphate (Maintain Color), Salt. Feb 3, 2015". (highlights are added by me)*

At McDonald's website about their French fries, the following pops up

> *"Golden on the outside, soft and fluffy on the inside. Made with quality potatoes and cooked in our Canola oil blend for zero grams of trans fat per serving. Now that's an epic bite. For information on food allergies, visit the Food Allergy and Anaphylaxis Network. For information on gluten and celiac disease, visit the Celiac Sprue Association."*

While they do list wheat in the ingredients on their website, it is not pasted all over their menu when you order, so a celiac never visiting the website will not know, and may indeed end up in the hospital from a single fry. Luckily for me, I have that "grain cough", and after eating a single bite of French fries I know there is grain in it. Soups, gravy, sauces, most crunchy stuff contain some grain. Also, most things that have golden color with caramel looking burnt edges (like French fries) also have sugar in them.

You need to know that grains are grasses that ruminants can eat—e.g., cows—they possess 4 stomachs and twisted squeezing intestines in order to handle the digestion of the cellulose that is filled with irritants to us but nutritional to them. There are some cultures where more adaptation has taken place over the past several thousand years toward some grains, such as rice, but these people are shorter, frailer, and have the highest stroke occurrence in the world[211].

Grains are among the highest glycemic index (GI) foods that are available. Most have a higher GI than sugar itself—most are very similar to glucose. Grains are among the most insulin-spiking foods there are, other than glucose itself! Even if you are not grain sensitive, consider what it does to your insulin and therefore to your migraines! As you read before, insulin spike means glucose entering your cells, leading to electrolyte imbalance. It is therefore a logical conclusion that those with migraines should quit grains.

Do we need vitamins?

This is a very controversial topic. Obviously, you may do as you wish but I hope you can benefit from what I have to say. A healthy digestive system transmits all necessary vitamins and minerals to the rest of the body, provided it is fed a nutritious diet and is capable of absorbing that nutrition. Many people take supplements without an identifiable need. And since many vitamins and minerals are dangerous in improper amounts[419,590,591], taking them can become a health hazard. Supplementation should only occur when there is a medically proven need, such as when one needs supplementation for something that her body cannot absorb. It is best to seek professional help and a blood test to see what you may need.

Let's talk about migraineurs and their possible (highly likely) nutrition absorption problems (caused by genetic variances), as well as their problems associated with our typical diet that can impair vitamin and mineral absorption. As you know by now, migraineurs come with a special set of genes that are different from those of non-migraineurs—this is discussed in great detail in Part IV. We also know that the very early human ancestors were carnivorous predators and ate every part of what they hunted—including organs—sea food when available, and insects. Organs are very rich sources of B, D, A, and E vitamins as is seafood and particularly cod liver oil, also rich in omega 3 DHA and EPA forms that humans can absorb. In my hypothesis, the assumption is that the prevailing brain type of the early humans – prior to any, even primitive, agriculture – had been the hyper alert migraine-brain. Today, the special set of genes that still facilitate the creation of migraine-brains in a segment of the human population also appears to include certain ancient digestive process determinants that have not kept up with the demands of modern dietary changes. Adaptations that are required to be able to efficiently absorb essential nutrients from fruits and vegetables have not taken place for migraineurs; at least not to the extent of the general population[190,191,592,593].

All migraineurs I so far treated have the MTHFR C667T genetic variance, implying methylation problems with folate and thus absorption problems with B vitamins. Taking a B multi vitamin is not going to help; the synthetic forms of B vitamins are not absorbable by migraineurs. Few doctors ever test for any condition involving B vitamins and for the signs of the potentially dangerous effects of inappropriate methylation ability, such as fatigue and neurological damage. Neither do most doctors test for potentially high homocysteine levels, their lack of clearance by B9 (folate) and B6 can lead to heart problems. In fact, of all the migraineurs I so far worked with, I can count on one hand how many even knew if their B vitamins had been ever tested. The few that had been tested found that their doctors had no understanding of the test results. In some public medical systems, such as in Canada or in the UK, it is not even possible to have certain B vitamins tested—except through a private doctor. I recommend that before you embark on taking any vitamins, you request the following blood tests, in batches if that way they can be carried out easier. Ideally, you can obtain them all. If not available through your healthcare provider, consider ordering these privately because the cost of prevention is always cheaper than the cost or an illness:

A

B1, B2, B5, B6, B9 (folate), B12 (Since B3 can cause type 2 diabetes[594], I don't recommend its testing; B3 is plentiful is food and easily absorbable)

D—they usually test for D3 and D2 or D25
Magnesium
Calcium
Selenium
Iron
Carnitine—tests how you can absorb fats
Carnitine, free—same but how much is floating in your blood?
Acylcarnitine, subs conc, ser/plasma—tests fatty acid oxidation
Homocysteine—tests how well you can methylate folate (B9)—migraineurs often have a problem
TSH, T3, T4 – these are test for your thyroid. You need all 3 tested
Lipid Panel (cholesterol): you need to only know triglycerides & HDL
Liver panel: you need to know how your liver is doing
Creatinine—muscle breakdown measure
GFR: glomerular filtration rate—how well your kidneys filter toxins
BUN: blood urea nitrogen—measures the amount of urea in your blood. Uric acid is held responsible for gout, a very painful condition—caused by fructose, alcohol, and glucose (not protein)
HbA1c—checks your glucose average for the past 3 months
Oral Glucose Tolerance Insulin test – similar to a standard oral glucose tolerance test but they (hopefully) also measure insulin—this is typically not available most anywhere; available privately
Protein—if you eat too much or too little or break it down inappropriately, this number will be off
Electrolyte panel: Na, K, Co2, Cl, and anion gap

Once you have these results, the following is important to be aware of. Homocysteine level over 6 is an indication that you are not able to methylate folate (B9) properly, even though they will tell you it is normal; it is not. High homocysteine levels build up from methylation deficiency. If your homocysteine is high, you will need to start taking a methylfolate (pre-methylated folate—B9) supplement. B12 values range between 200 and 950 but note: you will need to be around 600-800 if you are able to methylate properly. Having a very high B12 level (over 1000) is not any better than having a reading below 200! You will have to start taking bioavailable B12—I list it at the end.

Vitamin D is a hormone. Our body can make vitamin D assuming that there is enough fat and cholesterol under the skin!!! All the low-fat foods we eat (and statins for those who take them) hamper our body's ability to make D, no matter how much time we spend on the sun. If you are taking a statin medicine, you must supplement D, since statins prevent your cholesterol and D production (to the detriment of your whole body). If you are chronically low in D, it is a sign of an adverse health condition, such as thyroid or nutrition absorption deficiency. Please tests further to exclude any health conditions that may be associated with chronic low vitamin D. If you must be on D, don't go on a massive dose, unless your doctor recommends you do.

If you are deficient in any of the above-mentioned vitamins or minerals, please purchase the bioavailable form I note below—brands are not mentioned so you can choose whatever brand you like. Important: I added notes to explain why I am very much against some vitamins:

A: The most bioavailable form of vitamin A is in cod liver oil. While many fruits and vegetables contain high amounts of vitamin A, the type they carry may not be absorbable by you. Vitamin A from cod liver oil is absorbable by all.

B vitamins:
B1: Thiamin HCL (can be sublingual)
B2: Flavin mononucleotide
B5: Pantothetic acid
B6: Pyridoxal 5-phosphate
B9: Folate as L-5-Methyltetrahydrofolate
B12: Methylcobalamin (sublingual)

Note I didn't recommend B3, niacin. It is understood now that B3 is a possible agent for causing type 2 diabetes.

C: It is not needed; take extra only if you are sick. We need minimal C.

D: If you take the cod liver oil I recommended for vitamin A, it naturally also contains vitamin D.

E: Avoid! It is a blood thinner and supports blood vessel growth for cancer cells! If you think you need to increase your E vitamins for whatever reason, obtain it from a food source. Have some nuts!

K: It is a blood clotting agent. Not recommended unless your doctor prescribes it.

Iron: Iron deficiency nearly always masks some other health condition. Rather than popping an iron pill, please have a checkup with a full blood work. Too high iron is also a concern.

Calcium: It is now understood that calcium supplements can lead to calcium deposits (atherosclerosis) in the arteries and in the carotids, presenting a stroke danger[419]. Please avoid them, unless you medically must take them because of thyroid issues. Furthermore, calcium is fat soluble. That means you need to take calcium supplements with some fat. If you can drink whole milk, you may solve your problem without having to take a potentially harmful supplement.

Carnitine (Acetyl L-Carnitine): If your test shows too low Carnitine levels or if the various carnitine types are broken up in the test results and some are high but others low, that may indicate inadequate fat and protein metabolism. Supplementation may be warranted.

Thyroid supplements (if not prescribed): Avoid. Thyroid needs iodine to function well. If you have an underactive thyroid and no Hashimoto's or Grave's disease, please supplement iodine in your diet—use iodized salt. Adults need 150 mcg (pregnant and nursing women 225 mcg). Have your thyroid checked regularly and likely you will see an improvement from taking iodine.

Selenium: Don't ever supplement!! Selenium can reach toxic levels within a short time. Instead, eat Brazil nuts (max 5 a day) or walnuts or similar. Brazil nuts can be fatal if you eat too many.

Omega 3: Many of us are told about and believe in the benefits of taking fish oil capsules for supplementing omega 3. Taking fish oil in a pill provides great blood thinning instead of the desired anti-oxidant effect. In fact, if you prepare for a surgery, you will be asked to stop taking fish oil, similarly to Aspirin or other blood thinners, because fish oil reduces your clotting speed and can be harmful. Those with low blood pressure, such as most migraineurs, will not benefit from further reducing their blood pressure by a blood thinner. Eating the skin of salmon will not cause internal bleeding from overly thinning your blood and for many people can be a much tastier option! Granted it is an acquired taste, but once acquired, the taste is wonderful! Another way to get omega 3 is from Cod Liver Oil, it is safe to take for migraineurs with their low blood pressure.

Magnesium: It is likely that this mineral has to be supplemented for migraineurs since it is essential for voltage gate operation. Magnesium is a very important electrolyte mineral. Since a migraine-brain is electrically more active than a non-migraine-brain, it uses more magnesium. There are many magnesium types so look for the types that work best for you. The most common magnesium types used by migraineurs are:

Magnesium glycinate: Provides energy to the cells.

Magnesium malate: It is the most absorbable elemental magnesium but it is also the most likely to cause diarrhea.

Magnesium taurinate: It helps with heart irregularities that some migraineurs have.

Magnesium citrate: It is the type most often used because it is the least expensive and it also has a high absorption rate.

There are many other types so search out what is best for you. Note: Magnesium pills are very large, so look for one that you can swallow! Here is a link that explains what elemental magnesium types are best for what conditions:

http://www.naturalnews.com/046401_magnesium_dietary_supplements_nutrient_absorption.html

Because most magnesium pills are huge, I designed small and easy to swallow magnesium capsules that contain glycinate, malate, taurinate, and citrate. The serving size is 4 capsules per day. You can find it here: https://www.healthbyprinciple.com/ Disclaimer: Although I designed the supplement, I receive no compensation for product sales.

Vitamins For Vegans & Vegetarians:

Eating tons of carbs causes a nutritional challenge plus prevents some vitamins and minerals from absorption[595]. Some vitamin families and minerals are only available in animal sources. The most important for vegans and vegetarians is to supplement essential amino and fatty acids, B1, B2, B3, B6, B9, B12, K2, omega 3 (DHA/EPA), calcium, iron, iodine, and D[596-598]. Surprisingly, vitamin C is a problem as well. Although vegans and vegetarians eat C containing foods all day long, vitamin C and glucose compete for insulin receptors[599,600]. Vegans eat a lot more carbohydrates and also a lot more vitamin C than the body can handle, plus the absorption of vitamin C is inversely related to the amount consumed[601]. Excess carbohydrates consumption increases blood glucose and thereby insulin release, and high levels of glucose is accompanied by low absorption levels of vitamin C[602]. Vitamin A absorption can also be a problem—this requires a genetic testing to see if the vegan or vegetarian can absorb vitamin A from vegetables and fruits (many cannot absorb in the form present in plants).

Herbs

Herbs in general are not compatible with Western medicine, we know very little about their chemistry. Many of them are also diuretic and some can interact with electrolyte by manipulating sodium and potassium levels[603]. They are definitely not migraine friendly—they don't help migraines and may, in fact, cause harm. Please consider stopping all herbs.

Essential oils

They do absolutely nothing other than smell great. If you like the smell, open a bottle and let it permeate the air. Do not eat or drink essential oils. They are so concentrated that they can be fatal to a small child! Please keep essential oils out of reach!

I searched everywhere for the cause and a cure. It turned out to be right here at home, in my very own kitchen.

Kristin Elizabeth Ingram
Member of the Facebook Migraine Group

How Long Does Recovery Take?

The recovery time assuming proper hydration and the required dietary changes vary depending on how long you have had migraines and what medicines you have been taking. If you are a relatively new migraine sufferer who has not taken medicines (particularly preventives), your recovery may be very quick. A couple of weeks of proper hydration with electrolytes and the quitting of all sweets (real, natural, and substitutes) may be enough to put your body back into harmony and balance. If you had migraines for several years and had been taking triptans, the recovery is likely to take a few months and you may have to fight off triptan rebound. If you were placed on preventive medicines, even if you only had migraines for a short number of years, your recovery will be longer. Age also matter: the younger you are, the faster the recovery. And finally, recovery is slow for those who followed the vegan diet for some period of time. In previous sections I have covered many of the key factors of recovery. Here, I am bringing them all together so you can estimate the length of your recovery.

There is no such thing as "I am hydrated, therefore I will not have a migraine today". You need to increase your water intake (most migraineurs drink very little water) very slowly—typically by half a glass of water maximum a day—and reduce teas to zero and coffees to just one small cup a day. Stop drinking soft drinks, juices, smoothies, shakes, teas (even herbal), and alcohol. This takes time! Sugar is very addictive; sugar substitutes and so called "naturals" are even more addictive. Many migraineurs also need to quit all grains (not just gluten but all grains) because their sensitivity to carbohydrates is simply too high.

Next, as migraines lessen, all migraineurs decide to come off of their medicines! This is not a requirement per se, but they all do since, when there is no pain, there is no need for pain medicines. The reduction (with doctor approval if possible) should occur very slowly, and can take several months, and even several years when a number of preventive medications are involved. Many abortives, like triptans, also cause rebound pains that need to be handled. As a result, full recovery from migraines can take anywhere from a month to several years! Keep in mind the sentence, quoted earlier, "if it took 20 years to break it, it will take more than a day to fix it".

Recovery from the state of constant migraines is great. However, don't forget that you are endowed with a migraine-brain. Your cautious nutrition choices, proper hydration, and healthy lifestyle are all essential to maintaining a migraine free life. This is not a cure but a process of constant awareness and adjustments that lasts a lifetime.

Section 6

Food Challenges Migraineurs Face

Migraineurs face many challenges when it comes to foods. They need help to see through the enormous amount of junk information on the internet and in the media, bombarding them all day long. Here I discuss the challenges associated with getting the right minerals and nutrients as part of a healthy migraineur diet. I also discuss insulin resistance. Besides repeating some already mentioned findings in a different context, here I analyze everything from a food-consumption point of view.

I have had migraine with aura for over 45 years. They would come sometimes 8-10 a month and other times daily for months and even years. I have been on many drugs for migraines, Botox, acupuncture, meditation, herbal remedies, chiropractic, and surgeries to stop the pain. I have had many blood tests, x-rays, CAT scans, and MRI scans to determine the cause, all coming out normal. At the point I found the Stanton Migraine Protocol, I had been having daily debilitating migraines for over six years with the last month completely bedridden, unable to eat or even lift my head without vomiting. The day I started protocol I saw immediate relief! I have never had another migraine above level eight migraine and only one above a level six (due to mistakes I made with protocol). Some people heal much faster but I have made a 90% improvement in two months! I believe my progress is a little slower due to my previous degenerative state concerning insulin resistance. Since starting protocol, my low blood sugar episodes continued to improve drastically and I have more energy *than I have ever had in my life. Each day I followed the protocol resulted in far less low sugar issues with the current result being none! I can look forward to events in my son's life without having to worry about whether I am going to have a migraine or be out-of-touch due to migraine medications. I have been working and not missing any work due to a migraine or nausea from the pain. I walk with the dogs now...I laugh again. I owe everything to Dr. Angela Stanton!! No one in my life has ever given me such a great gift as my life back!*

--LORI WINKLER POTTS
MEMBER OF THE FACEBOOK MIGRAINE GROUP

What Are You Eating and Drinking?

There are lots of nutrition and diet books out there and this is not one of them. I am using some food examples because you can relate to those with ease—in a later section you will also find the do's and don'ts of diets. Food at the biochemical level looks very different from what you see before you put something into your mouth. Everything we eat or drink has some nutritional characteristics that, when they are digested and absorbed, may help or hinder cells and neurons in their ability to function. You recall my example of the Granny Smith apple earlier. Eating a small apple is like eating several spoonsful of sugar—3.9 teaspoons to be exact. For comparison, in a small table I compared a small Granny Smith apple versus a serving of cheesecake (125 g), 4 apricots, and a cup of raspberries[231]. Which would you rather eat from the table below in terms of sugar? What about in terms of potassium? How about vitamin C? It is interesting to note the zero vitamin C in the Granny Smith apple (USDA database).

food	serving size	fiber	net carbs	sugar (ts)	potassium	protein	vitamin C
Granny Smith	small	4	15.6	3.9	173	0.63	0
Cheesecake	125 g	0.5	31.38	7.845	112	**6.88**	0.5
apricots	4 fruits	2.8	12.77	3.1925	**363**	1.96	14
raspberries	1 cup	**8**	6.69	**1.6725**	186	1.48	**32.2**

Table 4. Nutrition comparison

The original USDA food guideline was created in 1996; some modifications were made in 2005, and again in 2015. The world has not stood still; our understanding of our body has grown. The USDA suggests that it is acceptable for a woman who eats 1600 Calories a day to consume 6 teaspoons (24 grams) of *added* sugar per day and a man with 2300 Calories a day may eat as much as 18 added teaspoons of sugar (72 grams); wow[231]. A different angle is presented by Robert H. Lustig, M.D., a pediatric doctor and researcher at UC San Diego—originally aired on the CBS program 60-Minutes in a conversation with Sanjay Gupta, M.D.[410]. Dr. Lustig calls sugar a poison, and recommends 0 grams *added* sugar, but sugar that naturally occurrs in food and is still attached to its soluble and insoluble fiber, is fine. The originator of his suggestions is John Yudkin, who wrote the definitive book on the harmful effects of sugar: "Pure, White, and Deadly"[407]. The third angle comes from tribal experience, such as that of the Inuit, who don't eat (or used to not eat) sugar in any shape and form, not even naturally occuring types, since they exclusively live(d) on fatty meat. They also lack fructose absorption enzymes so any added sugar and even fruits can harm them. Their sugar intake is truly zero, albeit they consume glucose that is stored in the liver and organs of the animals they eat. The

Nordic diet also contains fermented moss[604]. Moss is very low in carbohydrate but highly nutritious, high in omega 3.

So what is the correct daily amount of added sugar? Many nutritionists tell you that we cannot live without eating sugar because sugar is essential for cell function, but in reality, our exogenous sugar need is zero. This was discussed in the macronutrient section.

To further complicate matters, as mentioned before, the word "sugar" is believed to be a single ingredient of just sugar, be it cane, or beet, or any other type. As a result, most people don't think that they are consuming sugar when they eat fruits, vegetables, seeds, nuts, and grains, each of which is either full of natural sugars or converts into simple sugars in the body (such as grains—including whole wheat)—and anything that is made with or from these foods like juices, milk substitutes, cereal, bread, pasta, pizza, sandwiches, cakes, and treats.

Food is the best medicine, so take advantage of it and eat right for your cells, and not for your looks or mood. If you eat right for your cells, there is a good chance your looks and mood will also be great. And this is true simply because all your body parts are made from cells. Keeping them healthy keeps you healthy, thereby necessarily making you look and feel healthy too. It does not follow that being healthy means you fit into a pair of size 0 jeans. Fitting into that size may be healthy for some and not for others. The stakes are much higher than that. Having healthy cells automatically means that you are operating at an optimal level, whether fighting off diseases, performing at maximum effort, or maintaining an appropriate body weight—which is not necessarily low.

To Eat or Not to Eat?

We often dine out celebrating a life event with food. There is hardly any festivity without a cake or some dessert. Many people eat ice cream out of the container without even noticing how much they eat while watching a movie at night. Let's face it: we love to eat and we love to eat sweets. The question I am asking you to ponder is: Are you eating for your sustained health and well-being by satisfying your hunger, or is food a reward for you?

While this question may sound odd at first, it is not imprudent. Our body is a hormone machine. Everything we do is based on hormonal activities. Hormones can make you feel pleasure when eating something you enjoy. Neurotransmitters released when eating certain foods activate specific neuronal receptors in the brain that make you feel satisfied and sated. I discussed before that eating sweets releases dopamine, and eating grains releases morphine. Food is a powerful stimulant. So, are we eating for the release of pleasure signaling neurotransmitters to feel good? Are we expecting food in our brain as a reward?

Or, are we eating food to give our body what it needs to be healthy, even if the food we need isn't going to release a reward hormone? To ask the question another way, are we eating to live, or are we living to eat? That is the question, and it's a very important one!

Food Is Not A Reward

In the US and some other countries, a lot of people consider sweets as reward. Food has lost its appeal as something necessary for living, and it has morphed instead into something to be enjoyed. Many people *live to eat* rather than *eat to live.* Proper eating and drinking for a healthy and migraine-free life is not about what we want to eat but rather what we need to eat. We must learn to appreciate the concept that food is not a reward but a necessity. Some members in the migraine group "mourn" their favorite foods that they can no longer eat once they start to reach baseline—foods such as sugar, or pancakes for breakfast with maple syrup. Although they don't realize it, this act of mourning is a consequence of their addiction. Understanding this will help you navigate through the labyrinth of misinformation and advertisements that are inviting you to eat or drink the wrong things. It is a lifestyle change that you need to make and embrace! So collect your energy. You will need it.

Foods initiate insulin release simply by looking at them, and since extra insulin in your blood makes you hungry, food commercials will likely make you hungry[605]. Companies that make and sell food want you to be hungry. Today, the least expensive ingredients are also the least nutritious, albeit the ones that trigger the greatest reward response when consumed. By reward I am referring to the brain's dopamine center, whose job is to release the reward hormone. Eating great tasting food, even if it is sugar coated paper with no nutritional value, will release dopamine and you will feel great—for about five minutes! Then you will crash, and crave yet more of the same. This cycle is what I refer to as eating for reward, or living to eat. This is not beneficial for anyone and for a migraineur it is particularly undesirable; inevitably you will crave the least nutritious but best tasting foods and you will pay the price with a migraine.

Foods to Eat

So, what about the famous grandma's chicken soup? Chicken soup is said to be a cure for colds, flu, whatever. It is a miracle food we are told, and for once we are told the truth! It is a perfect food for electrolyte replacement. It is not the kind you buy in a can or in powder or bouillon form or the ones with lots of noodles and just add water. Those prepared types are great to give you lots of salt but seriously lack potassium and other nutrients. So avoid the prepared ones, especially the ones with noodles (avoid pastas and noodles altogether), and make your own soup. Freeze some in individual containers to make it handy to reach for when you need electrolyte.

There are foods that are superfoods for migraineurs because they are high in potassium, have sodium, protein, and other nutrients. Some are high in carbohydrates while others are low—try for the lower carbohydrates types:

- Whole milk is the perfect electrolyte as we discussed it in an earlier section on electrolytes.
- Many people love yogurt. Yogurt is great food but not all yogurts are made the same way. Live cultured yogurt has much of the lactose already broken up in the container, and

so whatever carbs amount is written on the container, that is the amount of carbohydrate you are eating. The same is true with any other type of fermented dairy. Avoid Greek Style yogurts. They are strained for very high protein content but in the straining process they retain very little nutrition.

- Low or zero carbohydrate and high potassium food examples: Salmon (fresh or frozen but not processed), romaine lettuce, zucchini, pasture raised beef of any kind, almonds, walnuts, avocado. Soak almonds in water for up to 2 days changing water several times—it will be yucky brown—to get rid of lectin; this is sprouting your almonds. Do it only with raw whole almonds.
- Higher in carbohydrate but also high in potassium: cauliflower, pistachio nuts, cashew nuts, squashes of all types, pumpkins of all types
- Very high in carbs but provide high nutrition: sweet potatoes, yams, legumes.
- Legumes are toxic if eaten raw—lectin is very high in legumes, so soak beans and other dried legumes in water for a day, replacing water several times, and preferably cook them in a pressure cooker, which destroys lectin. Often, in the low carbs nutritional literature, legumes are not recommended, yet legumes provide great nutritional value. They are highly insulinogenic—meaning they increase insulin—so check your response to them 3-4 hours after you ate them. Every person reacts to the glucose and insulinogenic value of beans differently. Some people, like me, have almost zero reaction

whereas others get a very large glucose increase from a serving of beans. Here are some examples of potassium content (per typical serving size):

Beans, Fava (raw): 418 mg potassium
Beans, Kidney (cooked): 717 mg potassium
Beans, Pinto (cooked): 746 mg potassium
Beans, Lima (cooked): 955 mg potassium
Split peas (cooked): 710 mg potassium

Note that legumes have very low sodium content so salt for taste and make sure to take extra salt afterward for carbs control!

Nuts and Seeds: Hands up, how many of you believe peanuts are nuts? The word peanut contains the word "nut", but in fact, peanuts belong to the legume family. So, technically I should not include peanuts in the nut category, but since just about everyone thinks of them as nuts, I might as well put them here. Note though that since they are legumes, they are high in lectin!! This may be what is behind the severe peanut allergy. It is unclear to me how to remove lectin from peanuts so eat any shape and form of it with care! Don't eat much of it! Here are the potassium contents of some nuts, including peanuts; each based on a 100 gr (3.5 oz) quantity, which is often the serving size, all unsalted:

Peanuts raw, all types: 705 mg potassium
Walnuts raw: 441 mg potassium

Pistachio nuts, raw: 1025 mg potassium
Sunflower seed, raw, shelled: 645 mg potassium

As you can see, nuts are a great source of potassium, but not so great when it comes to sodium. These nuts and seeds are not overly excessive on carbohydrates (like walnuts are very low carbs) but you may need to control the quantity you eat in order to manage the carbs intake. Make sure you balance the high potassium with the proper sodium amount or eat salted nuts.

There are many fruits and vegetables that we often eat without thinking what they do with respect to our migraine condition. For example, one whole large avocado contains 975 mg of potassium and only 14 mg of sodium. If you just gobble up an avocado without any salt, expect a major migraine. Make sure you match the potassium with the proper ratio of sodium in every meal!

One of the most nutritious fruits is cantaloupe! A wedge of a large cantaloupe contains 272 mg potassium and just under 8 grams of carbs, so just under 2 teaspoons of sugar equivalent. However, it is so full of other nutrients (very rich in vitamin A if you can absorb fruit/vegetable A) that, from a wedge, you can obtain most vitamins you need.

Quinoa is a recent "super food" that many believe to be a grain but it is not. It is a seed (pseudo cereal) that contains a ton of carbs and very little anything else—except potassium. It is not much of a super food for migraineurs, though it does have a bit of protein and fat (beats white rice!). Eat quinoa only in small quantities and follow with salt treatment. It is salt deficient so take care to monitor how much you eat and also how much salt you add. Uncooked quinoa, per 100 grams (3.5 oz) has 563 mg potassium, so it does provide nutrition, only a tad too much carbohydrate for comfort.

Foods to avoid

All foods below are listed with their net carbohydrates. Net carbohydrates are total carbohydrates listed in the USDA database under "carbohydrates by difference" minus the fiber.

- Rice (white is worse but they are all not for migraineurs—it is a grain) is bad. It is refined carbs so the moment you eat it, it turns into glucose (in your mouth). 1 cup of raw white rice contains 213 mg potassium but measures in at a hefty 145.51 net carb gr, which is over 36 teaspoons of sugar. There are no vitamins in white rice.
- Apples: one average regular apple with skin on has only 2 mg sodium and only 195 mg potassium but 21 gr carbs or 5 teaspoons of sugar!
- Banana (medium about 7 inches long): 1 mg sodium, 422 mg potassium. A banana has 24 gr or 6 teaspoons of sugar. Bananas are also known to make people feel sluggish. I don't recommend bananas for migraineurs.
- Blueberries (1 cup) contains nearly 18 gr carbs or 4.5 teaspoons of sugar. For that you receive only 114 mg potassium.

It has minimal vitamin C (14 mg) and all its flavonoids (antioxidants) are also minimal and never make it past our digestive system. That blueberries are good for us is one of the biggest marketing distortions we have been told. Blueberries are sugar bombs. Avoid them.

- Grapes are a very poor fruit choice. 100 gr (about a typical serving size) has 16.25 net carb grams (over 4 teaspoons of sugar) with only 191 mg potassium and next to nothing in vitamin C. They are also sugar bombs.
- Raisins are one of the worst things you can chose to eat. A half a cup contains 62.3 net carbs grams, that is 15.6 teaspoons of sugar, 615 gr potassium, with nearly zero vitamin C. Avoid.
- Dates: One date (a SINGLE medjool date) has 16.33 net carb grams or over 4 teaspoons of sugar and 167 mg potassium.
- Watermelon is poor in nutrition; high in sugar and water. An average 10-ball serving of watermelon contains 137 mg potassium and almost 8 gr carbohydrates, so 2 teaspoons of sugar.

Preferably avoid all of the above foods but if you choose to eat any of them, please make sure you salt after eating any of the above and similar food items—please check the USDA database. Take only salt and no water.

Dried fruits are amazing when it comes to their potassium content but they are extremely high in sugar. Avoid them as much as possible.

This section on what not to eat may have been depressing. Indeed, it is depressing. Many of these fruits have been bred and grown for extra sweetness that for migraineurs are harmful. The list of nearly all foods sold in the US and their ingredients can be found here:

https://ndb.nal.usda.gov/ndb/search/list

I have my life back after being a prisoner to migraines for most of my life! Dr. Angela Stanton discovered the answers to having a migraine free life without drugs! Thank you for my life back!

--Ruth Artz
Member in the Facebook Migraine Group

Nutrition Density and Calories

Numerous new food issues face all of us. There has never been so much fast and automated access to foods and drinks, particularly those heavy in carbohydrates, at any hour of the day and in any season. When it comes to food production there are no longer geographical barriers of soil and climate type. If something is out of season in Colorado, USA, the other side of the planet is experiencing its spring and summer and can ship to Colorado fresh fruits, vegetables, and meats of animals that are not even raised or live in Colorado. Our food may also contain preservatives, color-change preventers, color enhancers, a ton of sugars and/or sugar substitutes, etc. As recently as a hundred years ago people ate only seasonal and locally grown whole foods. There was no need for preservatives, color enhancements, fast food outlets, and refrigerators were not yet universally available. Families usually ate home cooked whole foods.

The problem is not only that we have too much food available but that foods have no "pattern" of availability in a way that our body is able to deal with them and metabolize them the proper way. Especially in regions where four seasons are the norm, it is not easy for the body to eat cantaloupe in the middle of winter, since high carbohydrate fruits provide a burst of energy that is better used in a season when one can run or play off the extra energy in an open field. Eating a cantaloupe in a heated room by the fireplace while sitting on the couch and watching TV does not provide the opportunity for the body to use the nutrition, and so it must store is as extra energy instead—and that means store it as fat. The human body stores all excess glucose and fructose as fat. This was discussed before in terms of insulin. Here I am looking at it from a different angle. We were born with a certain number of fat cells—this is genetic—and everyone is different. Think of a fat cell like a mini pouch (it looks like that) that can be filled up with fat. How much fat is in the pouch is the question and not how many such pouches one is born with[606]. The level of fat storage ability is genetic but genes represent an "option" and not a "fate."

The body has a layer of insulating fat under the skin (subcutaneous) brown fat—as discussed earlier. This fat is healthy and is essential. Mammals seasonally grow different sickness of this fat depending on temperature; the body uses this as insulation. Humans wear clothing and so the importance of this fat's insulating function is reduced.

Much of the food we eat out of season often provides us with white fat, which is stored for future energy. Seasonally, winter foods didn't used to contain fructose much, only starches: dry legumes, tubers like potatoes, nuts and seeds. These provided an insulating layer of fat and fuel to burn in preparation for the dead of cold. There were no available winter fruits in most places without storage and refrigeration though in some locations citrus fruits ripen in the winter. Although these provide fructose, as long as we didn't eat much, they were not harmful. Also, we do much better as long as we eat fruits and veggies whole rather than drink them as juice[409,439,453,607]. Now with summer fruits available in the middle of winter, not to mention the latest fad of juices, smoothies, and shakes, we have drastically changed the amount of fructose and glucose induced visceral fat we preserve and we do so all year around. This is not normal for our insulin use.

Prior to winter we should be insulating and increasing subcutaneous fat beneath our skin. In pre-consumerization days, people would "fatten up" for the winter to better tolerate the cold. This meant building up the layer of subcutaneous fat. However, with access to all kinds of summer fruits in great quantity during the winter and with the availability of winter clothing and heated homes, we changed our need for fat. No amount of exercise will remove visceral fat. This fat requires some form of starvation as it was built up to sustain our energy of leaner times in the winter.

One need not be fat or obese to have very high visceral fat. Visceral fat is also found on people who are very thin. This is called "thin fat" or TOFI (This Outside Fat Inside). Building up visceral fat is a sign of insulin resistance and it increases the risk for metabolic syndrome, cardiac disease, and obesity[483,538,608]. It is essential to reintroduce seasonality into our lives and eat only foods that are locally grown and eat them at the time they are available.

CALORIE COUNTING? WHY?

A Calorie is a unit for measuring energy, so the Calorie count of a food item represents how much energy a particular food produces in the laboratory under extremely controlled conditions. Officially, a Calorie is defined as the amount of energy required to raise the temperature of a liter of water by one degree Celsius at certain standard environmental conditions. The moment we change anything in the environment, such as take that same amount of water 500 feet higher up, or change the humidity in the air, or introduce a bit of wind, the amount of energy required to heat the water by 1C will change. For instance, you are probably familiar with having to boil eggs longer in higher altitudes.

If you look at how much energy it takes to increase the temperature of that same amount of water by 1C inside your body, you will be greatly surprised that it is not even close to the measurements in the controlled environment of a chemistry lab. For one thing, there is no fire in us to heat the water. Instead, we have milliard of steps by a huge number of cells to achieve that 1C rise in temperature, or actually its equivalent increase of energy. There are many factors in the human body that modify the amount of energy created and used, based not only on environmental variables but also on the kind of fuel available and how we metabolize that fuel. The human body has 3 fuel types it can use: carbohydrates, protein, and fat; these are the macronutrients we covered earlier. A single Calorie worth of each of these macronutrients is metabolized completely differently and in a very different number of steps in the body.

The basic tenet on which nutritional guidelines have been based on for many decades is the simple chemistry lab energy definition: whatever Calories one ate must equal the Calories expended or else weight gain occurs. Which macronutrient provides the Calorie, how this Calorie is burnt by the body (metabolic process, use of oxidation), and with what level of efficiency, has not been considered. There is a large group of establishment scientists and medical professionals still pushing the simplistic "Calorie in – Calorie out" interpretation but they are losing ground.

Food does not burn in a clear and controlled open flame in our body as it converts to energy. Every single macronutrient we eat has a unique metabolic pathway that needs to be considered[523,609]. As I described before, eating an apple with the skin on will bypass the liver and head to the gut so we do not metabolize the fructose from the fruit when it is attached to the insoluble fiber (the skin). But remove the skin or drink that fruit as a juice or smoothie and the metabolic path changes completely;

the same apple now becomes ethanol, and then as triglycerides it gets deposited into our fat tissue. Not only did the apple not burn with the same energy, it burned in a different oven and with a completely different type of flame. The two processes are not comparable.

To make this more interesting, assume that instead of the 15 net grams of carbs of a small Granny Smith apple delivering 84 Calories of energy, we eat 1 net gram (no fiber) of carbs of a small piece of mozzarella cheese also delivering 84 Calories. Which one would you choose the apple or the cheese? They are equal Calories on paper, but are they equal in terms of how they are used inside the body? Does one nourish your cells better than the other? Since most of the Calories in the apple come from carbohydrates, the body will burn them as sugar fast and you will be hungry soon after. The Calories in the cheese come mostly from fat and some from protein; your body will burn them as fat and protein—fat and protein are a lot more sating than carbs are. The two burning processes are extremely different. Carbohydrate burning takes many more steps in the body than fat burning and protein takes even longer than carbohydrates since some of the protein must convert to glucose. Carbohydrate burning metabolism is less energy efficient and crates more free radicals via the pyruvate process—something fat processing doesn't include. So in sum, after eating that apple of 84 Calories, you will be hungry in a short time but after eating the 84 Calories in cheese you will not be hungry for perhaps 3-4 times longer.

Counting Calories also ignores "nutrient density". Nutrient density refers to the value of the nutrition (micronutrients (vitamin, minerals) and macronutrients) in the food you eat. As shown earlier, an apple is very shallow in vitamins and minerals and its biggest substance, carbohydrates, is not an essential nutrient. By contrast, cheese is nutrient dense because it is low in carbohydrates but high in essential macronutrients (fatty and amino acids) and also contains minerals.

What matters is the nutrition density of the Calorie you eat, what it becomes in your body, and how it is burned or stored—a more nutrient dense food (like the cheese) provides plenty of essential fatty and amino acids and it is therefore satiating, whereas the apple provides nearly no nutrition at all and you will remain hungry. This is one way of showing that counting Calories is quite meaningless.

Sugar and Sugar Substitute Challenges

The challenge goes farther than correctly understanding Calories or cutting sugar or sugar substitutes out of our diet. As of this date, sugar appears under 35+ different names on food labels, most of which we don't even recognize as sugar. Sugar in crystal, powder, syrup, honey, or any other shape and form (table below) contains all the basic sugar types. Here is the list of sugars under their various names as of February 17, 2017:

Barley malt	Dehydrated cane juice	Golden sugar	Molasses
Barbados sugar	Demerara sugar	Golden syrup	Muscovado
Beet sugar	Dextran	Grape sugar	Panocha
Brown sugar	Dextrose	High fructose corn syrup	Powdered sugar
Buttered syrup	Diastatic malt	Honey	Raw sugar
Cane juice	Diatase	Icing sugar	Refiner's syrup
Cane sugar	Ethyl maltol	Invert sugar	Rice syrup
Caramel	Free flowing brown sugars	Lactose	Sorbitol
Corn syrup	Fructose	Malt	Sorghum syrup
Corn syrup solids	Fruit juice	Maltodextrin	Sucrose
Confectioner's sugar	Fruit juice concentrate	Maltose	Sugar (granulated)
Carob syrup	Galactose	Malt syrup	Treacle
Castor sugar	Glucose	Mannitol	Turbinado sugar
Date sugar	Glucose solids	Maple syrup	Yellow sugar

Table 5. Sugar Names

I earlier explained the hazards associated with sugar substitutes. Finding them on food labels is not easy and the list is growing by leaps and bounds every day. Sugar Substitutes List (their sweetness relative to how many times sweeter they are than sugar, which is in parentheses if known):

Acesulfama potassium (200)	Advantame (20,000)
Amino Sweet - Aspartame	Aspartame (160-200)
Curculin (550)	Cyclamate (banned in the US)
Erythritol (0.7)	Glucin (300)
Glycyrrhizin (50)	hydrogenated starch hydrolysate (0.4-0.9)
Lacitol (0.4)	Lead acetate
Mabinlin (100)	Maltitol (0.9)
Monelin (3000)	Osladin P-4000 (4000)
Neotame (8000)	Salt od Aspartame-Acesulfame (350)
Saccarin (300)	Splenda - made from Sucralose
Sorbitol (0.6)	Sugar alcohol
Sucralose (600) - Splenda	Xylitol (1.0)
Thaumatin (2000)	Alitame (2,000)
Brazzein (800)	Dulcin (0.5)
Glycerol (0.5)	Inulin, Isomal (0.45-0.55)
Luo Han Guo (300)	Malto-Oligosaccharide
Monatin	neohesperidin dihydrochalcone (1500)
Pentadin (500)	Sodium Cyclamante (30)
Stevia (250-300)	Tagatose (0.92)

Table 6. Sugar Substitutes and their strength relative to sugar.

As you can see, just finding out what you are really eating is not easy. Sugar and sugar substitute names are difficult to locate on food labels. Make sure you have a magnifying glass since they are often hidden quite well. Also keep on updating your knowledge as new substitutes are added regularly.

We are getting very confused messages from dietitians, doctors, advertisements, and food packaging on store shelves. Those who manufacture sugar tell us it is harmless, and that sugar substitutes are bad[461]. Those who manufacture sugar substitutes tell us that sugars are bad[365,366]. Those who produce grains tell us that grains are essential and heart healthy, but research and the US health history, ever since the grain-heavy food pyramid was introduced, seems to prove it otherwise[552,584,610]. We are very gullible and believe that if something costs more or is advertised more, it must be better[611,612].

The food industry is taking advantage of the general populace's lack of understanding about antioxidants using the power of suggestion in their advertisements. Blueberry producers want to sell their blueberries, so they will advertise to sell more and not to make you healthy. Do blueberries contain antioxidants? Sure. Can the body actually use them for anything? No, not really[613]. But most of us don't know that and fall for the gimmick.

The 2017 Super Bowl was sponsored by Coca-Cola Zero®, a soft drink of "zero sugar" nicknamed Coke Zero. People well educated in the sciences may know that this is a trick but what can we expect from those not having about a clue what "zero sugar" means when the drink is somehow still sweet? Coke Zero is not so harmless. As per the Huffington Post:

> "*Coca-Cola Zero's nutritional information reads 0 Calories, 0g Fat, 40mg Sodium, 0g Total Carbs, 0g Protein.*
>
> ***Artificial sweetener***: *Aspartame and acesulfame potassium*
>
> ***Ingredients***: *Carbonated water, caramel color, phosphoric acid, aspartame, potassium benzonate, natural flavors, potassium citrate, acesulfame potassium, caffeine*"[614].

Diet sodas and other diet drinks that use sugar substitutes of any kind all cause major health problems, including obesity, metabolic syndrome, type 2 diabetes, and even atherosclerosis; discouragingly, most advertisements aim at the young[462,615,616].

Expecting mothers wanting to do good for their unborn child, who eat sugar or sugar substitutes in various "health" products or drink their daily vitamin C in unsweetened cranberry juice, may predispose the child to type 2 diabetes in early childhood[617]. This is an indication that not only are sugar and sugar substitutes bad for us but also for our unborn children. This can spiral into what is called an epidemiological change, which is a genetic change as a result of environmental factors that last several generations! So, a pregnant mom consuming sugar substitutes can affect her great grandchildren's health—this is not a trivial concern!

Sugar substitutes of all kinds (including stevia) also activate dopamine and are therefore addictive just like sugar[618]. Both sugar and sugar substitutes increase blood pressure, cause obesity, metabolic disorders, and heart disease[225,235,275,366,403,411]. As a side note, I find it interesting that concern about stevia's bitter taste hasn't led to efforts to remove the toxic component that is responsible, instead, food scientists have focused on simply masking the bitter taste—stevia is nearly always mixed with other sweeteners. Researchers are also considering masking the bitter taste of stevia by targeting our taste buds responsible for detecting that bitter taste—they modify how we will perceive the taste of bitter (not necessarily exclusive to the bitterness of stevia), a representation of toxic elements! Stevia scientists will change YOUR tongue's bitter sensors by deactivating "two receptors, hTAS2R4 and hTAS2R14, [that] mediate the bitter off-taste of steviol glycosides" so you can enjoy stevia[619].

Food & Insulin Resistance

With all this talk on sugars and sugar substitutes and foods without seasonality, you may be wondering why all of these things are more likely to create insulin resistance in migraineurs than in non-migraineurs.

As by now you know, migraineurs are glucose intolerant and have genetic variances associated with glucose solute transport. The longer glucose stays at higher than normal concentration in the blood, the more likely a person develops insulin resistance. The brain has its own insulin sensitivity, which is distinct from that of the rest of the body[620-622]. The brain is not the only organ with its own insulin sensitivity; muscles also have their own[623], as does the liver[624,625], and also our fat[626,627]—as noted earlier, insulin resistance is compartmentalized in each of our organs separately[628]. Because insulin resistance can be in one organ and not systemically in the whole body, by the time a blood test identifies insulin resistance, every organ has already have been affected—a systemic condition. Unfortunately, this means that a very large percentage of people with full blown diabetes slip past the common glucose fasting or hemoglobin A1C (HbA1C) tests, without their insulin resistance ever being detected—this is particularly true for those migraineurs with reactive hypoglycemia. The recommended test is the Kraft insulin in-situ test but I never see it applied anywhere[335] and most doctors have not even heard of it. Often doctors offer an oral glucose tolerance test, which is a 2 to 3-hour long test, with 2-hour being the standard—the longer test is reserved for potential gestational diabetes. First, they test fasting glucose for baseline measurement. Next, they hand you a bottle of 50 gr or 75 gr glucose solution to drink up in 5 minutes, and then they check your blood glucose 1.5 hours after you finished the glucose solution.

Glucose tests tell nothing about insulin; only indirect correlations can be guessed at. The most critical problem in any glucose test for finding out about insulin resistance is that glucose spike is not dose specific but insulin spike is, and thus there is no relationship between the spikes of glucose and insulin[629]. Yet rather than measuring insulin, there are three formulas that may be chosen from for use in establishing insulin from glucose test[630-633]. The assumption that there is a constant relationship between glucose and insulin is incorrect, invalidating the oral glucose tolerance test for insulin measurement. Furthermore, it is interesting to find in the cited article that there are normal fasting glucose type 2 diabetics—this further indicates the case for speculative insulin assessments without direct measurements[630].

Another problem is the possibility of a missed delayed glucose response. For example, a non-US member of the migraine group recently had an oral glucose tolerance test taking readings at only fasting and at 1.5 hours after the she finished consuming her glucose (the 2-hour standard test). I asked her to take another reading 3 hours after her glucose intake at home. Her fasting blood glucose was 99 mg/dL, which is the very top of normal. 1.5 hours after glucose intake her blood glucose dropped so sharply that it raised an eyebrow in the lab; it was still in the normal range of 88 mg/dL but well below her fasting level and that is not normal. As she continued to measure her blood sugar at home per my request, by the end of the 3rd hour her blood sugar dropped below the normal minimum of 70 mg dL, indicating reactive hypoglycemia, a form of type 2 diabetes. Had she continued to at least 3 hours in the lab, her test would have shown reactive hypoglycemia to her endocrinologist. Unfortunately, even though most migraineurs face some form of insulin resistance, many are too thin to be considered at risk.

Medical professionals tend to ignore thin people and don't test them for potential metabolic syndrome. This oversight can lead to more serious complications later.

Migraineurs beware! You are predisposed to insulin resistance. Check for it, accept it, and live accordingly by changing what you eat. There is a great open access review about insulin resistance[318] and read an article I wrote online:

https://www.hormonesmatter.com/insulin-resistance-time-bomb/.

Insulin resistance is not caused by obesity, in spite of the fact that most doctors believe it is. One can have insulin resistance while being quite thin (TOFI), or not have insulin resistance while being quite obese[634,635]. Certain medicines can also cause insulin resistance and migraineurs get many such medications[330,636,637]. Any medicine that contains or promotes the creation of serotonin (most medicines migraineurs are prescribed are of this variety) can initiate insulin resistance[449] because serotonin uses insulin receptors, blocking glucose from being delivered to the interstitial fluid[638-640]. Another drug often prescribed is the most well-known for causing insulin resistance, which is corticosteroid[311]. Corticosteroid occupies insulin receptors, thereby backing glucose up for a long time in the blood. Beta blockers that are often prescribed are well-known causes of insulin resistance[641,642].

After these depressing preliminaries let's look at foods. Which foods increase or decrease your odds of developing insulin resistance? First the ones that increase; I just list the categories, with a few items as samples--avoid these foods:

- Sugar (white, brown, beige, pink, black, … any kind)
- Honey, maple syrup, and any other syrup that is sweet
- Sugar substitutes
- Natural sweeteners, including Stevia
- Juices, sweetened or not! This includes vegetable juices, nut juices and nut milks as well.
- Milk substitutes (soy milk, almond milk, etc.,)
- Reduced fat anything
- Smoothies and shakes
- Refined grains (rice, bread, pasta, tortilla, popcorn, etc.,)
- Non-refined grains (oats, rye, whole grain, colored rice, etc.,)
- Starches (tapioca starch, corn starch, potato starch... etc.,)
- Processed foods (frozen meals, all canned foods, all boxed prepared foods, in-container prepared foods, deli mixes, processed mixed meats like hot dogs, etc.,)
- Dates, bananas, raisins, persimmons, all tropical fruits, blueberries, grapes, golden kiwi, apples, peaches, cherries, watermelon, etc.,
- Vegetable oils of any kind (except olive oil or avocado oil that you can eat cold and coconut oil you that can use for medium heat cooking or cold)
- Margarine or any other partial or full hydrogenated nonsense
- Sweetened and flavored yogurts
- Regular potatoes

Reduce the following foods to small amounts:

- Tubers (sweet potatoes and yams)
- Root vegetables (carrots, onions)
- Pears, cuties (small tangerine or mandarin), cantaloupe, green kiwi, wild small sour apples, nectarines, apricots
- Greek style (strained)unsweetened whole fat yogurt
- White meat poultry
- Legumes
- Butternut squash

Eat freely:

- Whole fat dairy (milk, cream, butter, cheeses, unsweetened, unstrained, and live cultured yogurt, cream cheese, mascarpone, etc.,)
- All fresh unprocessed fish and crustaceans (fresh frozen OK)
- All fresh unprocessed meats (fresh frozen OK)
- Organ meats
- Whole eggs cooked in any way you like
- Dark leafy vegetables as much as you like
- Fruits that we call vegetables (zucchini, bell peppers of all color, tomatoes of all kinds, squash of all kind (other than butternut squash), pumpkin of all kinds, eggplant, avocado, etc.,)
- Other vegetables like cauliflower, broccoli, etc.,
- Fungi (mushroom of any kind)

- Bone marrow and broth (home cooked, full fat—don't use bouillon cubes)
- Some berries (raspberries, blackberries and strawberries)
- Some root vegetables (radishes, kohlrabi, garlic)
- All animal fats
- Olive, avocado, and coconut oil

Special Note on Blood Sugar Measurement

Over the past several years, it has become clear that most migraineurs have never measured their blood sugar and when they first try, they show insulin resistance, prediabetes, reactive hypoglycemia, or full-blown type 2 diabetes already. Insulin resistance is 100% reversible. Conditions of prediabetes through type 2 diabetes all are possible to place into remission—perhaps reverse as well but there have been no studies to confirm that. I now recommend to all of the migraineurs in my group to invest in a blood sugar measuring kit and monitor their status. Most migraineurs find out that they need to work on reversing their insulin resistance and this is quite a project.

Section 7

Diets

We are all familiar with the plethora of diets that are available in the market for weight loss, for workouts, and even for migraine cure. Dieting for weight loss is a very bad idea for migraineurs because simply eating less (with a few exceptions that I detail under Real Migraine Diets) can be harmful. Not only can they initiate migraines, but can also harm some of our organs. In this section I briefly identify various diets and nutritional plans that can be harmful for migraineurs, and at the end I describe nutritional plans that are safe and healthy for them.

I am a chronic migraineur & for years was seeing doctors, taking meds, but sick 25 days a month & had to quit work. I tried 30 different "cures" that did not work. Dr. Stanton's Migraine Protocol has given me my life back! It is the only approach I have found in my quest for wellness that actually works! Dr. Stanton, a neuroscientist migraineur herself, understands exactly how migraines work & how you can fix them. This book is a must read for families and sufferers of migraine. Welcome to a real path of wellness!

-- Fran Coleman
Member of the Facebook Migraine Group

Avoid These Diets or Nutritional Plans

There are lots of diets and nutritional plans that are meant for people who wish to lose or gain weight or who have other health related issues. Here the focus is on those nutritional approaches (hate the word "diet" but that is what they are called) that are purported to work for migraine prevention but end up causing more harm than good. I explain why some of these diets do not work for preventing migraines but may work for other concerns.

Elimination Diets

The diets I am first crossing off the migraineurs' list of "good eating" are the elimination diets. They are not harmful (perhaps) but they cut a lot of food groups out of your diet because, as they suggest, the eliminated foods are the ones that trigger migraines. On the surface it makes sense: if peanuts give you migraines, just don't eat them. But, what will you do if you are triggered by most foods? Will you starve?

As ridiculous as it may sound, this is the most often heard complaint from people who apply the elimination method: they are running out of things to eat (and they still have migraines). While the authors (and many doctors) of these nutritional plans understand that some foods trigger migraine, they lack the knowledge of *why* they do so.

Cleansing, Detoxing, & Juicing

These days one can't help but hear about the cleansing, detoxing, or juicing diets—actually they all mean the same thing. For the record: we do not need any cleansing or detoxing! Our kidneys and liver do this job quite nicely[643]. Cleansing and detoxing diets can be harmful. Heavy juicing loads the liver up with ethanol from the fructose in the fruits that are juiced. Ethanol converts to triglycerides (fat)—not exactly what you want[409].

Weight loss Diets

Weight loss diets are everywhere. They are probably great for temporary weight loss; undoubtedly people lose weight. But, the moment they stop, they gain it all back. The business model of these diets it to keep people on them for life. These diets are full of processed foods void of fiber and minerals. Processed foods are also heavy in grains and contain sugar and and/or substitutes. As noted before, sugar and substitutes spike insulin causing insulin resistance[365,366,644]. These diets also contain little fat, and the fat they do contain is the wrong kind[645,646,647,648].

Whole30

Whole30® restricts some of the foods migraineurs should not eat (such as sugar and other simple carbs) but it also restricts some that migraineurs should eat, like dairy. The Stanton Migraine Protocol® excludes fruit juices, smoothies, and shakes whereas Whole30® permits them.

Low FODMAP Diet

The Low FODMAP Diet (Low Fermentable Oligo-Di-Monosaccharides and Polyols diet) eliminates certain food groups based on their metabolic processes and the food's fermentation quality that support certain types of undesired gut bacteria. It does not consider the sugar content per se, only the type of sugar. Unfortunately, for migraineurs FODMAP is not sufficient.

Paleo Diet

I know many people who follow the Paleo Diet but there are so many forms of this diet that I have yet to find two people with the same understanding. The original Paleo Diet is restrictive in its adherence to what is believed to have been available to Paleolithic humans. Most critically for migraineurs, it does not allow enough *fat* and *salt* because the belief is that our modern meats and vegetables contain the same amount of these vital nutrients as in the Paleolithic era. Since this is incorrect, this diet can be harmful for migraineurs.

Vegetarian

Being a vegetarian means that most of one's diet is carbohydrates—the very thing migraineurs need to reduce. While some fish, eggs, or dairy are permitted in some forms of vegetarianism, in truth the amount of essential fatty and amino acids, as well as micronutrients like B vitamins and alike, are too low for maintaining good health. Additionally, a vegetarian diet is very low in salt. Since migraineurs should not drink water with and after a carbs meal, and since most meals of a vegetarian are carbs, there is a problem with the drinking schedule.

Vegan

Unfortunately, being a vegan means that your entire food repertoire consists of carbohydrates. This diet lacks essential amino and fatty acids, as well as many micronutrients. It is impossible to eat enough salt to help a vegan to reach proper hydrated state. Because of the inherent carbohydrate sensitivity of the migraine-brain, being a vegan and wishing to remain so means migraines will stay with you for life. I cannot be of help.

Junk food or no Junk Food

I am sure you are 100% convinced that junk food is bad for you. I agree with you and I wish I have never been tempted by it. But if I am about to get a migraine, and I am away from home or office and the only thing within reach is a junk food place, I will, in fact, prevent or treat my migraine by eating junk food. A cheeseburger (without the bun or fries or soft drink) provides a high potassium meal, just add mustard or salt. Choose to drink water or milk instead of a soft drink. Although junk food seems to be "just right" in terms of its mineral intake, do not forget that it has a lot of other, less than ideal, ingredients, including the unhealthy choice of fats used in the cooking. All in all, do not make a habit of eating junk food but if you have no choice, in an emergency, is way better than a nasty migraine!

After less than one month on Angela's protocol, I was able to stop 6 years of propanol use, 80 mgs, t i d... I was on more blood pressure meds, than my dad, who has had 5 heart attacks, a quad bi-pass, and triple stents. I'd lost about 10 lbs as well. My only problem was too much sodium in my blood work, and I've learned to reduce when necessary, and push more water, to equal balance. This protocol works, if given the opportunity. Once someone has had enough pain, and is ready to put forth a little effort when saying that they'll "do anything to make the pain stop", well it's simple. Follow the protocol. Paleo diet just doesn't allow for certain dietary needs for our brains. We need more of one, less of another. I'll stick with Angela, any day!

--BLTN
A MIGRAINE GROUP MEMBER

Real Nutrition for Migraineurs

Of the many nutritional programs and diet types only a very few are supportive of the migraine-brain. The reason for this is that the migraine-brain is an ancient brain that has never adapted to foods rich in carbohydrates and has no means to deal with the ensuing electrolyte disruption. The migraine-brain's genetic variations are vast in scope, with major variances associated with the ionic voltage gated channels that are supposed to manage glucose transport and absorption, and with electrolyte balance. The migraine-brain has problems with keeping up with the constant, heightened level of stimulation of modern life, and ends up with damaged myelin. The nutritional plan of choice must be designed to meet the specific needs and abilities of the migraine-brain. There are several choices.

Low Carbs High Fat Diet

If you search the internet, chances are you will run across several different versions of "low carbing." The Low Carbs High Fat (LCHF) diet is a nutritional solution with low carbohydrates, moderate protein, and high fat intake (usually 60% of the Calories from fat and 20% from protein and 20% from carbs). The LCHF diet is not a reduced Caloric diet but it excludes food groups that are harmful: sugar, all sweets of any kinds, all sweetened foods and beverages, all grains, and usually most starches like potatoes, rice, corn, and similar. A proper LCHF diet can be very suitable for migraineurs. The Stanton Migraine Protocol® has its own diet plan called the Stanton Migraine Diet™, which is very similar to the LCHF diet. It also eliminates sugar substitutes but permits small amounts of starches, such as sweet potatoes or yams. The LCHF diet is also often used as a subfamily within the ketogenic diet[649], usually as a stepping stone to getting to the full ketogenic diet.

The Ketogenic Diet

This is a metabolic process and not a diet. It is being misunderstood and misused by the public as a weight loss diet. It is also misunderstood by doctors as a health danger that leads to diabetic ketoacidosis—a consequence of not having insulin (as in type 1 diabetics) and having too much glucose in the blood together with ketones. Its name does include the word "diet" and it has the side effect of weight loss but it need not induce a weight loss. It is a therapeutic and medical nutrition plan that has been used (recorded in literature) since 500 BC to prevent or treat some brain disorders—mainly seizures in the ancient times[650]. Today it is used for many neurological conditions, including seizures, and is under evaluation for treating neurological and autoimmune diseases like Parkinson's, Alzheimer's, MS, cancer, and autism; so far with very positive results[196,214,651-654]. Just recently it was also found that it can reverse kidney disease[543]. The ketogenic diet is especially useful for reversing insulin resistance and to place type 2 diabetes into remission. Because of the coincidental weight-loss side effects as a result of visceral fat burning, it can also reverse obesity[655,656]. The ketogenic diet is not a calorie restricted diet; it is a carbohydrate restricted diet only.

The benefits come from many areas. One super benefit is that a fat burning body doesn't use glucose as fuel for most of the body, so it doesn't use much insulin for glucose transport. This helps migraineurs, who are glucose sensitive, to recover their insulin sensitivity and return their body to its homeostasis. For an ancient brain, the ketogenic diet is likely the default, original diet. It is also the human basic metabolic process even today. This is shown by newborn babies having been born in a ketogenic state and nursing infants remaining in ketosis[657]. It is natural for the body to go back and forth between ketosis and glucose burning as the opportunity or need arises for each, consistent with the history and evolution of human diets.

"You are what your ancestors ate. There is tremendous variation in what foods humans can thrive on, depending on genetic inheritance... vegetarian regimen of India's Jains, the meat-intensive fare of Inuit, and the fish-heavy diet of Malaysia's Bajau people. The Nochmani of the Nicobar Islands off the coast of India get by on protein from insects. 'What makes us human is our ability to find a meal in virtually any environment,' says the Tsimane study co-leader Leonard... Studies suggest that indigenous groups get into trouble when they abandon their traditional diets and active lifestyles for Western living. Diabetes was virtually unknown, for instance, among the Maya of Central America until the 1950s. As they've switched to a Western diet high in sugars, the rate of diabetes has skyrocketed. Siberian nomads such as the Evenk reindeer herders and the Yakut ate diets heavy in meat, yet they had almost no heart disease until after the fall of the Soviet Union, when many settled in towns and began eating market foods. Today about half the Yakut living in villages are overweight, and almost a third have hypertension, says Leonard. And Tsimane people who eat market foods are more prone to diabetes than those who still rely on hunting and gathering."

(http://www.nationalgeographic.com/foodfeatures/evolution-of-diet/)

As you can see, glucose intolerance has a genetic background, and is an ancestral inheritance for migraineurs as well. The migraine-brain experiences no migraines on the ketogenic diet. More will come soon on the subject of ketogenic diet, especially for migraineurs, in my next book "Keto Mild: The Ketogenic Diet for Migraine Prevention". If you are interested in the ketogenic diet, and if you are no longer on any migraine preventive medicines, please join us:

https://www.facebook.com/groups/156925271342382/

Special Nutritional Needs

Many members of the migraine group are not migraineurs. There are hundreds of people using the Stanton Migraine Protocol® who never had a migraine in their lives. You may find this odd. A healthy migraineur's nutrition and hydration habits are optimal to all people—migraineur or not. Several people with out-of-control high blood pressure use the Stanton Migraine Protocol® with tremendous success. On average, within one month, assuming all requirements were followed, and baseline status is met, their blood pressure drops back to normal and many start tapering off their heart medicines, some stopping them completely. Members with extremely high triglycerides (one starting the program with over 300) achieve amazing results in a short time (this person in one year dropped 300 triglycerides points). Several diabetics and hypoglycemic patients are using the Stanton Migraine Protocol® or Keto Mild™ and are working to reverse their insulin resistance and hypoglycemia. The Stanton

Migraine Protocol® does not cure diseases such as brain cancer or replace a missing kidney but it seems to reverse many lifestyle-caused health conditions.

The Skeptics Diet

Undoubtedly many of you shake your heads and are skeptical of some of the material you have read so far about the nutritional approaches presented, particularly if you have been following the SAD. Not being an impulse buyer of goods or services is definitely wise. In fact, the many migraineurs I deal with often express their skepticism at the time of joining the migraine group, particularly with respect to glucose, fat, and salt. When their doubts sneak in, I encourage them to eat their sweets and other favorite foods. I recommend they eat their filling of cakes, candies, fruits juices, smoothies, soft drinks, pastas, sauces, white rice and bread to test how they feel. When they do, without exception they come down with a migraine. This usually takes care of their skepticism.

Section 8

Frequently Asked Questions

If you're a migraine sufferer, this is the book for you! Dr. Stanton is truly a genius! Through her own groundbreaking experimentation and knowledge, she has discovered how to treat the root cause of this debilitating disorder from the inside out. The Stanton Migraine Protocol has given me my life back! I'm eternally grateful to Dr. Angela Stanton for sharing her journey along the way and for helping so many who suffer with migraine... It is life changing and liberating!!! And it's time for the medical community to catch on!

--Alle Russo Dean
A Member of the Facebook Migraine Group

After I published the 1st edition of this book, I received lots of questions; some with merit and needing serious responses, others more interrogative (many not so nice). For answering the negative questions some diplomacy was required and I admit I was not always successful—hostile attitudes are not easy to change. With this in mind, I have decided to try to recall as many questions as possible, no matter how odd, and answer them here.

Q: How come we cannot find your migraine solution in scientific literature?

A: Although you *can* find my migraine solution in scientific literature[17,228,390], it has not been published in well-credentialed academic journals. To understand why, read about it in detail in Part IV. It is not easy to gain quick acceptance of advancements that fly in the face of entrenched scientific and commercial interests. Gradually, as more and more scientists become familiar with my ideas, the publishing environment will change.

Q: You are not an MD, how can you tell me to drink more, stop sugar, etc.?

A: There are two answers to this question:

1. I don't tell anyone to do anything. This book is to inform and educate you based on my experience and research. It is completely your choice if you follow any of the examples. The people in the migraine group do everything voluntarily—they can leave any time and stop following the

experience of thousands of migraineurs. What you read here is the migraine recovery of those who decided to try what I did and succeeded; you may or may not try it.

2. I am not an MD (Medical Doctor) but I am a PhD (Doctor of Philosophy). A PhD is a 10-year degree followed by an oral test, tremendous research, a dissertation (book), defense, and the mandatory publishing of the dissertation. The dissertation must contain something genuine and new that no one has ever thought of before. To be a PhD is to discover new things; to invent. To be an MD is to apply in practice what a PhD invented. MDs and PhDs work together best in a research environment.

Q: The Stanton Migraine Protocol® is just a bunch of quackery (this is not a question but a statement).

A: If migraineurs are taking many prescription medications and still have migraines, wouldn't you call that quackery? By contrast the Stanton Migraine Protocol® doesn't involve taking any medicines, supplements, or herbs; nothing is sold—and migraineurs end up migraine-free. Where is the quackery?

Q: Why don't you have a clinical trial?

A: A great question and I wish I could. There are several stumbling blocks in creating a clinical trial for something that may take years to achieve. It would require migraineurs to spend months to years (depending on medicines taken) under hospital care, with 24/7 observation, and with a diet that is fully controlled and monitored. It is practically impossible to take the most representative age group under consideration for a clinical trial since they are mothers with young children. Many researchers favor the recruitment of college volunteers but they are not a representative cohort for chronic migraineurs. It is also important to note that in a properly conducted clinical trial, the researcher modifies one thing and holds all other variables unchanged. In migraine prevention there are several variables that need to be modified at once: increasing (or decreasing) water, stopping all refined carbs, reducing complex carbs, increasing salt, keeping potassium and sodium in a particular ratio, changing when and how to drink after eating carbs, and increasing fats. This could not ever be considered a *clinical trial* since there are too many variables to control. It is also impossible to have a placebo group that receives the same food without migraine treatment since the food is the migraine treatment. And finally, the treatment group will have to come off all their medicines, as would the placebo group—therefore the researcher knowingly causes pain without treatment. This would never be considered ethical and would never be approved by any ethical board—and I would not do it even if approved. It was suggested to collect data instead—well, I have. By now the Migraine Group's archives contain an immense data base of migraineurs' authentic life and treatment histories and their self-reported accounts of failures and successes.

Q: How come some migraineurs recover within a week and others take months or years to become migraine free?

A: There are several reasons for the time difference it takes to fully recover.

1. Recovery is greatly age dependent. Neurons that have experienced lots of migraines and have not seen electrolyte balance for many years will need to be repaired. A younger person may replace cells with greater frequency but neurons only get replaced once every 50 years or so. Research is underway for neuronal regeneration[658].
2. Recovery is greatly dependent on how long a migraineur has suffered with migraines. Some migraineurs started as early as age 2, others started in their teens, yet others in their 20's or 30's, all the way to migraineurs starting migraines in their post-menopausal years. The longer a migraineur has had migraines in her life, the longer the recovery will take
3. Recovery is contingent upon the medications taken prior to beginning the protocol, as well as while being already on the protocol. Those migraineurs who don't take any medicine will neither have to quit a drug nor experience withdrawals ("discontinuation syndrome"). Since they take no medications, they will not have any rebound effects either. In addition, when not taking any medicines, the brain tries to activate its own pain reducing system. Thus, migraineurs who never used medicines of any kind have a much easier start to recovery.
4. Migraineurs commonly are given triptans, vasoconstrictors that increase blood pressure and serotonin in their brain and

intestines. The brain is highly adaptive and the more it receives of something, the less it will want to make it on its own. Taking triptans, i.e. serotonin, means that the brain may end up with a reduced capacity to make serotonin on its own. Hydration is also blocked by triptans because of their vasoconstriction effect, and thus the body has a harder time becoming and remaining hydrated, placing stress on the kidneys and electrolyte homeostasis.

5. Many migraineurs take preventives that block either serotonin reuptake (SSRIs) or voltage gated sodium or calcium channels, or all three. These drugs can cause permanent damage to the brain[659-662]. Migraineurs taking these medications may face a life-long struggle to regain important brain activity, such as the release of neurotransmitters, memory recovery, and similar. Because of the negative consequences of all these medications, it is important that migraineurs titrate down their medications (with doctor's care), until they are off completely. Since recovery is not complete as long as medications are still taken, this represents both a challenge and a delay in full recovery. To avoid side effects accompanying sudden discontinuation, some medications can take over a year to slowly reduce.
6. For many migraineurs it takes months to just increase their water intake to the level where they need to be—they simply don't drink enough water (some drink literally no water at all). The kidneys cannot change from a 0 glass of water a day routine of many years to working with 8+ glasses the next

day without major trouble. Recovery may be significantly delayed by the length of time required for reaching the necessary hydration level.

7. And finally, there are several restrictions for migraine prevention: no refined carbs, no sweeteners of any kind, reduced complex carbs, drinking unflavored water, maintaining a proper potassium and sodium balance, and increasing fat. Every person has a different level of self-discipline. A single "cheat" can throw a migraineur back in recovery time significantly.

Q: How can we be sure that what the migraineurs experience is not a placebo affect?

A: This is extremely easy to debunk with this simple logic:

If A > B AND B > C then A > C

Where > means "better than". This applies to pharmaceuticals since their clinical trials for medicines are always placebo tested. Therefore, migraine medicines 'M' are proven to be better than placebo 'P', or M > P. Let's call Stanton Migraine Protocol® treatment 'SMP'. Given that the 'SMP' treatment has been successful for thousands of migraineurs who had quit taking all their migraine medicines – they use 'SMP' instead of 'M' and remain migraine free, we can state:

If SMP > M and M > P then SMP > P

proving that the Stanton Migraine Protocol® is much better than placebo.

Q: Oh, she is just out to make money

A: The book is not free. I spent countless hours writing it without salary—the cost of the book is more than reasonable, it is probably less than the copay of a single week's supply of one migraine medicine. The Facebook service is entirely free. Consider the help you receive, which includes my time, and the time of several admins who also give their brainpower to help you full time to become migraine free, and the many members who do the same, as our contribution to your health.

Q: How come I spend my whole day with my partner, eat exactly what he does, drink exactly what he does, do exactly what he does, and I wake up with a migraine and he doesn't?

A: By now you have read the book and understand that migraine is only possible for those with a migraine-brain. Your partner doesn't have a migraine-brain and so he will not get a migraine.

Q: "How come my doctor doesn't tell me about this protocol?"

A: While there are some doctors who already prescribe the Stanton Migraine Protocol®, many are restricted by their organization's and insurance company's codes that requires treatments to be medicinal. The Stanton Migraine Protocol® is not medicinal, and so there is no medicine to prescribe. In most large healthcare organizations doctors have to follow treatment guidelines established by the organization's Compliance Panel. With that said, some doctors have sent their patients to our group—many of these doctors were migraineurs themselves who had also been treated in the group. On occasion doctors also ask for entry into my group to observe what they may be able to apply in their practice to help their migraine patients.

Q: If migraines run in our family, can your protocol work for all of us or is the migraine a more complicated problem?

A: All migraines have the same cause and there is no reason for the solution to work for one person and not the other. It is also perfectly safe for kids.

Q: I've noticed that the protocol helps other conditions like chronic fatigue syndrome and fibromyalgia, high blood pressure, and I no longer have pre-diabetes, etc. How does it do that?

A: Many health conditions benefit from reducing carbohydrates and maintaining a healthy electrolyte homeostasis.

Q: I suffer from an eating disorder and some people said your migraine treatment worked for their eating disorders. How?

A: The answer is more in the disciplined approach toward healthy eating habits. Additionally, when migraineurs feel "normal" again, they are more likely to tackle other issues in their life successfully. We are also a very large support group providing support for all who need it.

Q: I'm diabetic - can I do this regime and still take my meds?

A: Absolutely. What you may find is that your insulin sensitivity will improve as you are removing those elements from your food that caused insulin resistance in the first place. This may allow you to reduce your medication—with your doctor's supervision.

Q: Can I partially do this regimen and still be successful? Do I have to do keto eventually?

A: You don't need to do keto if you feel fine with applying the Stanton Migraine Protocol®. Most migraineurs (so far) stop there and don't start keto. However, you must stick with the restrictions of the Stanton Migraine Protocol® for life—don't forget, it is a lifestyle change—your brain remains the same.

Q: What may I experience physically, mentally, emotionally when beginning and during this regime?

A: Since the regimen starts with quitting all sugar and sugar substitutes, teas, alcohol, smoothies, juices, and for some also quitting all grains, the changes can place you on an emotional rollercoaster at the beginning. Physically you may or may not experience pain (depending on how your body tolerates change), but while your body gets used to the lack of sugar, you may feel a bit more tired.

Q: My doctor prescribed me the Cefaly for my migraines. Why is this not a good method for migraine treatment?

A: Cefaly generates voltage in your brain without providing essential minerals. When you take it off, the electrical stimulation stops and you will be back to having migraines. It is a symptom treatment without addressing the underlying cause.

Q: Why is mental health treatment so ineffective in treating migraines, yet so often pushed by doctors?

A: Migraine is not a mental illness. Prescribing medicines, frequently employed in mental health treatment, for migraines is an ineffective stab in the dark at best and a dangerous practice in general. Doctors don't have enough information about migraines and they are in the dark trying to help you.

Part IV

For scientists & physicians

Section 9

Where is the Science?

The human understanding, once it has adopted opinions, either because they were already accepted and believed, or because it likes them, draws everything else to support and agree with them. And though it may meet a greater number and weight of contrary instances, it will, with great and harmful prejudice, ignore or condemn or exclude them by introducing some distinction, in order that the authority of those earlier assumptions may remain intact and unharmed.

--Francis Bacon, Novum Organum, 1620

Since the nearly four years of this book's first edition was published, thousands of migraineurs have joined our Facebook migraine group. The feedback migraineurs have provided effectively compelled me to recognize a more complete spectrum of migraines and helped me sort out what works and what does not. After a while it became necessary and obvious to give a name to the lifestyle changes the emerging system of migraine prevention required. The collection of dos and don'ts, step by step recommendations, and general advice has become known – and then trademarked – as the Stanton Migraine Protocol®. Stanton Migraine Protocol® works – and has worked – for 100% of those migraineurs whose migraine is a primary headache and who are not vegans. Vegans diet is 100% carbohydrate-based and migraineurs are carbohydrate intolerant[13,14,663,664]. Those with secondary migraines caused by some underlying health condition, such as brain trauma, sport injury, pinched nerve, or even medicines that inflict migraine-like pain, all improve by the use of the protocol but the pain cannot always be prevented. With this said and done, migraine is not just a pain since many migraines are pain free.

Because the actual for-certain diagnosis of migraine would require an fMRI scanner – not readily available in physicians' offices – that can visualize the migraine-causing cortical spreading depression in action, the diagnosis is completed by elimination of other conditions. "If it is nothing else, it must be migraines" is the current diagnostic method. Many non-migraineurs who are chronic pain sufferers end up being misdiagnosed and treated by doctors as migraineurs—cluster headaches, chronic stress headaches, trigeminal neuralgia, occipital neuralgia, and cervicogenic headaches are often categorized and treated as migraines incorrectly. There are many medications in the market used for migraine treatment and prevention—see Section 12 on Drugs of Shame—but none works consistently and long term, although some may work for some migraineurs occasionally and temporarily.

A large number of pain sufferers – overwhelmingly women – turn out to have cluster headaches instead of migraines—either comorbid with migraines or with other forms of headaches, such as cervicogenic or occipital neuralgia[665]. Consequently, the accuracy of statistics about gender distribution of cluster headaches is highly questionable. Current statistics suggest that cluster headache is more likely in men than in women, and that only about 200,000 cases of cluster headache sufferers are recorded in the US, while approximately 40 million suffer from migraines[666]. Misdiagnosis is extremely easy so doctors should collect more information from their patients before judging a condition to be migraine. This is not a trivial matter. Many medications prescribed for migraines have headache as a side effect. Distressingly, these medications are frequently prescribed to chronic headache sufferers regardless of the type of headache they have. Often more than one medication is prescribed, which can cause drug interaction, therapeutic duplication, or serotonin syndrome[640,667-677]. It is important to point out that the most prominent symptom of migraines is not the pain in the head, so diagnosing purely on pain can mislead the medical professional. All patients joining our Facebook migraine group must answer a questionnaire. One of the questions is "what are your prodromes?". I often get the answer "what are prodromes?" or "I have no prodromes". These people are clearly not migraine sufferers yet have been diagnosed with migraine.

Given the success of the migraine group using the Stanton Migraine Protocol®, I wanted to publish my findings in academic journals and conferences. This is when I hit the well-known brick wall of scientific publishing: where is the double blind controlled randomized clinical trial? Where is the grant? What about the ethical board approval? A Facebook group does not fit the mold of any of these—it is just anecdotal evidence and doesn't count. The findings and conclusions of my work with over 4000 migraineurs are impossible to publish in an elite scientific journal but it is not all doom and gloom. Because of the difficulty of publishing in top tier academic journals, scientists like me now turn to article repositories or become scientific bloggers to spread the information even faster and wider than it is possible with peer-reviewed academic journals. I have recently also presented my findings at conferences. Publishing in open access, higher ranking journals are expensive; a single article may set the author back by between US$2,000-US$8,000; an insane charge for information dissemination to a limited audience. Furthermore, it is well known that the peer review system doesn't work well and that junk often gets published[678-681]. Many journals have lost their reputations. Do I cry over not being able to publish in these journals? Not really.

Understandably, there are many critics and skeptics of a new scientific concept or theory; for acceptance, a randomized double blinded controlled clinical trial is the standard process. However, few think about the *applicability* of these trials. For example, do we need to have such rigorous scientific evidence to show that eating food satisfies hunger, or in many cases it prevents a headache? Not everything needs a rigorous scientific experiment to be shown valid or to prove that it works. Nevertheless, some credible proof is required for consideration, and the acceptance of a new theory or practice.

There are two schools of thought on proof: evidence based and science based. I am not the first one to point out that in the world of healthcare, and to some degree pharmacopeia, evidence based proof carries the day, while in research scientific circles only science based proof is taken seriously. The two are incompatible.

Evidence-Based Medicine

Evidence based medicine is defined as "the conscientious, explicit, and judicious use of *current best evidence* in making decisions about the care of individual patients" (emphasis added)[682]. In case of migraines, *current best evidence* about what migraine is and how to treat it leads to a dead-end. There is no current evidence of anything that has been proven to work for migraine, work permanently, and without terrible side effects. Yet this has not prevented the application of the available treatments and medications, even in light of the lack of evidence for their effectiveness and the very serious side effects associated with their use for migraines. This is an unacceptable compromise; a copout. Moreover, when it comes to prescribing psychotic medications, migraines do not have exclusivity in receiving this half-baked interpretation of proof in medical science. Each medication prescribed to migraines is also prescribed for a host of other health conditions like neuralgia, depression, seizures, and even dementia. A medicine prescribed to health conditions with no similarity to migraines seems out of place because the cause of these disparate illnesses is different.

Just consider the great number of new medicines coming to market. In a very short time many end up receiving FDA warnings about additional adverse effects that were not originally reported. Often medicines are black-boxed, receiving a severe restriction for use. This is called "post clinical experience." In some cases, such adverse effects are not visible at the time of the drug trial because the subjects selected had no interfering health conditions and were not taking other medicines. In these cases, the "evidence" provided is inaccurate and incomplete. In other cases, the evidence found is not what has been hoped for, and the negative evidence is swept under the rug in order to secure the coveted FDA approval[683]. The FDA encourages fast trials and only a limited number of successes are required before they approve fast-to-market those drugs that helped a few patients[684,685]. The number of patients not helped is not reported in these trials. The number of patients not helped or hurt by a drug is reported in a special way: Number Needed to Treat (NNT). NNT represents the number of people needed to be treated in order to help a single person[686,687]. Here is a glaring example, 100 people will not benefit (may get hurt) from the use of statins for 1 person to benefit[688]. The clinical trial controls and the statistical methods used in evidence-based medicine frequently rely on false science, with results that are often manipulated, so evidence-based medicine is inappropriate for new discoveries[689-691].

Another good example of the failure of evidence-based medicine is the debate over the connection of blood pressure variation to dietary salt change. There are many scientific papers that show why this finding is wrong but let me refer to a paper I published[390] because it purely looks at how statistics are misunderstood in understanding how dietary sodium affects blood pressure. Many similar articles have been published[50,235,242,243,246,250,253-255,692-694]. While most journal articles that state the variation of blood pressure as a result of increased dietary sodium show that, indeed, there is a correlation of sodium intake change to blood pressure change, the lack of understanding of what that finding actually means is scary. The statistical significance that these papers present refers to the *direction of changes* only, and not the magnitude of those changes. The directional changes only have statistical meaning to show that the change was not caused by random events but it says nothing about the magnitude, or the importance of that change. Sodium-induced blood pressure change's relevance to normal daily blood pressure variations is always missing.

The daily normal variation in systolic BP for a healthy individual is in the range of 39 mm Hg[18,695-698] (between 100 and 139 mm Hg). No two blood pressure measures separated by as much as a heartbeat or a breath taken will ever be the same. Taking a deep breath lowers BP[699] and feeling pain associated with a very firmly applied BP cuff increases BP[700,701]. There are significant variations of BP if taken on the left arm vs right arm[702], through clothing or bare arm[703], leaning back against the chair and having the feet on the floor, etc[704]. BP after eating is higher than before eating[705,706]; weather changes our BP as does our mood and all of these changes occur without any changes in dietary sodium[705]. What the person ate the day before the test also influences the result, since sugar consumption greatly affects BP, often with a time delay[235,254,275-279,411,707]. Thus, while BP did increase for most everyone with increased dietary sodium, did that increase also correlate with eating sweets the day before? Mood changes? How much the participant slept[708]? No one checked. Most studies did not control for conditions such as diabetes mellitus or existing heart conditions or if the subject took their medicines or not, yet each has a very different response to increased sodium in their diet[694].

Thus, we are facing many problems since BP is not a constant, stable number. To make a statement that dietary sodium increases BP, we must have a stable baseline that remains identical at all times when no changes in dietary sodium are present. The fact that the baseline is a moving target is ignored in almost all of the studies, yet this alone invalidates all statistical analyses.

However, putting all these experimental challenges and errors aside, here is the real crucial factor usually not discussed: if 39 mm Hg variation a day is normal, what level of variation in BP should be considered *abnormal* and a concern with respect to increased dietary sodium?

Studies show that increased dietary sodium raises systolic BP by about 2 mm Hg in a healthy individual and up to maximum 6 mm Hg in hypertensive individuals. Relative to the normal BP variation of 39 mm Hg, a change of 2 mm Hg seems very tiny and may not even be connected to dietary sodium increase at all[709,710]. Does such a small BP change warrant any concern if a 39 mm Hg doesn't? In hypertensive individuals, the BP change in response to increased dietary sodium was (on average between the many papers) 6 mm Hg. How significant is 6 mm Hg relative to the normally acceptable 39 mm Hg daily variation?

Furthermore, how do medicines that lower BP work relative to dietary sodium reduction? Recent research finds that reduced dietary sodium is more dangerous than increased dietary sodium and that dietary sodium has nothing to do with increased BP[242,248,249,256,710,711]. The *insignificance* of BP rise in response to increased dietary sodium questions the health benefits derived from the reduction of dietary sodium[235,712]. Yet, evidence-based medicine still applies the dogma of reduced dietary sodium. Evidence-based medicine fails because it doesn't apply its own principles[682,713-715].

Science-Based Medicine

Science-based medicine ignores "what is" and instead looks to "what may be." Scientists don't just observe but examine the "evidence" trying to prove it wrong. The key expression here is "prove it wrong"; the official scientific principle. Evidence-based medicine attempts to prove things right, whereas science based medicine attempts to prove things wrong. In short, "science-based" investigation plays the devil's advocate and has a far better chance of discovering new science and revealing the truth.

Science based medicine encapsulates scientific findings regardless what those findings mean relative to the hypothesis. By this I mean the evaluation by skeptical eyes using placebo treatments or control groups, making the scientists blind to who is receiving and what particular treatment. Unfortunately, to conduct many types of research projects in the gold standard "double blind" manner is impossible. Cancer, tuberculosis, certain infectious diseases, etc., are a few examples. This has been a major stumbling block in my efforts as well for disseminating the findings of my migraine research.

To illustrate what I mean, some time ago I submitted my findings to JAMA (Journal of the American Medical Association), one of the most prominent journals in the field. I received a letter from the editor stating that "Very interesting but we would like to see a clinical trial." OK. So how do you create a double blind clinical trial with placebo and a control group for a migraine study on the effectiveness of a protocol that uses no medicines, changes the participants' diet to be completely sweetener free (not even artificial sweeteners allowed), increases dietary sodium, increases water consumption, advises against all juices, smoothies, shakes, teas, pastas, etc., and all subjects must be in a controlled environment for minimum a month (if they are not taking preventives) or for a minimum of a year (many preventives take a very long time to quit) without any outside influence at all? As migraineurs who receive treatment also come off all of their medicines once they are pain free, those in the placebo group would also need stop all preventives and abortives. Both the placebo and the treatment group would then not receive any preventive and abortive medicines to treat pain. The many disabling conditions migraineurs may get in the placebo group during the trial will likely preclude an ethical board's approval. It is one thing to know what would be good to be done and an entirely different thing to apply it in a scientific experiment in real life with real people.

We also face the issue of figuring out how one creates a placebo for a sweetener free food that has sweet taste but no sweeteners (not even artificials or naturals). Since the placebo and the treatment group must eat the same tasting food such that they don't know who is in the placebo group and who is not, the treatment group would have to eat a slice of cake with absolutely no sweet ingredients. Do we still believe this can be done as a double-blind study? You may say "ok, so let's not give them cake." Fine, let's talk about some other carbs, say an apple. Everyone gets an apple. The treatment group needs to finish that apple by taking a salt pill or a small amount of loose salt and also fatty protein, such as perhaps a slice of cheese. The placebo group cannot get that. Any idea where one may find a placebo equivalent of salt and cheese?

Migraineurs, as earlier described, need to eat more salt than non-migraineurs do and they start and end the day with salt or salt pill. Simple enough, we give migraineurs a salt capsule and a glass of water both first thing in the morning and last thing at night. What do we give to the placebo group? Normally a placebo capsule is a sugar pill or a flour pill or something similar. In this case, however, both sugar and flour changes electrolyte, the very thing whose quality we don't want to change for the placebo group. Also, since the diet of the two groups must be identical in looks, it would be very hard to increase the water amount of one group and not the other—the treatment group would have to drink a calculated amount of water based on weight, activity, age, etc., whereas the placebo group would continue drinking whatever they were drinking. Thus, we are facing serious technical difficulties. Therefore, providing the required clinical trial to meet the prerequisites of serious academic journals is impossible. I did publish my findings in a number of, less well-known journals[17,227,228,258,390]; these journal articles without funding, grant number, and ethical board approval – critical details for being considered sufficiently credible – do not have the chance to attract widespread attention.

A trial that only contains test subjects who know exactly what they are receiving is biased and carries the possibility that the treatment works because of suggestions. This is quite true for all types of treatments, including our migraine protocol in the migraine group. However, I have managed to acquire some confirming information precluding the placebo effect. Migraineurs, once they already are completely migraine free, often break the rules and go for some sweets as a result of forgetting that they are migraineurs—this happens to nearly every single migraineur in the migraine group. Without exception, every single one comes down with a migraine. Yet even this can be said to be a placebo effect since they realize they did something they were not supposed to do.

The proof for the lack of placebo effect is as follows:

$$\text{If } A > B \text{ AND } B > C \text{ then } A > C$$

For our comparison we are going to utilize pharmaceuticals since their clinical trials for medicines are placebo tested. Abortive migraine medicines, M, have been proven to be better than placebo, P. Meaning M > P. The Stanton Migraine Protocol®, a medicine-free treatment is SMP. Given that the SMP treatment has been successful for thousands of migraineurs who also quit taking all their migraine medicines and remained migraine free (SMP > M), we can state:

If SMP > M and M > P then SMP > P – that is the Stanton Migraine Protocol® is better than placebo.

Nearly all migraineurs upon joining our migraine group report taking at least one migraine preventive medicine. All also take abortives that are used upon the first feel of a migraine. The abortives are various triptans, such as Imitrex or Maxalt. There are several types of preventives: some work with vascular control such as Verapamil,

Propranolol, or Nortriptyline, some are SSRIs or SNRIs such as Zomig, Celexa, or Prozac, some work as triptan but are also serotonin agonists that work on a vascular way such as Replax, or SNDRs such as Effexor, or TCAs such as Elavil. Many take Keppra, Gabapentin, Pregabalin, or Topamax—these are voltage gated calcium channel blockers, etc. See the list of the most frequently prescribed drugs under the Drugs of Shame section. The number of medication types that is prescribed for migraineurs is staggering.

Let's label the taking of medicines by migraineurs at the time they join the migraine group *Treatment A*. *Treatment A* (all medicines taken) have had their clinical trials against placebo and they all have tested better than the placebo. So what happens to migraineurs participating in our protocol? Once their migraines start to disappear, all migraineurs slowly come off all their migraine preventives (completely voluntarily) and don't need abortives. In other words, the Stanton Migraine Protocol®, which is *Treatment B* is so much more effective than *Treatment A* that all migraineurs stop *Treatment A* and only use *Treatment B*. Migraineurs remain migraine free since they have learned how to apply *Treatment B* both preventively and abortively in a way that their life remains pain free.

Treatment A that migraineurs dispose of is not just medicine but some have surgically implanted neuronal stimulators as well. So far all have had them surgically removed in favor of *Treatment B* alone and remained medicine and migraine free.

This is the most valuable conclusion in our "clinical trial". A treatment that is proven to be better than placebo in clinical trials, when replaced by a different treatment that is more effective than the clinically proven treatment, is better than placebo by a compound degree.

The question then becomes: can an empirical trial such as this be considered a valid scientific evidence of the Stanton Migraine Protocol®'s effectiveness for preventing and treating migraines better than medicines? I suggest we look at the results. When over 4000 migraineurs use the Stanton Migraine Protocol® instead of their medications (or neuronal stimulators) for maintaining a pain free life, we can say we have results-based evidence of efficacy. We are not talking about migraineurs switching off medicinal life in exchange for a restricted or compromised life. We are talking about migraineurs – with their pain and brain fog lifted – being able to think again, plan again, attend family events, reclaim their jobs, go to church, go hiking, go diving, and run Marathons.

Healthcare vs Disease-care

In the dictionary this is how "Healthcare" is defined:

> "...the field concerned with the maintenance or restoration of the health of the body or mind." (dictionary.com)

Healthcare thus means *the care and maintenance of the health of the healthy,* and *to make again healthy those who were once healthy*. The problem with this is that the healthy don't need medical care, and an industry that creates healthy from the sick is left with no patients to care for. The healthy need no healthcare for maintaining their health—instead it is the sick who do. We must look at the "active" meaning of the term, and we find that healthcare should mean caring for those with a disease. Therefore, the correct term is "Disease-care". The primary function of the disease-care industry is to manage the sick, not to get rid of diseases. That is what our doctors, pharmaceuticals, hospitals, and medical insurance companies do: they manage disease, not health, and by so doing, they also profit. There is no incentive to cure because of the conflicting profit motives. They cure nothing; the actual curing is performed by the human body. Effective medical care is that which is supportive of the body in healing itself. Healthcare therefore should be redefined as "Assisted Self-Healthcare".

However, since disease management is a profitable business, managing disease is here to stay and health is in the hands of those individuals who read books like this for self-help! It is not in the interest of the medical industry to have the sick become healthy without the need for medicines, further visits, and treatment—after all, financial gain is the underlying motivation to be in business. It follows that disease management is a permanent profit model for doctors, hospitals, pharmacies, and pharmaceuticals. There is nothing wrong with that, business is business, only it is not for the benefit of the ill.

As an illustration, let's examine the current case of hepatitis C treatment. It now has a predicted "cure" rate (remission is an equivalent statement to cure in this case) for certain genotype viral disease forms. The medication costs over $1000 per pill per day and the shortest treatment takes 12 weeks, which means $84,000 minimum. And even a treatment like this does not come with a 100% guarantee; it is not a cure of Hep C for all the people with even the target genotype! As we mentioned earlier, the true cost of the medicine is hidden in NNT. In this case, NNT represents the number of patients that received the new Hep C treatment but for whom it failed (they died or had to stop for various complications), in order for 1 person to be cured. A 2014 paper reported that for a particular group receiving the new Hepatitis C medication, the NNT declined from 1052 to 61[716], meaning that with the previous drug the true cost of treatment of one cured patient whit 1052 uncured ones was US$84,000x 1052 = $88,368,000 and when the NNT declined to only 61 with the new drug, the true cost of the new medicine for the one cured patient changed to $84,000 x 61 = US$5,124,000. This demonstrates two important facts:

1. The industry makes money regardless of the effectiveness of the treatment, based on NNT earnings
2. The majority of patients doesn't get cured from the medicines they take.

You may think I pulled an extreme case out of the hat so let me show the NNT for statins, the well-known cholesterol lowering medicines. A study evaluated pharmaceutical clinical trials and listed the NNT for statins to be minimum 30 and in some cases over 100[688].

How about NNT for aspirin for the prevention of CHD? It was 44 or 77 in 2001 based on the type of prevention it provided[717]. In other words, the pharmaceuticals making Aspirin or its generic equivalence collect earnings from 44 to 77 patients even if it only works for just one person. To state this another way, 44-77 people may get zero benefits or even get hurt from taking Aspirin but one will be better from taking it—though 44-77 pay for Aspirin.

Another reason for the failure of our healthcare system is well described with an expression used by a JAMA Neurology article: "McDonaldization of Medicine"[718], which explains why the healthcare patients receive is so poor. McDonaldization refers to a business model in which the healthcare industry has to provide fast, efficient, and cheap care to the sick with good financial returns, without a lot of concern for quality: quantity is of higher importance. Sort of like "drive through" medical help. Amazingly (and perhaps coincidentally) this article was released on the day of National Fast Food Day, a day we celebrate fast food. I have no clue why we need to celebrate fast food. The honesty of the article shocked me. Given how patients are viewed by the professionals who care for them, we stand a limited chance of finding a doctor we can trust with our health.

Since all healthcare professionals use some profit model, it can be said that no doctor really needs to expend the energy to decipher what a migraine is and what it represents in order to remain in business. Nor do they need to understand what is special about migraineurs so that they could treat the underlying cause rather than control symptoms. There are plenty of individual exceptions to the above attitude, like the doctors who help support patients' becoming well on the Stanton Migraine Protocol®; those who send their patients to the group; those who read my book for their patients' recovery. I even have a few MDs in my group who joined to understand what I do so they can help their patients. There are a few gems!

In the case of migraine, controlling symptoms is not nearly as useful as when someone has the flu! Controlling symptoms of a flu will not cure it; the body cures the flu. Controlling the symptoms may help you relax so your immune system can work more efficiently. Controlling flu symptoms also has value in an epidemiological context (other people may be less likely to get it). Controlling the symptoms of migraine means much less. Migraines are not just accompanied by pain but by several symptoms, each one requiring a different symptom treatment. In truth, there are no medicines to treat even one of them successfully. For example, one set of migraine symptoms includes cramping, gases and urgent bowel movement with pain (also called irritable bowel syndrome, or IBS). However, unlike a disease of "just" IBS, it is not possible to treat the symptoms of IBS during migraines because the underlying cause of the IBS accompanying a migraine is the same as the underlying cause of the migraine itself, which is different from a cause in case of a person with IBS alone. Thus, the migraine related IBS will not respond to standard symptom treatment of the standard IBS. Because medicines that are generally prescribed for IBS don't work for IBS that accompany migraines, doctors often reach for off-label medicines in desperation. Off-label medicines are those that are used for the treatment of a condition other than the primary conditions for which they were approved; more on this later.

Section 10

The Genetic Connection

Brain activities are directed at the ionic level as organized by expressions of the DNA. Many of the conditions that lead to or are associated with the migraine-brain originate in the genes as variances. Each person possesses a set of genes that belongs to that person only. It is not possible to state what the default genetic makeup is for humans; we can only look at phenotypes (observable characteristics or traits) and the genetic makeup of what, on average, we are today. We use the average of these genetic commonalities to establish the default from which each person differs to some degree. How we interpret what we end up with using such averaging is a serious question that directly relates to understanding migraines.

The genetic commonalities of today's humans (our average genome) cannot be identical to the long-ago genomes of ancient humans, since this would imply that evolution is somehow not applicable to humans. Indeed, time to time some characteristic or trait shows up as a result of atavism (an evolutionary throwback). We consider it a mutation (in a negative sense), different from the current norm that needs to be medically treated. While in many of these instances treatment is clearly desirable and justifiable, in some other cases intervention is not warranted. Migraine is one of the latter ones.

Migraine is considered to be a neurological disorder[719,720] that is treated with dangerous drugs that don't cure migraines, only try to reduce symptoms, all the while leaving migraineurs with permanent side effects. Migraineurs are very sensitive to their environment because their sensory organs (scent, sight, hearing, touch, taste) are more sensitized[228]. Such hyper-sensitive sensory organs and the associated hyper sensitivity[3] are sometimes considered to be childhood disorders[721-723] or phantom hallucinations in adulthood[724-726] that need medical treatment. Yet this is not an exclusively childhood condition, nor is it hallucination. Hyper sensory organs are more sensitive to stimulation and detect scents, sounds, sights, tastes, and touches more vividly than those without such sensitized neurons. Unfortunately, migraine also comes with disabling prodromes, pain, and postdromes that place migraine into a disorder category. Research is focusing on downregulating the brain's sensitivity. Instead, why don't we focus on the *cause* of and *reason* for the pain? After all, this highly sensitized brain must have yielded some evolutionary benefit to have become the 3rd most prevalent condition in the world[727], representing 15%[728] of the (diagnosed) population.

Did the hyper sensory "on alert" brain of migraineurs or the less sensitive brain of non-migraineurs come first? This question aims to establish an important timeline. Is the original (default) brain the hyper sensitive brain? If so, we have a few things to ponder.

We consider evolutionary adaptations those genetic changes that improve the survival chances of the organism. The nervous system that smells, hears, and sees better – particularly in the dark – does have a survival advantage. In ancient times, it was important to smell a lion in the bush miles away, or feel weather changes ahead of time, or notice the movement of a single leaf. The hyper sensitivity of the migraine-brain is similar to the hyper sensitivity of the wild mammalian brain, where not being alert is equal to becoming food. Alertness is not just mammalian—all wild creatures have hyper sensitivity to their environment. My theory is that the brain of migraineurs is the original brain and those without migraines have had the good fortune to adapt to changing life circumstances as a result of a series of genetic variances. Does genetics support my hypothesis?

Migraine-Brain Genetics

The migraine-brain is genetic variance(s) initiated. There are a number of variances that are associated with a hyper sensitive on-alert brain, a migraine-brain. Looking at the near identical phenotypes of all migraineurs, regardless of migraine type, it is logical to suspect that migraineurs have a certain critical set of genetic variances in common.

You need to be a member in my migraine group to appreciate how much migraineurs are like siblings. Sometimes we run surveys that are either initiated by me or by members out of curiosity. Before I introduce two recent surveys, an important fact to note: migraine has 1069 SNPs[208] (SNP is genetic variance of a single nucleotide) at the time I write this book—this is a moving target.

So here are two specific survey questions:

1. How many of you have Ehlers-Danlos Syndrome of any kind?
2. How many of you have Raynaud's Disease?

The answers surprised me. Several hundred migraineurs responded within 2 days for these informal surveys posted in the migraine group in the standard Facebook survey format where people can click into a given option to state "I have it", or add additional options if the answer they wish to give does not fit any of the presented choices. The outcome of these surveys is automatically calculated by Facebook, so getting percentages is simple.

1. Ehlers-Danlos Syndrome (EDS)[141], a condition associated with hyper mobility and vascular differences of several types. The results of this survey were fascinating and informative. EDS is very rare; the most common form is found in only 1 out of 5000[729] (0.02%) people in the US. Yet over 60% of the surveyed migraineurs have at least one type of EDS

(there are ten types). EDS has 121 SNPs[208]. The overlap between EDS and migraine SNPs is highly significant: 43% of EDS SNPs are common with migraine SNPs. The two conditions must be related—perhaps by a common ancestor.

2. Raynaud's syndrome, a rare disease, is present in 1 out of 20 people (5%) in the US[730]. Yet over 70% of the migraineurs surveyed have Raynaud's. The SNP count for Raynaud's is 88[208] and 68% of the Raynaud's SNPs are common with migraine SNPs. The two conditions must also be related—perhaps by a common ancestor.

The SNPs of EDS and Raynaud's also overlap with each other; 16% of the SNPs in Raynaud's are also in EDS and 12% of the EDS SNPs are found in Raynaud's—the disparate percentage numbers represent the different absolute SNP numbers in each. It appears that the two conditions are related and both are related to migraine. I can reasonably speculate on the evolutionary benefits of the genetic adaptations for both Raynaud's and EDS. They both are adaptations to specific environmental pressures on predecessor mammalian species, like small mammalian predators, such as today's cats (both wild and domesticated kind). Their body is very flexible having extremely elastic cushioning disks and joints, and the shoulder blades are not connected to each other; they are attached to the rest of the body by muscles and not bones. This gives the shoulders freedom and a need for only tiny collarbones that allow squeezing through tight openings similarly to many mammals, like rodents, and very unlike most modern humans[731]. Such flexible joints also need a flexible blood vessel structure and thin flexible skin, possessing easier stretching ability, with many smaller vessels instead of a few larger ones that may get hurt—I just described the survival benefits of both EDS and Raynaud's. I don't think this has ever been examined; most papers describe the vascular nature of EDS only from the angle of the associated modern complications, no connection has been made to the extent of how blood vessel numbers and sizes differ from the general population[732].

The challenge here is to understand which variance group presents a survival benefit adaptation versus a survival disadvantageous negative mutation. Neither Raynaud's nor EDS nor migraine is a negative mutation; they each presented a survival benefit that over time turned into important and necessary adaptations. By recognizing that migraineurs' hyper sensitive brain is an adaptation with an evolutionary benefit, we have to ask why this adaptation has lost its benefits causing pain in our modern world? During the olden days when the hyper sensitive migraine-brain, EDS, and Raynaud's were important and beneficial, there were no soft drinks, smoothies, sugary sweets, breads, and pastas on every corner. Perhaps the problem is with the modern environment and the kind of food migraineurs are exposed to!

Today, many of the benefits of a migraine-brain are not necessary for survival. Eating a modern diet, migraineurs are subject to a host of health conditions because their ancient brain is not able to handle electrolyte variations caused by a carbohydrate-rich diet. Migraineurs have genetic variances associated with inability to tolerate glucose[14] and fructose[733,734]. These lead to metabolic syndrome[8,10,735,736] for migraineurs. By getting rid of most glucose and fructose providing carbohydrates in the migraineurs' diet, together with providing a higher-level mineral-enriched electrolyte to retain high concentration mineral balance, migraine can completely be prevented. Migraine pain is fully preventable without any medicines by proper nutritional choices alone.

Some Specific Migraine-Brain Genes

We already know that proper hydration is the basis of maintaining electrolyte homeostasis but how does that work at the cellular and the genetic level? And how does that work in the case of the migraine-brain with its hyper sensory organs that require a more mineral dense electrolyte? Clearly a hyper sensitive organ must use more energy to retain its alertness. What does that mean in terms of the electrolyte homeostasis, and the mineral and nutrient need in the electrolyte? And more importantly, what is in the migraine-brain that causes the pain in terms of genetic variances? How does this puzzle fit together?

The migraine-brain has 1069 genetic variances relative to what we today would call "normal" brains—the non-migraine-brains. Of this number, there are several that are very specific to electrolyte maintenance and glucose intolerance (by glucose intolerance I mean glucose malabsorption)—here is a small sample of the variances generalized: CACN (calcium voltage gated channel), ATP1 (ATPase, Na^+/K^+ transport), SCN (sodium voltage gated channel), NOTCH3 (white matter—myelin—abnormalities), KCN (potassium 2-pore domain), DRD (dopamine receptors), INS, IRS1, INSR (insulin), ACE and ACE2 (angiotensin), several SLC (solute carriers), LEP (leptin), GYS (glycogen synthase), GCG (glucagon), GHRL (ghrelin), APP (amyloid beta precursor protein), etc.

There is some evidence that migraine populations in still isolated geographical locations present similar genetic variances to people with migraine-brain elsewhere, and that in isolation, with fewer options for genetic mixing, the percentage of migraineurs is much higher as well[181]. This provides support for the genetic nature of migraine-brain and also strengthens the suggestion that the migraine-brain is the default brain.

The question "why migraine hurts" has several answers. The first one is simple: pluck a group of people with a special adaptation from its natural habitat and place it into a different environment, and what was an advantage suddenly becomes a disadvantage. There are many examples for this in nature.

As noted in an earlier section, Greenland Inuit[483], Canadian Inuit[737] and the Native American populations[738] all have glucose and fructose intolerance SNPs associated with their genes[739]. Migraineurs are also endowed with many glucose and fructose malabsorption SNPs. From SLC11A1 through SLC6A4 solute carrying genes nearly all are typical migraineur SNPs, including SLC2A1 (GLUT1 glucose transporter) SLC2A2 (GLUT2 glucose transporter), as well as many other solute caring variations that in some way connect to glucose processing or creation: GBA (an intermediate in glycolipid metabolism), G6PD (a carbohydrate metabolic condition that is characterized by abnormally low levels of glucose-6-phosphate dehydrogenase[740]), GSK3B (Glycogen Synthase Kinase 3 Beta), INS (insulin), INSR (insulin receptor), GCDH (oxidative decarboxylation of glutaryl-CoA to crotonyl-CoA and carbon dioxide), GLUD1 (nitrogen and glutamate metabolism and energy homeostasis), and SLC1A3 (glial high-affinity glutamate transporter), NPS (appetite control) among many others[208]. The inability to carry solutes to their destination causes a major problem for migraineurs—as it apparently also does for many isolated native populations. The inability to digest sucrose can cause diarrhea[741] but can also be undetected for life and may just presents itself as a burden in other forms—perhaps as a type of metabolic syndrome, such as insulin resistance and diabetes mellitus. The INSR (insulin resistance) gene has many SNPs that are very specific to insulin resistance of migraineurs.

The inability to metabolize glucose and fructose properly is referred to as malabsorption in modern parlance. If so many people are born without the ability to absorb these sugars[742], and so many subpopulations are known to lack the specific genes and therefore the enzyme for sucrose absorption, can we still suggest it is a *malabsorption*? Or is sugar absorption an *adaptation* that occurred later in time and thus not being able to eat sucrose may be the default? I am not the first one to ask this question[743].

Migraineurs with genetic testing all show variations of the MTHFR gene—uniformly the C667T polymorphism, in addition to several other SNPs[744,745]. The variations of this gene are associated with myelin damage as well. Migraineurs all seem to have this mutation. One may speculate that these variations also play a role in myelin damage in the brain of migraineurs[190,192,592,593,746,747]. Interestingly, this particular deficiency is very easy to remedy by supplementing proper bioavailable forms of B vitamins but I hear from most migraineurs that they have to fight to get a blood test checking for their B vitamin levels, as well as for higher than average homocysteine levels that the presence of MTHFR C667T variance can lead to by the migraineur's inability to methylate folate (B9). Sometimes life-changing solutions are a simple blood test away.

Why do migraineurs have such difficult time maintaining electrolyte homeostasis? The answer lies in the voltage gated sodium-potassium pumps, sodium channels, potassium channels, calcium channels, and ATPase, where SNPs affect functioning[113,114,118,119,748-750]. While this seems to be a negative variant potential, it is not likely to be the case. If we examine the nutritional habits of humans in ancient times when the hyper sensory alert brains provided their benefits as discussed earlier, the foods consumed included little if any elements that would disrupt electrolytes, such as today's carbohydrates do. You may not recall why carbohydrates disrupt the electrolyte so I post the quote from the medical manual—particularly since in my discussions with scientists and doctors I have found that many remember this wrong: "*...serum Na^+ falls by 1.4 mM for every 100-mg/*

dL increase in glucose, due to glucose-induced H_2O efflux from cells"[39] (page 4). This implies that as glucose enters the cells, water and sodium both get expelled if one is experiencing a diabetic increase of 100 mg/dL. While this is not expected from a non-diabetic, it is completely normal to have such a huge glucose increase from a small serving (10 pieces) of cherries for a glucose intolerant person (such as a migraineur like me) with genetic variants that don't support glucose metabolism, who is not diabetic and has no insulin resistance. Thus such increases are not reserved for diabetics alone. Sudden glucose increase is the ultimate electrolyte disruption. Migraineurs, many native culture members, and diabetics cannot deal with such electrolyte changes and end up with major disruptions.

In the ancient times, there was nothing that could disrupt the brain's electrolytes to the extent today's nutritional lifestyle can. Here again, I refer the reader to "lack of adaptation" rather than mutation. I offer a series of hypotheses to summarize the salient details of my theory:

Hypothesis 1: If you look at mammal species in the wild today, you find they are always on alert for predators. If they are not on alert, they are likely to become food. For them, the hyper-sensory alert brain is the default. The migraine-brain is a hyper-sensory alert brain.

Hypothesis 2: If hyper-sensory alert brain can be the default, then such a brain, the migraine-brain, is the default mammalian brain that all human ancestors must have had at one time. Since this brain is still very prevalent in the human population (15%[178]), it must have represented a significant survival advantage in ancient times. Today, however, the majority of humans do not have this brain type.

Hypothesis 3: While the majority of humans were able to adapt to more modern lifestyles and food supply, some could not; their brain remained unchanged, still holding onto the ancient traits and retained hyper sensory organs. These then are today's migraineurs.

Hypothesis 4: The tendency for electrolyte imbalance is a sign that the migraine-brain is greatly compromised under modern nutritional challenges. While the majority of humans adapted to the use of carbohydrates for fuel during our recent evolution, migraineurs did not. Up until about 10-15,000 years ago carbohydrates formed only a minimal part of the human diet.

Hypothesis 5: The ancient brain (in some of its traits) may go back as far as the Euarchontoglires (100 million years ago), the first common ancestor to all mammals and primates. The early mammals had a few special traits that appear to be connected to the migraine-brain. Two of these are the Ehlers-Danlos Syndrome (EDS) and Raynaud's Syndrome. Both of these are highly connected to migraine and to each other and are ancient traits that some mammals still carry today—and apparently a very large percentage of migraineurs do as well, although in the general population their percentage is miniscule.

Hypothesis 6: Migraine is a neurovascular condition (not a disease) that is similar to an evolutionary throwback. *Neuro* because it is a neuron voltage energy generation problem, *vascular* because of the different vascular structure migraineurs have from non-migraineurs, and because of how electrolyte disruption affects vascular pressure. Both EDS and Raynaud's are vascular in nature and EDS is also associated with hyper mobility and being disjointed, which were very important adaptations in early mammals and still are in many contemporary ones, such as cats, for example, with floating shoulders. Having a more intricate vascular system allows for increased flexibility without suffering vascular damage.

Hypothesis 7: Migraineurs probably have a very different vascular system from non-migraineurs, the vasculature segments are likely shorter and more numerous. This can often be seen through the skin of people with EDS because they also have very thin, transparent, and flexible skin. Shorter vascular regions and flexible skin and joints allow more flexibility for those afflicted with EDS and Raynaud's.

Hypothesis 8: The precursor version of the human migraine-brain evolved in an era when being disjointed and having different vascular system were evolutionarily beneficial. Looking at the combination of these traits as an evolutionary throwback, explains why migraineurs are glucose and carbohydrates intolerant. Back then exogenous glucose from carbohydrates was not consumed.

Let's try to examine the evidence – as much as possible.

By visiting the GeeneCards database[208] and searching for the genes associated with migraine, then organizing the "score" (relevance to the condition) starting with the most important ones contributing to migraines, one can clearly see a pattern (this table is from the time this book is written, relevant percentages and the order of some genes may change):

Order	Category	Function	Score
1	CACNA1A	Calcium Voltage-Gated Channel Subunit Alpha1 A	84.08
2	ATP1A2	ATPase Na+/K+ Transporting Subunit Alpha 2	80.67
3	SCN1A	Sodium Voltage-Gated Channel Alpha Subunit 1	67.55
4	NOTCH3	Notch 3 (pain sensory)	47.15
5	PRRT2	Proline Rich Transmembrane Protein 2	45.81
6	KCNK18	Potassium Two Pore Domain Channel Subfamily K Member 18	45.5
7	EDNRA	Endothelin Receptor Type A	35.86
9	HTR1A	5-Hydroxytryptamine Receptor 1A	34.08
12	CALCA	Calcitonin Related Polypeptide Alpha (blood calcium)	25.46
14	MTHFR	Methylenetetrahydrofolate Reductase (B vitamin methylation)	22.09
16	SLC2A1	Solute Carrier Family 2 Member 1 (GLUT1 glucose)	21.3
17	SLC6A4	Solute Carrier Family 6 Member 4 (sodium-dependent serotonin transporter)	18.96
18	HTR1D	5-Hydroxytryptamine Receptor 1D (vasoconstriction)	18.81
20	SLC1A3	Solute Carrier Family 1 Member 3 (insulin signaling)	18.56
21	ATP1A3	ATPase Na+/K+ Transporting Subunit Alpha 3	18.28
22	DRD2	Dopamine Receptor D2	18.21
23	HTR1B	5-Hydroxytryptamine Receptor 1B (5-HT1B serotonin receptor)	17.83
24	HTR3A	5-Hydroxytryptamine Receptor 3A (5-HT3A serotonin receptor)	17.19
25	HTR2C	5-Hydroxytryptamine Receptor 2C (5-HT3A serotonin receptor)	16.95
26	MAOA	Monoamine Oxidase A (an MAO-A enzyme inhibitor, prevents apoptosis in melanoma cells)	16.65
27	HTR2A	5-Hydroxytryptamine Receptor 2A (5-HT2A serotonin receptor)	16.43
28	TAC1	Tachykinin Precursor 1 (vasodilator and secretagogue)	15.69
29	HTR1F	5-Hydroxytryptamine Receptor 1F (5-HT1 seotonin receptor)	15.65
30	PRDM16	PR/SET Domain 16 (development of adipocytes in brown & white adipose tissue)	15.33

Table 7. Top 24 Gene variances of migraine

In the above table 24 highly correlated migraine genes are shown out of the top 30—I removed those SNPs that represent aura or other migraine types in general and only highlighted those that represent variances in key functions that are present in migraineurs. These 24 clearly demonstrate that the migraine gene variants are grouped around the important electrolyte ionic gates and channels. Note the MTHFR (methylenetetrahydrofolate) reductase, TAC1, HTR1D, and NOTHCH3 genes all encode for vascular conditions of the smooth muscle, brain vascular structure, and amyloid β precursor--an Alzheimer's associated condition reflecting (potentially) the myelin damage. By recognizing the most important feature that migraine-brain genes cluster around the electrolyte homeostasis maintenance function, glucose transport variations, and vascular variances, we can appreciate that migraineurs face a problem with carbohydrate consumption. Insulin is also heavily on the list, INS, INSR, IGF1, IGF1R, IGF2, IGFBP1, IGFBPP3 with placements from 226 through 650 from the 1069 variants.

Of course, pharmaceutical researchers have known for a long time that ionic channels are important gene variants in migraineurs, as all current preventive medicines are aimed specifically at downregulating voltage gated channels, rendering them nonfunctional. Yet a non-migraineur individual has all these voltage gated channels fully functional and so obviously, these channels are there for a reason. Stopping something from working is not fixing it. Changing the migraineurs dietary habits so they can function without pain makes much more sense than downregulating otherwise perfectly healthy gates and pumps, necessary for proper brain operation that simply cannot work in a glucose-rich environment. Rendering excitable voltage gated channels useless shows lack of understanding and ignorance. Being genetically different should not mean to have to be made dysfunctional at the detriment of the migraineur's abilities and life. The drugs prescribed downregulate everything to the point that even the body's thermal controls stop working and most migraineurs suffer permanent brain damage[751].

Why Don't Migraineurs Get Genetic Tests?

The reader may wonder why I have spent so much emphasis on the genetic basis of migraines. The answer is really a question: why don't migraineurs get tested for some of the obvious genetic differences via simple blood tests? For example, testing for the functioning of the MTHFR C667T gene variance is a simple blood test of all B vitamin levels and homocysteine levels, providing the answer for folate methylation. Of course, the problem is twofold: understanding what tests migraineurs should receive and then being able to interpret the results. For example, in my entire medically-known and confirmed migraine history of over 40 years, I had my homocysteine levels checked twice, once at my request! Why? And if my test result comes back at 15 or 5, for example, would a medical professional know what either of these numbers means? Similarly, the range of B12 is given as 200 to 950 (variable to some degree by labs). If my result comes back at 201 or at 1000, will my doctor know what these numbers mean? In my personal experience and in the experience of many migraineurs when vitamin B12 levels are either below or above the norm (and the norm should really be between 500 and 700), doctors have no idea what to do. Migraineurs with B12 level below the norm are sent to take a B multivitamin complex (which they cannot absorb for lack of methylation), and migraineurs with higher than normal B12 are sent home with "all is great"; yet it is a sign that they cannot methylate and their B12 is high because it is unused. All is not great!

I am not an MD and don't intend to become one but I do have the expectation that an MD would recognize an under or over methylation problem and would know what to do about it. I also expect that an MD would know that homocysteine levels that are high (big confusion over what it should be[752]) represent cardiac, cancer, and stroke danger because it is a sign of the inability of proper folate absorption[753-755]. Would my doctor know that if I also have MTHFR C667T mutation (of course not, it is not tested!), I am at a high risk for cardiac events[756,757]? Doctors think that people in general get enough B vitamins but migraineurs are a special breed. No doctor I know has ever mentioned that there may be an absorption problem that is genetic—do they know[758]? Migraineurs with the MTHFR C667T mutation need to take active bioavailable B vitamins; each separately, or consume organ meats regularly—organ meats are not only not seen commonly in modern diet but are also discouraged by the prevailing dietary guidelines. With this section I hope I have been able to open some minds for the importance of certain blood tests and potentially even genetic tests. They can save many migraineurs from chronic pain and dozens of unnecessary medicines.

Section II

The Migraine-Brain Difference

Mutation is random; natural selection
is the very opposite of random

--Richard Dawkins

In this section I provide a brief summary of the migraine-brain difference highlighting some of the key evidence for its incorrect medicinal treatments. It is meant to guide medical practitioners in understanding why medicines don't work and why piling one medicine on top of another or increasing the dose not only fails but is harmful. The goal is to help migraineurs live a better life and be able to rely upon their doctors and not fear them.

Migraine Cause–Advanced Explanation

Throughout the book, I have been emphasizing the futility of migraine research efforts focusing on migraine pain rather than causation. Here I show how such faulty research fails. I explain in detail my thoughts on the true cause of migraines. Chronic migraine is considered to be a disabling neurological disease[286,759-761], treated with dangerous[751] and often brain damaging[762] medicines[763,764]. A good summary of recent findings labels migraine as "an inherited, episodic disorder involving sensory sensitivity"[765]. While crucial findings like this have been made, and even with the medical community's understanding and acceptance of the previous section's genetic explanation, research of dietary factors is still missing. Why? There are several reasons but one of the fundamental ones is the belief that migraine is a disease.

Research showed long time ago (1951 to be precise) that migraineurs excrete 50% more sodium in their urine than non-migraineurs do and have "busy brains"[144]. These findings suggest an important clue for the mechanism of migraines even without the understanding of the genetic connection. This clue led me to the recognition of a promising hypothesis, namely, the possibility that in some manner sodium depletion is involved in migraine onset and persistence. As far as I could ascertain, the question of "Why sodium is depleted?" has not been asked—though some resent research found support for an inverse relationship between migraines and the amount of dietary sodium consumed: the more sodium was consumed, the fewer migraines appeared[226,241,257,258].

The anatomy of migraine is visible in scanners[60,168,766-768]. Regions in refractory state, zones of CD, are unable to generate energy for action potential[55,60,79,168,767]. Healthy regions send a voltage shockwave of a CSD that is also visible in scanners[55,60,79,766,767]. Deep-brain electrical stimulation of the CD regions in patients in the state of depression or migraine yields complete resolution, the re-activation of the CD region, and the elimination of symptoms[769-774]. Additionally, it is known that blood flow changes occur in the brain preceding and during a migraine[768,775-777]. The white matter in migraine-brains, critical for voltage transfer and myelination, is different from non-migraineurs and changes during a migraine attack; the entire brain anatomy is different in migraineurs[5,165,778-780]. Even voltage activated brain regions differ for the same stimulus between migraineurs and non-migraineurs[5].

Migraineurs are much more likely to have metabolic disorders than non-migraineurs[8-12,139,140]. This is connected to electrolyte disturbance caused by glucose[39], based on the migraineurs' response to carbohydrate intake. The extreme response is caused by genetic variations of glucose transporters, ionic channels that manage electrolyte homeostasis, and associated proteins[14,118,119,299,781-784]. Migraineurs appear to genetically be predisposed to other forms of metabolic diseases as well[13,14,114,220,304]. For them, the COMPT gene is usually different, interfering with dopaminergic and noradrenergic functions[785]. Frequent genetic variants are also present, such as MTHFR C677T (mentioned earlier[186,190,192,593,786]), MTR and also MTRR, representing a host of variations associated with general health status, including insulin resistance, obesity, and cardiovascular risks[787,788]. Numerous findings point to the ACE Angiotensin I Converting Enzyme's influence as it reduces the RAAS from balancing electrolytes properly, influencing key elements in metabolic syndrome and cardiovascular diseases in addition to migraines[789,790]. That the ACE Angiotensin I Converting Enzyme negatively influences RAAS makes sense once it is brought in the context of the glucose transport variant, indicating that consuming carbohydrates may not have always been a substantial part of nutrition during human evolution, and all traits associated with carbohydrate-based glucose metabolism must have been adaptations. A body that consumes no carbohydrates has no need to regulate electrolyte, since the disruptive element is the sudden increase of exogenous glucose.

Additionally, migraineurs' neurons seem to operate at a higher voltage level with a bigger response pattern and in different brain regions for the same stimulus than neurons of non-migraineurs do, indicating that a migraine-brain is "always on," confirming the "busy brain" hypothesis of the 1951 paper noted above[4,6]. Migraineurs have a higher voltage reaction than non-migraineurs do to the same sensory stimulus, supporting the model that migraineurs have hyper sensitive sensory organs that are over stimulated[3,791]. Hyper sensitive sensory organs result in more receptor connections among sensory neurons[3,7,63,792,793]. Thus, brains containing hyper sensitive sensory organs with multiple receptor connections need more voltage for generating action and resting potentials, and need well-balanced electrolytes with higher mineral density to accommodate the demands of the extra activity and increased amplitude of their action potentials. The excretion of 50% more sodium in the urine is indicative of increased sodium use by such active brains. Combined, these findings suggest an increased need for sodium and other electrolyte minerals for migraineurs—proving the conclusions of studies on inverse correlation between dietary sodium intake and migraines.

Voltage is generated by the interaction of a proper ratio of sodium (Na^+), potassium (K^+), and chloride (Cl^-) ions through neuronal membranes. Glucose entering cells hampers the preservation of electrolyte homeostasis, interstitial fluid, and blood volume in the brain. Furthermore, in the case of migraineurs whose genetic test results I have had access to and could review, I always find the ANK2 gene (associated with diabetes mellitus, metabolic syndrome, and heart arrhythmia) and the INSR gene (associated with insulin resistance of migraineurs with or without aura), strongly suggesting that migraineurs have gene variants predisposing them to just about every single metabolic disorder possible, likely as a result of glucose and fructose malabsorption issues. These issues can be identified by genetic testing once migraine genes have expressed[739,742,743,794]. The populations of many Inuit nations lack certain enzymes and while they are on their native diets, converting glucose only from protein or organ meats, they are completely healthy[483,737,738]. Similarly, migraineurs on the ketogenic diet, which is carbohydrate poor, who are not on any preventive or abortive medication, remain migraine free.

While plenty of research support the hypothesis that migraineurs are intolerant to glucose[8,9,11,138], I found only one reported research finding that shows – indirectly – the glucose absorption problem; this is the only research that tested what happens if migraineurs consume simple glucose[663]. My own findings in the migraine group show that migraineurs, pressing their luck after a period of being migraine (and sugar) free, always come down with a migraine after consuming sugar, and they also stand a good chance of getting a migraine if they exceed a carbohydrate level of approximately 12 net carbohydrate grams per meal. Since glucose disrupts electrolyte balance by removing sodium and water from the cells, dietary glucose's connection to the frequently found coupling of metabolic disorders with migraines, the changes in blood flow, and the lack of action potential in brain regions[8-13,138-140,736,795] is clearly established.

Misapplied Medicine

Serotonin plays an unintended part in glucose intolerance, particularly due to the widespread medical practice of prescribing triptans and other serotonin providing or generating medicines[449,636,637,639,796-800] for migraine treatment. Serotonin occupies the available insulin receptors, causing glucose backup, initiating insulin resistance[620,639,801,802].

Serotonin medications in the form of triptans or SSRIs are the most frequently prescribed medications to migraineurs, causing trouble with insulin resistance to an otherwise already predisposed sub-population[140,640]. High levels of blood glucose over extended periods lead to insulin resistance[620,636,801,803-805]. Moreover, unless the sodium that was removed by glucose is replaced, excess urination ensues, similarly to diabetes mellitus[371,806,807]. Excess urination, typically void of color, is a very typical migraine prodrome[719,808]. The energy required for action potential generation is hampered without the replacement of the lost sodium, leading to regions of CD and then to CSD, and the start of migraine pain. Consequently, migraine is preventable by the decrease of carbohydrate consumption and the increase of dietary sodium – particularly after carbohydrate consumption – to reestablish electrolyte homeostasis and action potential generation. In addition, greatly reduced carbohydrates and increased animal fats and cholesterol in the migraineurs' diet is beneficial, since they support the necessary fat and cholesterol concentration in the white matter, providing protective myelination[809-811]. Serotonin medicines make recovery from a migraine more difficult by taking up insulin receptors.

Many medicines that migraineurs are prescribed make glucose intolerance worse by occupying insulin receptors in a way that glucose cannot clear from the blood fast enough[636,812]. The brain also has insulin receptors and thus glucose absorption can be problematic, resulting in serotonin activated insulin resistance[813-815]. In insulin resistance testing, we are unable to differentiate among insulin resistance in the brain, in lipids[5], in the liver; and its effects in individual organs versus its systemic effects in the body as a whole. By the time insulin resistance shows up in conventional tests it is systemic, and specific organ centered insulin resistance—such as in the brain—may already have been present for many years[620,816,817]. While the hemoglobin A1c test is extremely popular for evaluating insulin resistance status, it doesn't measure insulin. It only measures average glucose levels over a 6-12 weeks period[345], from which insulin is interpolated[630,632,633]. The only accurate insulin resistance test is the Kraft insulin in-situ test that I have never personally seen being administered by any doctor so far[335]. Relatedly, Kraft has also shown that a decent percentage of full blown diabetics is capable of passing the hemoglobin A1c test in flying colors — a very inaccurate test[346,818].

One of the reasons why the HbA1c test misses its mark is the average blood sugar. A hypoglycemic individual whose blood sugar changes between 50 and 146 every day is a sick patient whose average blood sugar is 98 and whose test will arrive at an HbA1C of 5%, passing with flying colors, yet she is diabetic.

Alterations of glucose absorption and migraineurs' general glucose intolerance may lead to Alzheimer's and other diseases, in which myelin damage is also an important contributing factor[819-821]. In addition to genetic predisposition, medicines that promote insulin

5 NMR lipoprofile testing can check insulin resistance in lipid management but NMR lipoprofile testing is not mainstream.

resistance in the brain may contribute to the frequently found connection between metabolic disorders and migraineurs[799,822]. Insulin resistance, by not permitting glucose to clear fast enough, is associated with and can prolong electrolyte imbalance and cause migraine as a result.

Try as you may, you will not find a single academic research article on the importance of electrolyte homeostasis associated with migraine prevention, yet just about every single hospital emergency room starts migraine treatment by the administration of a saline IV. The need for proper hydration is mentioned often in general but not in association with migraines[352-354]. I asked a prominent doctor from the Mayo Clinic (via email) why – in their ER – they could not stop and refrain from any additional treatment or medication after the administration of saline IV, in order to see if the migraine has been eased or eliminated. His answer was "we never thought about it." Indeed, there is not much money in providing only saline IV to an ER patient.

The anatomy of a migraine-brain was detailed in part III. Please refer back to some of the details there. It is assumed that those reading this part of the book are familiar with the anatomy of the brain and the differences between a non-migraine-brain and a migraine-brain with its hyper sensory organ sensitivities. In the previous section an explanation for the cause of migraine was provided detailing my new non-medicinal prevention regime of migraines. In this section I revisit the concept at a neuronal level for clarity. I hope that reading this section will make it crystal clear why medicines cannot and do not work for migraines.

What Stops Neurons from Functioning

Chemically, neurotransmitters are identical to hormones. The difference is that neurotransmitters stay within the brain and hormones play various regulatory roles in the body. But before neurotransmitters can perform their function of information exchange, a neuron must deliver an electrical signal across its own structure to the synapse shared with another neuron, the intended recipient. The electrical signal – in the form of a voltage spike train – has to travel through the neuron's axon. Importantly for our subject, the axon is insulated with myelin to prevent voltage leaking to other nearby neurons. Myelin can get damaged by glucose and insulin—as discussed before[285,567,823-827].

Neurons have some basic important functions in terms of migraines, and though they have lots of other functions, we will only focus on the migraine related ones here.

A neuron has an outside layer (lipid bilayer, membrane) to block everything from entering or leaving it, unless conditions are just right for facilitating an ionic exchange. Alternatively, small, electrically neutral molecules can also transit the membrane. For example, water molecules are tiny so they can float through channels in the membrane between the intracellular space and the interstitial fluid.

Nevertheless, most nutritionally essential molecules have to be in an ionic form to enter or leave the neuron, and they do so through specialized protein structures of the membrane, the voltage gated pumps and channels. It is essential to keep neurons' voltage gated pumps and channels (also referred to as voltage dependent) fully operational for the neurons to work. A critical function of a neuron is the generation of alternating action and resting potentials for the voltage gated pumps' proper operation. There is also a refractory period, during which the neurons do not generate either action or resting potential, therefore no pumps can operate. All of this activity takes place at regions called Nodes of Ranvier, unmyelinated regions on the axon, and only here is voltage generated via the axon's spike train. Without the axon's spike train there is no neurotransmitter release in the neuron's synapses. If at any Node of Ranvier the spike train stops, the action potential is terminated.

Inability to Generate Voltage

Influx of sodium is necessary to generate an action potential to open voltage gated pumps. Of course, if a neuron is not able to generate action potential as detailed above – there is no neurotransmitter release. This is exactly the strategy with many medicines that block the generation of action potentials in neurons. Other medicines block the release of neurotransmitters directly at the synapses, or they force the neurons into working 24/7 by inhibiting neurotransmitter reuptake sensors. However, if neurons cannot create action potential or release neurotransmitters, they may go "offline" and stay in a refractory state, which can be seen as a region of CD[79]. Regions where there is no ionic exchange as a result of CD, don't release neurotransmitters. The lack of neurotransmitters alerts connected neurons. They initiate a CSD, a kind of wake-up call, that is seen in scanners as a slow-moving wave of energy (2-5 mm per minute), with its goal of restoring the CD-affected neurons to their healthy operational state[49,55,56,70,79,828,829]. If this wave of electricity is not followed by the recovery of the CD region, resulting in action potential generation, the CSD continues all the way to the dura where nociceptors start the migraine pain[830].

There is a constant exchange of sodium, chloride, and potassium ions between the intracellular and extracellular space to maintain action and resting potentials. These essential minerals are in charge of creating a balance through chemical interactions, the very biochemical balance that is one of the main subjects of this book. This balance allows the neurons to function properly. The actual physical opening and closing action of the voltage gated pumps is based on sodium ions and potassium ions entering and exiting the neuron, in a timely manner, together with chloride, magnesium, and ATPase. Magnesium and ATPase provide the energy for the pumps to open[783,831-834]. The direction to which the pumps may open is based on the charge difference between the inside and the outside of the membrane[422,835]. There is a threshold voltage value for opening the pumps in each direction[836]. Not having enough sodium, chloride, or potassium ions reduces the ability of the pumps to create a large enough action or resting potential to open or close the gates[837].

This can create a catch-22 situation, where less voltage causes even lower voltage by lowering the number of ions coming and going. Falling below a certain voltage threshold, ion exchange may be halted completely, preventing the pump from opening in any direction, causing an extended refractory state that leads to the earlier mentioned CD[838].

While numerous studies from the 20th Century claim that too much sodium is bad for a person because it increases blood pressure, in fact, it increases blood volume, causing hypervolemia. Hypovolemia is a migraineurs' trademark[839,840]; many migraineurs develop Postural Tachycardia Syndrome (POTS) as well[239]. An increased sodium diet increases blood volume for migraineurs, which for them is highly desired.

Mineral imbalance affects electrolyte homeostasis. Someone with hypokalemia could end up with hypernatremia, retaining too much water, potentially leading to pump failure. The opposite is also true: hyponatremia leads to hyperkalemia, thereby dehydration. Hyperkalemia may lead to seizures, epilepsy, or death[132,841,842]. Ca, Na, K and ATPase related genetic variants likely play a part in the circuitry variants that cause problems for migraine-brains and their metabolic sensitivity[114,118]. Migraineurs, who enhance their electrolyte mineral density and homeostasis (see part III) by increased dietary sodium, reduced carbohydrates, and use of the Stanton Migraine Protocol® for safe carbohydrate consumption, are able to prevent all their migraines.

Hypovolemia with Hypo- or Hypertension

We need to elaborate on the difference between *blood volume* increase and *blood pressure* increase. Blood can have hypovolemia that is associated with hypotension and represents a dehydrated state—I have found that most migraineurs typically have sub-clinical hypotension (systolic below 90 and diastolic below 50)[18-20], with severe hypovolemia (some migraineurs drink no water at all). Confusingly, sometimes migraineurs present with hypovolemia and hypertension at the same time, particularly under high stress, anxiety, and pain but without shock. In a hypovolemic non-migraineur patient, cardiac output decreases and this decrease initiates the sympathetic nervous system to raise blood pressure by systemic vasoconstriction that typically represents cardiogenic shock[39,843]. In migraineurs, the same process is hormone driven by adrenaline release and is part of a prodrome cascade. This is never recognized in emergency rooms where migraineurs often turn for help with uncontrollable pain.

Hypovolemia also comes with fewer but larger red blood cells in those migraineurs who shared their blood test results with me. I would recommend that doctors check MCV for the size of red blood cells in migraine patients. The healthy range of MCV is between 81 and 99 but I often see migraineur MCV higher than 99 and even if not out of range the value tends to get very close to the higher limit of normal. This changes as the migraineur starts increasing her hydration to the proper level at all times. Larger red blood cells, in addition to blood clot danger, also carry another negative factor. Larger red blood cells are necessary for hypovolemic migraineurs because they need to carry more oxygen; there are fewer red blood cells to travel the approximately 60,000 miles of blood vessels through the body[844]. This indicates that with hypovolemia, the red blood cell size has to increase to be able to ferry adequate levels of oxygen, as less blood circulates and at a reduced rate, as a result of the lower blood pressure and pulse rate. Hypovolemic hypertension is extremely common for migraineurs during a migraine. There is much literature on migraineurs sporting hypertension but all of those papers examine migraineurs only during a pain period[11,18,170,238,845]. Although hypervolemia is generally undesired, in the case of migraineurs, temporary hypertension reduces migraine pain[846]. Indeed, one of the reasons why triptan-use may seem helpful is not that the migraine responds to serotonin but that it responds to vasoconstriction. In our migraine group, migraineurs who are hit by a migraine episode after quitting all their medications are instructed to have a cup of coffee, successfully aborting the pain. Unfortunately larger red blood cells under vasoconstriction may increase stroke danger[847].

Hypervolemia typically coincides with higher than normal blood pressure, representing an over hydrated state. While we work hard to increase blood volume for all migraineurs, we manage to avoid hypervolemia by calculating the precise water amount a migraineur needs to drink every day. A normal blood volume is one which is neither low nor high and that corresponds to optimal red blood cell size. I call normally hydrated blood *volumized* blood. Volumized blood allows for the enriched electrolyte homeostasis and proper neural function migraineurs need, without increase or decrease in blood pressure and with normal blood cell size. After several months on properly maintained volume controlled hydration, migraineurs experience a reduction in red blood cell size. This also reduces blood clot danger. Blood pressure sometimes reaches a normal-low range of systolic 100-110 and diastolic 60-70 but more often remains as before, 90/50 on average.

Carbohydrates Convert to Cholesterol

As noted previously in the genetic section, migraineurs share a specific glucose transport variance and are extremely sensitive and intolerant to carbohydrates. Most carbohydrates have both glucose and fructose, of which the excess is converted to triglycerides by the liver. High blood triglycerides contribute to heart disease and atherosclerosis[225,235,254,259,274-279,403,406,408,411,440,444,461,467,468,848-851].

Migraineurs carbohydrate metabolism disrupts their electrolyte homeostasis[9,11,13,138,140,184,663,735,781,788,852-855]. Many migraineurs end up with what is considered to be high total cholesterol (a debate on its own whether this means anything) and doctors feel obligated to place them on cholesterol lowering statins.

However, statins are more dangerous for migraineurs because the migraine-brain needs more cholesterol and fat than the non-migraine-brains of the general population. Statins reduce the brain's ability to produce cholesterol, thereby increasing the possibility of a weakened myelin sheath, preventing proper axon operation[856]. As we discussed earlier, myelin performs a very important insulating function around the axons of neurons. Damaged myelin may be one of the causes of misfiring in the brain (seizures), loss of motor functions (Parkinson's, MS), and voltage leaks (migraine)[857]. It is clear, therefore, that the maintenance of the myelin sheath is vital to a healthy brain. Prescribing a medicine that prevents myelin repair is detrimental to migraine-brain health and it is not defensible in light of the questionable cardiovascular benefits it might provide. Recently, the National Headache Foundation published an article "Statins a Possible Treatment for Prevention of Migraine" that sounds like an oxymoron to me. Nevertheless, a trial of this treatment was announced with the combination of Vitamin D[858,859]. I hope nobody will get hurt.

Section 12

Drugs of Shame

This is a very special section in which I collected a lot of useful information for capable doctors and scientists to review, discuss, and learn from at their discretion and leisure. I am desperate to help change the sad world of migraineurs whose lives are destroyed by misinformed care and prevalent ignorance. It is time for healthcare professionals to pay attention to migraineurs as if one of their own family members was a migraineur. Would they also just prescribe whatever off-label drug comes to mind to their family member?

I found Angela's protocol after a 4-month episode of chronic migraine. I had suffered for over 20 years with the monster. I didn't try much medication as the few I did try did nothing for me. In fact, medication seemed to make it worse. I had near instant relief as I began implementing the protocol. I could not believe it. And, here I am, two years later, migraine free. I still witness the undeniable joy of new members who join the fb group as they find their way to being pain and migraine free ♥

--Terri Haas Corley
Member of the Facebook Migraine Group

Medication Challenges

Migraine is quite challenging in many other ways in addition to the pain. Unfortunately, the industry only works on pain reduction. There are two main classes of medicines prescribed for migraineurs: preventives that need to be taken every single day and abortives that are taken on demand. I briefly describe the types of drugs within these two classes, first focusing on preventives and then abortives.

Some of the most common preventives are voltage gated calcium channel blockers (Topamax for example), serotonin modifiers (SSRIs or SNRIs or antidepressants), beta-blockers (blood pressure medicines), in addition to narcotics, muscle relaxants, and several other types. Many migraineurs complain about using voltage gated calcium channel blockers; they don't work and the adverse effects are horrendous—often permanent even after the medicines are quit—usually a much slower titration method is required than what is recommended by the pharmaceutical company. Some of these drugs have a special name by doctors: they call Topamax "Dopamax" because they make the person act and feel as if they were doped. The users of these drugs complain that these drugs do make them "stupid and dumbed down". I write for the HormonesMatter.com science blog where one of my articles, "Topamax: The Drug with 9 Lives"

https://www.hormonesmatter.com/topamax-drug-nine-lives/,

has gained much interest. Many Topamax users have commented about the damage this drug has done to them. Voltage gated calcium channel blockers are very dangerous for migraineurs. The NNT for an antiepileptic such as Topamax, even in combination with another drug to reduce epileptic seizures by 50%, can be as high as 24 or more[860]—I could not find NNT for migraines with the use of anticonvulsants. We must point out that migraine is not equivalent to seizure. Prescribing anticonvulsant drug therapy for someone without seizures is questionable at best, even if the FDA approved it for such use.

Another favorite drug class for migraine treatment is SSRI and SNRI. These can lead to serotonin syndrome, which can be fatal—and often is, since doctors don't recognize the symptoms. A true story I wrote (about my mother's death from serotonin syndrome) explains how SSRI's work. Lamentably many doctors don't have a clue. Please read "Silent Death – Serotonin Syndrome;" it can be found here:

https://www.hormonesmatter.com/silent-death-serotonin-syndrome/

SSRIs and similar reuptake inhibitors block the natural inhibitory responses of the neurons that normally allow them to "STOP making serotonin now". Making serotonin 24/7 assures an oversupply of serotonin. Such neuronal burnout may be behind the many adverse reactions that end in cognitive decline from the use of SSRIs[861-864]. SSRIs were found to exacerbate migraines[21].

Another preventive migraineurs receive is the TCA class of antidepressants—though I have yet to see a single depressed migraineur. In addition to not working for migraines at all, some, like Amitriptyline (Elavil), damages healthy hearts[865]. Amitriptyline is one of the "dirty drugs" that implies its broad effect on many organs—yet exact mechanism is unknown—and it interacts with hundreds of other medications.

Blood pressure medications seem to pop up very often for migraine prevention—though migraineurs have extremely low blood pressure to start with. The most frequently prescribed heart medicine is also a dirty drug: Propranolol (Inderal) that most migraineurs find impossible to reduce and quit. Those who cannot quit end up with heart trouble since this drug is well-known to damage the heart, particularly by causing toxicity to those who had no heart trouble prior to taking it[866]. To add insult to injury, Propranolol also crosses the blood brain barrier, potentially causing trouble in the brain as well.

The abortive class of drugs specifically target pain on those days when pain is not controlled by preventives (which is apparently every day based on the 4000+ migraineurs I had worked with). There are several classes of abortives: triptans (serotonin), steroidal anti-inflammatory medicines (corticosteroids), non-steroidal anti-inflammatory medicines (NSAIDs), narcotics, and caffeinated pain killers. Triptans are handed out like candy—they increase blood pressure, increase bowel movement, reduce nutrient absorption, and cause IBS-like symptoms. Moreover, they can kill the migraineur by serotonin syndrome if used when an SSRI or TCA is already taken. All of the abortives also cause rebound pain when an attempt is made to quit them, and can exacerbate migraines by becoming addictive and extremely hard to quit[21].

From the list of medicines my migraineurs take at the time they join the group, it is clear that most doctors have no idea that once a serotonin-type preventive is prescribed, a triptan cannot also be prescribed. 100% of those migraineurs who joined taking some preventives were also prescribed triptans—often many different types! Furthermore, in my experience, having used triptan in pills and in nasal spray form, the actual chance that triptans helped my migraine was about 25-30% because in order for serotonin to have any effect, the brain region in CD needs to be the one that is not able to make serotonin.

Approximately 30% of the migraineurs are prescribed either SSRIs or SNRIs or antidepressant and about 30% are prescribed voltage gated calcium channel blockers. On average, 50% of these migraineurs get both prescribed. This is a very serious problem. Studies show the seriousness of the situation but I suppose doctors don't read once they leave med school[867-870].

One of the biggest challenges healthcare providers face today is that most people want a pushbutton pop-a-pill solution for everything. I used to find people joining the migraine group who appeared to be interested in the biochemical balancing process. But when the next migraine pain hit they were chatting with migraineurs in other groups, asking what pills they used to take the pain away—these migraineurs were always removed from the group. Some people strongly prefer a pill solution even if they know that on the long run they may get hurt by it. I suppose it is a question of having the willpower to change a lifestyle. However, it is a dilemma for doctors who don't want to prescribe medicines. Not receiving any medicines may make many patients unsatisfied and feel that they have not been taken care of. While doctors seem to be in a rather hard spot of being damned if they do and damned if they don't prescribe, their oath of *Do No Harm* requires them to observe patient-safety over patient-wish.

Much of the blame about pill-popping goes to the pharmaceutical companies and doctors that have been giving pills for just about everything that could otherwise be naturally treated. The speed with which changes occur in our lives does not afford much time for long-term testing, analysis, and confirmation to see if something is harmful or healthy, and many medications are pulled off the shelves or are black-boxed a few years (sometimes few months) after they were released, on account of the many adverse effects that have initiated lawsuits. It has also come to the public's attention that many clinical trials only report a fraction of their findings; usually only the successful cases[679,871-873], making clinical trial results questionable.

It is also a problem that the Food and Drug Administration (FDA) overseeing all phases of medicine testing and administration has no power for enforcing a limitation they place on drugs, such as a black box. If a doctor decides to ignore the rules – and this happened to me in an ER – the average patient is helpless. No regulatory office can stop a doctor from prescribing the wrong medicine if he or she believes it to be helpful, even if the FDA doesn't agree. An FDA representative told me the following "*we create the rules but have no power to enforce them.*" There is also the problem of advertising prescription medicines to patients on TV. Prescription medicines should be within the realm of the prescribing doctor without any coercive influence by pharmaceuticals.

As long as any doctor has the right to override FDA rules, there is not much incentive for proper and ethical conduct on the part of the participating researchers and pharmaceuticals either. I have found that a good 90% of all medicines prescribed for migraineurs are prescribed off-label without the knowledge of the patient. While off-label prescriptions are legal, I personally question the right of any doctor to conduct an experiment without the express written consent of the patient, and a full disclosure that the treatment is off-label and experimental.

If I applied for a permit to run a clinical trial for the Stanton Migraine Protocol®, I would have to obtain an ethical review board approval, which can take over a year to receive. Thus, while a medical provider can experiment with an off-label medicine without receiving any ethical permit and patient consent, a researcher cannot. I personally find this very distasteful and sneaky.

An additional problem is that the FDA approves drugs without proper testing and also removes warnings that the patients (and doctors) should know! Here is an example:

> *"On June 21, 2016, the FDA announced the approval of a supplemental New Drug Application (sNDA) modifying the REMS for Sabril [a new medicine]. The FDA determined that, although the risk of vision loss with Sabril still exists, the REMS should be modified to remove certain elements.*
>
> ***Sabril was approved with a risk evaluation and mitigation strategy (REMS) to ensure that the benefits of Sabril outweigh the risks of vision loss and of suicidal thoughts***

and behaviors. Sabril can cause permanent bilateral concentric visual field constriction, including tunnel vision that can result in disability. In some cases, it also can damage the central retina and may decrease visual acuity. *Since approval, the REMS has required periodic visual monitoring results to be documented through submission of ophthalmologic assessment forms (OAFs).*

The FDA has determined that requiring submission of OAFs as an element of the REMS is no longer necessary to ensure the benefits of Sabril outweigh its risks. *Prescribers should continue to follow the vision monitoring recommendations described in the prescribing information for Sabril. As a condition of certification in the REMS, prescribers must agree to ensure that periodic visual monitoring is conducted as described in the product label,* ***but they will no longer be required to submit OAFs as a part of the REMS.***

The FDA is also modifying the REMS to remove additional education requirements about the risk of suicidal thoughts and behaviors because this risk is adequately communicated in the Warnings and Precautions section and the Medication Guide of the current FDA-approved prescribing information.

In addition, the FDA is eliminating the patient registry as an element of the REMS because the related postmarketing

> ***study*** [understand: off-label use]***, which is a postmarketing requirement (PMR), is a better mechanism for further characterizing and assessing the risk of vision loss associated with Sabril.***
>
> ***Finally, the REMS is being modified to allow for inpatient pharmacy certification in order to alleviate delays in initiating treatment with Sabril and interruptions in treatment during hospitalizations.*** *" (emphasis added by me)*
>
> *(http://www.fda.gov/Drugs/DrugSafety/PostmarketDrugSafetyInformationforPatientsandProviders/ucm507990.htm?source=govdelivery&utm_medium=email&utm_source=govdelivery).*
>
> (Last accessed in this form on 9/21/2016)

Sabril is an anticonvulsant, used to treat seizures. Given the number of seizure medicines already available, an accelerated green light for a drug with known major side effects that can cause permanent vision loss and suicide is highly questionable, particularly as it ignores even the subsequent analysis of efficacy. Note that here the FDA bypassed all its own regulations, even though the medicine in question causes very serious, debilitating, permanent damage, and even fatality. Why did the FDA go against all its own earlier regulations? One can only speculate… and I do.

Sabril is an anticonvulsant medicine, and although migraines are not the same as seizures, a very large percent of migraineurs are put on anticonvulsants (none works of course) with horrendous adverse effects and permanent brain damage. I just know that I will have to save the lives and sights of hundreds of migraineurs who will be put on this medication. Why would they be put on this medication instead of others? Simple: brand name medicines bring more money to doctors, medical facilities, hospitals, pharmaceutical companies, and pharmacies, and rest assured that the pharmaceutical company producing Sabril had put great pressure on the FDA to get the approval, and will also put great pressure on doctors to prescribe this drug.

On the positive side, there are doctors who stick to their oath. Here is a testimonial I received from one of my members with a funny twist at the end, when her doctor prescribed the Stanton Migraine Protocol® to be continued as a treatment:

> *"So, I went to see my PCP today… I told him all about Dr Stanton's protocol. He could not believe I was off my topamax, botox and zomig. I explained that I went from 25 migraines per month to an occasional [one] which unfortunately [this time] was really bad only because I gambled with carbs. I could tell by his facial expression that he thought it was crazy when I mentioned [the Stanton Migraine Protocol]. After I explained, he said he was very interested in this. I said that I know this is*

against everything he probably learned in med school but sugar is the enemy, not salt. I showed him my salt pills. He said that the proof was in the fact that undeniably, it's working. He wrote down the name of the book. And he typed on his laptop on my chart 'to continue Stanton Migraine Protocol salt therapy'. Next, the nurse who came in was so intrigued she asked for the name of the book because she had been struggling all day with a migraine."

--CS

Drugs Prescribed to Migraineurs

In my desire to incorporate other sufferers' symptoms and issues while writing this book, I learned a lot from the migraine group members about the medicines they use and the problems those medicines cause. The following section introduces the readers to the medicines that migraineurs are most often prescribed. Most of the medicines listed here set off severe adverse effects that are often so permanent that even after quitting them, though free of migraines, the migraineur may sustain debilitating lifelong brain or heart damage. I have added this section of the book specifically to inform doctors who prescribe these drugs, so they fully understand the kind of harm they cause. I strongly advise all migraineurs to refuse all of the drugs listed in the next section. Since most doctors are not migraineurs, they may honestly have no idea what these medicines do, and they certainly don't recall how they work and what they may interact with. Furthermore, I also want to highlight a problem that doctors or pharmacists should be aware of but they seem to ignore: drug interactions. Check for drug interactions at:

https://www.drugs.com/drug_interactions.html

The quantity and variety of medications migraine sufferers are taking — often like candy — is shocking. Often one medicine can cancel the effects of another one already prescribed, or amplify or duplicate (therapeutic duplication) another one, thereby overdose the migraineur. Some medicines, when taken with other medicines, can be fatal—the killing need not be instantaneous but over time the migraineur's body will simply give up. I have seen doctors prescribing a variety of medicines to migraineurs that cause severe side effects even in low doses, yet doctors keep on increasing the dose anyway, even when the patient says the medicine is not working and/or is making them ill. While the intention of "more is better" maybe good for some things in life, medicine is not one of them. Not only am I against certain medicines but I am also against irresponsible doctors who prescribe them. Often little mistakes can cause serious side effects and even permanent damage. Doctors should know better.

This section is not going to be pharmaceutical friendly. Medicines have their place in life but migraineurs do better without medicines if given the proper care for their special brain.

The five medication types most often prescribed are as follows.

1. Anti-seizure medications – voltage gated calcium channel blockers
2. Reuptake inhibitors (SSRIs, SNRIs)
3. Simple serotonin meds (triptans)
4. Beta blockers – heart medications
5. Opioids, narcotics, and barbiturates

There are of course other types of medicines migraineurs may receive but not as often as the ones on this list. Rather than review the medicines in these categories, I am posting them in the order of prescription frequency per the migraineurs' reports and records in the FB migraine group. For simplicity, the general description of the medicine is either taken from Wikipedia or from the FDA; my personal comments and explanations are added here and there.

Section 13

The Drugs of Migraine Shame

America does not have a health care system; what modern medicine has created is an illness maintenance system.

--Morris Hyman, M.D.

In this section I list 30 medications that are most often prescribed to migraineurs; all of them are harmful. Many of these are prescribed off label but since medicine status changes I only incorporate that note on a few. I excluded most triptans; it goes without saying that there is no diagnosed migraineur on the planet for whom at least one type of triptan has not been prescribed. I also didn't include all narcotics and barbiturates since there is also hardly a migraineur without receiving at least one. I only selected here the top 30 that I find the most unnecessary, the most unlikely to work, and the most likely to cause harm. If you are a prescribing doctor, please take note: do not prescribe any of the following medications to your migraineur patient. Chances are you will be hated and exchanged for another doctor at the first opportunity as the migraineur starts to have the side effects of these drugs or if she decides to reduce and quit them.

Topamax (Topiramate)

Topamax is unique because it is a fructose derivative (recall that fructose is the sweetest part of sugar that converts to triglycerides), which is unusual for a medicine that is prescribed for so many health conditions. As with many other medicines provided to migraineurs, this medicine falls into the category of "we don't know how it works". What we do know is that it blocks high voltage gated calcium and voltage gated sodium channels that are essential to the function of brain cells [874,875]. It affects the whole body because it is systemic and doesn't differentiate between cells. It also affects GABA-$_A$ receptors – major inhibitory neurotransmitters in the brain. When activated, the $GABA_A$ receptor pushes negatively charged chloride Cl^- through the membrane, causing hyperpolarization (makes the cell more negatively charged). This prevents action potential, which is the critical element in opening voltage gated pumps. It also blocks AMPA/kainate (glutamate) receptors and carbonic anhydrase, an enzyme that converts carbon dioxide and water to bicarbonate. Beyond the general mental deterioration, the most significant adverse side effect is a change in the thermal maintenance of the body. Many migraineurs taking Topamax are not able to regulate their body temperature and thus cannot go on the sun or go out in the winter. For some this had become a permanent adverse effect even after stopping treatment. Read all about it here:

https://www.hormonesmatter.com/topamax-drug-nine-lives/

Known adverse effects as per clinical trial:

- Acute myopia and secondary angle closure glaucoma: Untreated elevated intraocular pressure can lead to permanent visual loss.
- Visual field defects: These have been reported independent of elevated intraocular pressure.
- Oligohidrosis and hyperthermia: Monitor decreased sweating and increased body temperature, especially in pediatric patients
- Metabolic acidosis: Baseline and periodic measurement of serum bicarbonate is recommended.
- Suicidal behavior and ideation: Antiepileptic drugs increase the risk of suicidal behavior or ideation
- Cognitive/neuropsychiatric: TOPAMAX may cause cognitive dysfunction. Depression and mood problems may occur in epilepsy and migraine populations
- Fetal Toxicity: TOPAMAX use during pregnancy can cause cleft lip and/or palate
- Withdrawal of AEDs: Withdrawal of TOPAMAX should be done gradually

- Hyperammonemia and encephalopathy associated with or without concomitant valproic acid use: Patients with inborn errors of metabolism or reduced mitochondrial activity may have an increased risk of hyperammonemia.
- Kidney stones: Use with other carbonic anhydrase inhibitors, other drugs causing metabolic acidosis, or in patients on a ketogenic diet should be avoided
- Hypothermia has been reported with and without hyperammonemia during topiramate treatment with concomitant valproic acid use

The most common adverse reactions at recommended dosing in adults and adolescents in controlled migraine clinical trials were paresthesia, anorexia, weight decrease, difficulty with memory, taste perversion, upper respiratory tract infection, abdominal pain, diarrhea, hypoesthesia, and nausea.

Adverse effects post clinical trial as reported by patients to the FDA: Dizziness, Weight loss, Paresthesia, Somnolence, Nausea, Diarrhea, Fatigue, Nasopharyngitis, Depression, Weight gain, Anemia, Disturbance in attention, Memory impairment, Amnesia, Cognitive disorder, Mental impairment, Psychomotor skills impaired, Convulsion, Coordination abnormal, Tremor, Lethargy, Hypoaesthesia, Nystagmus, Dysgeusia, Balance disorder, Dysarthria, Intention tremor, Sedation, Vision blurred, Diplopia, Visual disturbance, Vertigo, Tinnitus, Ear pain, Dyspnoea, Epistaxis, Nasal congestion, Rhinorrhoea, Vomiting, Constipation, Abdominal pain, Dyspepsia, Dry mouth, Stomach discomfort, Paraesthesia oral, Gastritis, Abdominal discomfort, Nephrolithiasis, Pollakisuria, Dysuria, Alopecia, Rash, Pruritus, Arthralgia, Muscle spasms, Myalgia, Muscle twitching, Muscular weakness, Musculoskeletal chest pain, Anorexia, Decreased appetite, Pyrexia, Asthenia, Irritability, Gait disturbance, Feeling abnormal, Malaise, Hypersensitivity, Bradyphrenia, Insomnia, Expressive language disorder, Anxiety, Confusional state, Disorientation, Aggression, Mood altered, Agitation, Mood swings, Anger, Abnormal behavior, Crystal urine present, Tandem gait test abnormal, White blood cell count decreased, Bradycardia, Sinus bradycardia, Palpitations, Leucopenia, Thrombocytopenia, Lymphadenopathy, Eosinophilia, Depressed level of consciousness, Grand mal convulsion, Visual field defect, Complex partial seizures, Speech disorder, Psychomotor hyperactivity, Syncope, sensory disturbance, Drooling, Hypersomnia, Aphasia, Repetitive speech, Hypokinesia, Dyskinesia, Dizziness postural, Poor quality sleep, Burning sensation, Sensory loss, Parosmia, Cerebellar syndrome, Dysaesthesia, Hypogeusia, Stupor, Clumsiness, Aura, Ageusia, Dysgraphia, Dysphasia, Neuropathy peripheral, Presyncope, Dystonia, Formication, Visual acuity reduced, Scotoma, Myopia, Abnormal sensation in eye, Dry eye, Photophobia, Blepharospasm, Lacrimation, Photopsia, Mydriasis, Presbyopia, Deafness, Deafness unilateral and neurosensory, Ear discomfort, Hearing impaired, Dyspnea exertional, Paranasal sinus hypersecretion, Dysphonia, Pancreatitis, Flatulence, Gastroesophageal reflux disease, Hypoesthesia oral gingival bleeding, Abdominal distension, Epigastric discomfort, Abdominal tenderness, Salivary hypersecretion, Oral pain, Breath odor, Glossodynia, Calculus urinary, Urinary incontinence, Hematuria, Incontinence, Micturition urgency, Renal colic, Renal pain, Anhidrosis, Hypoesthesia facial, Urticaria, Erythema, Pruritus generalized, Rash macular, Skin discoloration, Allergic dermatitis, Swelling face, Joint swelling, Musculoskeletal stiffness, Flank pain, Muscle fatigue, Metabolic acidosis, Hypokalemia, Increased appetite, Polydipsia, Hypotension, Orthostatic hypotension flushing, Hot flush, Hyperthermia, Thirst, Influenza like illness, Sluggishness, Peripheral coldness, Feeling drunk, Feeling jittery, Learning disability, Erectile dysfunction, Sexual dysfunction, Suicidal ideation, Suicide attempt, Hallucination, Psychotic disorder, Apathy, Lack of spontaneous speech, Sleep disorder, Affect lability, Libido decreased, Restlessness, Crying, Dysphemia, Euphoric mood, Paranoia, Perseveration, Panic attack, Tearfulness, Reading disorder, Initial insomnia, Flat affect, Thinking abnormal, Loss of libido, Listless, Middle insomnia, Distractibility, Early morning awakening, Panic reaction, Elevated mood, Blood bicarbonate decreased, Neutropenia, Apraxia, Circadian rhythm sleep disorder, Hyperesthesia, Hyposmia, Anosmia, Essential tremor, Akinesia, Unresponsive to stimuli, Blindness unilateral, Blindness transient, Glaucoma, Accommodation disorder, Altered visual depth perception, Scintillating scotoma, Eyelid edema, Night blindness, Amblyopia, Calculus ureteric, Renal tubular acidosis, Stevens-Johnson syndrome, Erythema multiforme, abnormal skin odor, Periorbital edema, Urticaria localized, Limb discomfort, Acidosis hyperchloremic, Raynaud's phenomenon, Face edema, Calcinosis, Mania, Anorgasmia, Panic disorder, Disturbance in sexual arousal, Feeling of despair, Orgasm abnormal, Hypomania, Orgasmic sensation decreased (Wikipedia).

As listed in the 06/29/2005 label posted at the Drugs@FDA website page 14, "conditions or therapies that predispose to acidosis may be additive to the bicarbonate lowering effects of Topiramate"[6].

Overdose: Fatalities have occurred as the result of multiple medicine exposure. (Most new migraineurs joining my group always take multiple drugs with Topamax.)

Symptoms of overdose: Agitation, Depression, Speech problems, Blurred vision, double vision, Troubled thinking, Loss of coordination, Inability to respond to things around you, Loss of consciousness, Confusion and coma, Fainting, Upset stomach and stomach pain, Loss of appetite and vomiting, Shortness of breath; fast, shallow breathing, Pounding or irregular heartbeat, Muscle weakness, Bone pain, Seizures. (Several migraineurs ended up getting seizures from Topamax.)

The latest information on Topamax:

http://www.fda.gov/Safety/MedWatch/SafetyInformation/ucm195797.htm

---

6 This I found especially interesting since many epileptic patients (particularly children) who are started on the ketogenic diet (high acidosis level for a reason) are usually concurrently kept on their anticonvulsant medication, including Topamax. It is noted by the FDA that such practice is dangerous but practitioners still maintain that the use of medicines like Topamax is necessary together with the ketogenic diet, which on its own is capable to treat and often cure seizures.

Gabapentin (Neurontin)

Gabapentin was originally developed to treat epilepsy, but it is now also used for neuropathic pain, migraine, and restless leg syndrome. Gabapentin mimics the chemical structure of the neurotransmitter gamma-aminobutyric acid (GABA), but is believed to act on different brain receptors. Gabapentin reduces calcium currents via blocking the voltage-gated calcium channels in the central nervous system. Gabapentin also halts the formation of new synapses—this is brain degenerative.

Adverse effects: dizziness, fatigue, drowsiness, weight gain, peripheral edema (swelling of extremities), sexual dysfunction, loss of libido, inability to reach orgasm, erectile dysfunction, renal impairment due to possible accumulation and toxicity, adenocarcinomas (cancerous cells), induce pancreatic acinar cell carcinomas, suicide. In 2009 the U.S. Food and Drug Administration issued a warning of an increased risk of depression and suicidal thoughts and behaviors in patients taking gabapentin. A 2010 meta-analysis confirmed the increased risk of suicide associated with gabapentin use.

Pregabalin (Lyrica)

An anticonvulsant drug used for neuropathic pain and as an adjunct therapy for partial seizures. It is a more potent successor to gabapentin and has anxiolytic effects similar to benzodiazepines.

Adverse effects: Blurred vision, diplopia, increased appetite, weight gain, euphoria, confusion, vivid dreams, changes in libido (increase or decrease), irritability, ataxia, attention changes, abnormal coordination, memory impairment, tremors, dysarthria, parasthesia, vertigo, dry mouth, constipation, vomiting, flatulence, erectile dysfunction, fatigue, peripheral edema, drunkenness, abnormal walking, asthenia, nasopharyngitis, increased creatine kinase level, depression, lethargy, agitation, anorgasmia, excessive salivation, sweating, flushing, hallucinations, myoclonus, hypoaesthesia, urinary incontinence, hyperaesthesia, tachycardia, myalgia, hypoglycaemia, neutropenia, muscle cramp, rash, arthralgia, dysuria, hypotension, thrombocytopenia, kidney calculus, first degree heart block, hypertension, pancreatitis, dysphagia, oliguria, rhabdomyolysis, suicidal thoughts or behavior.

Pregabalin blocks voltage-dependent calcium channels, thereby decreasing the release of neurotransmitters including glutamate, norepinephrine, substance P and calcitonin gene-related peptide. Pregabalin is a Schedule V drug, and is classified as a CNS depressant.

Withdrawal symptoms include insomnia, headache, nausea, anxiety, diarrhea, flu syndrome, nervousness, depression, pain, convulsion, hyperhidrosis and dizziness.

Nortriptyline (Sensoval, Aventyl, Pamelor, Norpress, Allegron, Noritren and Nortrilen)

A second-generation tricyclic antidepressant (TCA). It is FDA approved for major depression and childhood nocturnal enuresis. For anything else, such as migraines, it is used off-label.

The FDA black-boxed Nortriptyline with the following note:

> *"Suicidality and Antidepressant Drugs Antidepressants increased the risk compared to placebo of suicidal thinking and behavior (suicidality) in children, adolescents, and young adults in short-term studies of major depressive disorder (MDD) and other psychiatric disorders. Anyone considering the use of Nortriptyline Hydrochloride Oral Solution or any other antidepressant in a child, adolescent, or young adult must balance this risk with the clinical need. Short-term studies did not show an increase in the risk of suicidality with antidepressants compared to placebo in adults beyond age 24; there was a reduction in risk with antidepressants compared to placebo in adults aged 65 and older. Depression and certain other psychiatric disorders are themselves associated with increases in the risk of suicide. Patients of all ages who are started on antidepressant therapy should be monitored appropriately and observed closely for clinical worsening, suicidality, or unusual changes in behavior. Families and caregivers should be advised of the need for close observation and communication with the prescriber. Nortriptyline hydrochloride is not approved for use in pediatric patients. (See Warnings: Clinical Worsening*

and Suicide Risk, Precautions: Information for Patients, and Precautions: Pediatric Use)" from FDA label found here:

http://www.accessdata.fda.gov/drugsatfda_docs/label/2007/014685s028lbl.pdf

"Prescribers or other health professionals should inform patients, their families, and their caregivers about the benefits and risks associated with treatment with nortriptyline hydrochloride and should counsel them in its appropriate use." From the same as above, which healthcare professionals rarely if ever observe. Furthermore, *"A subset (3% to 10%) of the population has reduced activity of certain drug metabolizing enzymes such as the cytochrome P450 isoenzyme P450IID6. Such NDAs 14-685/S-028 individuals are referred to as "poor metabolizers" of drugs such as debrisoquin, dextromethorphan, and the tricyclic antidepressants. These individuals may have higher than expected plasma concentrations of tricyclic antidepressants when given usual doses. In addition, certain drugs that are metabolized by this isoenzyme, including many antidepressants (tricyclic antidepressants, selective serotonin reuptake inhibitors, and others), may inhibit the activity of this isoenzyme, and thus may make normal metabolizers resemble poor metabolizers with regard to concomitant therapy with other drugs metabolized by this enzyme system, leading to drug interactions."*

Based on this, patients who are prescribed Nortriptyline should be tested for the genetic mutations of P450 isoenzyme P450IID6, which I have yet to see happen. Of the clinical trial adverse reactions, one type of adverse reaction is worthy to note: "*Cardiovascular--Hypotension, hypertension, tachycardia, palpitation, myocardial infarction, arrhythmias, heart block, stroke.*" Nortriptyline can cause irregular heartbeat, and both increase and decrease blood pressure. Nortriptyline thus damages the heart. Migraineurs in general have low blood pressure and healthy hearts before taking Nortriptyline.

Additional adverse effects include dry mouth, sedation, constipation, increased appetite, mild blurred vision, tinnitus, euphoria, mania. Nortriptyline should not be prescribed to those with thyroid problems treated with thyroid medications; to those with a history of cardiovascular disease, stroke, glaucoma, or seizures. Most importantly, nortriptyline blocks sodium channels thereby preventing hydration. This can cause migraines, making its prescription for migraines a very bad choice.

Escitalopram (Lexapro)

An SSRI that can cause serious serotonin toxicity in people who take more than one kind of serotonin—including triptans.

Adverse effects: Headache, Nausea, Ejaculation disorder, Somnolence, Insomnia, Dizziness, Paresthesia, Tremor, Decreased appetite, Increased appetite, Anxiety, Restlessness, Abnormal dreams, Libido decreased, Anorgasmia, Sinusitis, Yawning, Diarrhea, Constipation,

Vomiting, Dry mouth, Excessive sweating, Arthralgia, Myalgia, Fatigue, Pyrexia (fever), Ejaculation disorder, erectile dysfunction.

Reduction causes serious brain zaps, loss of memory, and brain freeze. Extreme slow reduction is recommended.

Elavil (Amitriptyline)

The second most prescribed "dirty drug" on our list. It is a serotonin-norepinephrine reuptake inhibitor (SNRI) that acts on multiple serotonin, histamine, mACh (acetylcholine), δ_1 (calcium signaling), and α_1-adrenergic (noradrenaline and adrenaline) receptors. It also inhibits sodium channels, L-type calcium channels, Kv1.1, Kv7.2, and Kv7.3 voltage-gated potassium channels. It also affects TrkA (nerve growth factor) and TrkB (brain-derived neurotrophic factor) receptors. It is a functional inhibitor of acid sphingomyelinase (a major element in the production of ceramide in the cellular response to stress, such as environment, pathogens, and other irritants). It crosses the blood brain barrier, thereby capable to affect many of the CNS receptors. An important note for those with genetic mutations of CYP2D6 and CYP2C19 enzymes (common in migraineurs): these mutations cause reduced metabolic speed of Amitriptyline and can cause more serious side effects than they do to the general population. To date, I have yet to see a doctor asking for a test of these two possible genetic mutations to find out if their patients could be at risk for major adverse effects.

Adverse effects: Poor coordination, Dementia, Decreased mucus production in the nose and throat, dry sore throat, Dry-mouth with possible acceleration of dental caries, Stopping of sweating, warm blotchy or red skin, Increased body temperature, Pupil dilation, Loss of accommodation (loss of focusing ability, blurred vision – cycloplegia), Double-vision, Increased heart rate, Tendency to be easily startled, Urinary retention, Diminished bowel movement, sometimes ileus (decreases motility via the vagus nerve), Increased intraocular pressure; dangerous for people with narrow-angle glaucoma, delirium, Confusion, Disorientation, Agitation, Euphoria or dysphoria, Respiratory depression, Memory problems, Inability to concentrate, Wandering thoughts, inability to sustain a train of thought, Incoherent speech, Irritability, Mental confusion (brain fog), Wakeful myoclonic jerking, Unusual sensitivity to sudden sounds, Illogical thinking, Photophobia, Visual disturbances, Periodic flashes of light, Periodic changes in visual field, Visual snow, Restricted or "tunnel vision", Visual, auditory, or other sensory hallucinations, Warping or waving of surfaces and edges, Textured surfaces, "Dancing" lines, "spiders", insects, Lifelike objects indistinguishable from reality, Phantom smoking, Hallucinated presence of people not actually there, seizures, coma, and death (rare), Orthostatic hypotension, Older patients are at a higher risk of experiencing CNS side effects due to lower acetylcholine production.

Fluoxetine (Prozac)

An antidepressant of the selective serotonin reuptake inhibitor (SSRI) class.

Adverse effects: abnormal dreams, abnormal ejaculation, anorexia, anxiety, asthenia, diarrhea, dry mouth, dyspepsia, flu syndrome, impotence, insomnia, decreased libido, nausea, nervousness, pharyngitis, rash, sinusitis, somnolence, sweating, tremor, vasodilatation, and yawning. Fluoxetine is considered the most stimulating of the SSRIs. It also appears to be the most prone of the SSRIs for producing dermatologic reactions (e.g. urticaria (hives), rash, itchiness, etc.), sexual dysfunction, including loss of libido, anorgasmia, lack of vaginal lubrication, and erectile dysfunction. Symptoms of sexual dysfunction have been reported to persist after discontinuing SSRIs, although this is thought to be rare. Fluoxetine has been found to act as an agonist of the σ1-receptor, with a potency greater than that of citalopram but less than that of fluvoxamine. Fluoxetine also functions as an anoctamin 1 channel blocker, a calcium-activated chloride channel. In addition, it acts as a positive allosteric modulator of the GABAA receptor at high concentrations, actions which may be clinically-relevant. A number of other ion channels, including nicotinic acetylcholine receptors and 5-HT3 receptors, are also known to be inhibited at similar concentrations.

Seroquel (Quetiapine)

An atypical antipsychotic approved for the treatment of schizophrenia, bipolar disorder, and together with an antidepressant to treat major depressive disorder—it is used off-label for migraines. Seroquel is a dopamine, serotonin, and adrenergic antagonist and a potent antihistamine. It binds strongly to serotonin receptors; the drug acts as partial agonist at 5-HT1A receptors. Some of the antagonized receptors (serotonin, norepinephrine) are autoreceptors whose blockage tends to increase the release of neurotransmitters.

> *"Approximately 10,000 lawsuits have been filed against AstraZeneca alleging that Seroquel caused problems ranging from slurred speech and chronic insomnia to deaths."*

Adverse effects: Dry mouth, Dizziness, Headache, Somnolence, High blood pressure, Orthostatic hypotension, High pulse rate, High blood cholesterol, Elevated serum triglycerides, Abdominal pain, Constipation, Increased appetite, Vomiting, Increased liver enzymes, Backache, Asthenia, Insomnia, Lethargy, Tremor, Agitation, Nasal congestion, Pharyngitis, Fatigue, Pain, Dyspepsia, Peripheral edema, Dysphagia, Extrapyramidal disease, Weight gain, Prolonged QT interval, Sudden cardiac death, Syncope, Diabetic ketoacidosis, Restless legs syndrome, Hyponatraemia, Jaundice, Pancreatitis, Agranulocytosis, a potentially fatal drop in white blood cell count, Leukopenia, Neutropenia, Eosinophilia, Anaphylaxis, a potentially fatal allergic reaction, seizure, Hypothyroidism, underactive thyroid gland, Myocarditis, swelling of the myocardium., Cardiomyopathy, Hepatitis, swelling of the liver, Suicidal ideation, Priapism, prolonged and painful erection, Stevens-Johnson syndrome, a potentially fatal skin reaction, Neuroleptic malignant syndrome (a rare and potentially fatal complication of antipsychotic drug treatment characterized by the following symptoms: tremor, rigidity, hyperthermia, tachycardia, mental status changes), Tardive Dyskinesia.

This drug changes dopamine, serotonin, adrenergic and histamine receptor sites in the central nervous system.

Propranolol (Inderal)

It is the number one drug recognized by medical professionals as a "dirty drug". It is a beta blocker originally created for heart conditions, such as hypertension and heart arrhythmia. Propranolol crosses the blood brain barrier and as a non-selective beta blocker affects the entire central nervous system (CNS). It blocks epinephrine (adrenaline) and norepinephrine (noradrenaline) at both β1- and β2-adrenergic receptors (it can create breathing difficulties and for those with asthma can be fatal). It indirectly affects α1-adrenoceptor as an agonist in addition to potent β-adrenoceptor antagonist actions. Furthermore, it may function as an antagonist of the serotonin receptors: 5-HT1A and 5-HT1B. It also blocks cardiac, neuronal, and skeletal voltage-gated sodium channels, triggering antiarrhythmic, and some undesirable CNS effects[876]. The titration of Propranolol is impossible without a step-down heart medicine, such as Atenolol (Tenormin), which controls heart arrhythmia and reduces the irregular blood pressure that follows the discontinuation of Propranolol. In many cases, those placed on Propranolol are unable to quit, yet it doesn't help migraines and it destroys the heart. Please do not ever prescribe this drug to a migraineur!

Adverse effect: nausea, diarrhea, bronchospasm, dyspnea, cold extremities, exacerbation of Raynaud's syndrome, bradycardia, hypotension, heart failure, heart block, fatigue, dizziness, alopecia (hair loss), abnormal vision, hallucinations, insomnia, nightmares, sexual dysfunction, erectile dysfunction, alteration of glucose and lipid metabolism, orthostatic hypotension, edema, sleep disturbances, insomnia, vivid dreams and nightmares, bronchospasm, peripheral vasoconstriction, hyponatremia, hyperkalemia, hypoglycemia, lowers plasma glucose, masks fast heart rate that serves as a warning sign for insulin-induced low blood sugar, resulting in hypoglycemia unawareness (known as beta blocker induced hypoglycemia unawareness). Beta blockers increase the risk of diabetes mellitus. Blockade of only beta receptors increases blood pressure, reduces coronary blood flow, left ventricular function, and cardiac output and tissue perfusion. Beta blockers are contraindicated in patients with asthma and should also be avoided in patients with a history of cocaine use or in cocaine-induced tachycardia.

Relpax (Eletriptan)

It is a second generation triptan. Eletriptan is *believed* to reduce swelling of the blood vessels surrounding the brain. Eletriptan is a selective 5-hydroxytryptamine receptor agonist. It is contraindicated in patients with diseases of the heart and circulatory system as well as in patients who had a stroke or heart attack in the past. It is also contraindicated in severe renal or hepatic impairment.

Adverse effects hypertension, tachycardia, headache, dizziness, and symptoms similar to angina pectoris.

Fioricet (Esgic)

A combination of butalbital with or without codeine, acetaminophen (Tylenol) and caffeine; indicated for tension headaches, muscle contraction headaches, and post-dural puncture headaches. It is often used off-label to treat migraines.

Adverse effects: Euphoria, Dizziness, Drowsiness, Intoxicated feeling, Light-headedness, Nausea, Vomiting, Shortness of breath, Sedation, Substance dependence, Abdominal pain, Stevens–Johnson syndrome, an adverse reaction to barbiturates. Fioricet is known to cause rebound headaches.

Frovatriptan (Frova)

Frovatriptan inhibits excessive dilation of arteries with a half-life of 26 hours.

Adverse effects: affects the heart with coronary artery vasospasm, transient myocardial ischemia, myocardial infarction, ventricular tachycardia, and ventricular fibrillation; and thus can cause major heart problems. It also causes major rebound headaches.

Venlafaxine (Effexor)

An antidepressant that is prescribed with amazing frequency and off label to migraineurs. It is a serotonin-norepinephrine-dopamine reuptake inhibitor (SNDRI). Venlafaxine is used primarily for the treatment of depression, general anxiety disorder, social phobia, panic disorder and vasomotor symptoms. Suicide is the most common side effect!

Adverse effects: Headache, Nausea, Insomnia, Asthenia (weakness), Dizziness, Ejaculation disorder, Somnolence, Dry mouth, Sweating, Constipation, Nervousness, Abnormal vision, Tremor, Anorgasmia, Hypertension, Impotence, Paresthesia, Vasodilation, Vomiting, Weight loss, Chills, Palpitations, Confusion, Depersonalisation, Night sweats, Menstrual disorders associated with increased bleeding or increased irregular bleeding, Urinary frequency increased, Abnormal dreams, Decreased libido, Increased muscle tonus, Yawning, Sweating, Abnormality of accommodation, Abnormal ejaculation/orgasm (males), Urinary hesitancy, Serum cholesterol increased, Face edema, Intentional injury, Malaise, Moniliasis, Neck rigidity, Pelvic pain, Photosensitivity reaction, Suicide attempt, Withdrawal syndrome, Hypotension, Postural hypotension (POTS), Syncope, Tachycardia, Bruxism, Ecchymosis, Mucous membrane bleeding, Gastrointestinal bleeding, Abnormal liver function tests, Hyponatraemia, Weight gain, Apathy, Hallucinations, Myoclonus, Rash, Abnormal orgasm, Urinary retention, Angioedema, Agitation, Impaired coordination & balance, Alopecia (hair loss), Tinnitus, Proteinuria, Syndrome of inappropriate antidiuretic hormone secretion (SIADH), Thrombocytopenia, Prolonged bleeding time, Seizures, Mania, Neuroleptic malignant syndrome (NMS), Serotonin syndrome, Akathisia/psychomotor restlessness, Urinary incontinence, Anaphylaxis, QT prolongation, Ventricular fibrillation, Ventricular tachycardia (including torsades de pointes), Pancreatitis, Blood dyscrasias (including agranulocytosis, aplastic anaemia, neutropenia and pancytopenia), Elevated serum prolactin, Delirium, Extrapyramidal reactions (including dystonia and dyskinesia), Tardive dyskinesia, Pulmonary eosinophilia, Erythema multiforme, Stevens-Johnson syndrome, Pruritus, Urticaria, Toxic epidermal necrolysis, Angle closure glaucoma.

It is metabolized in the body into desvenlafaxine, which is an antidepressant under the brand name Pristiq. There is a high suicide rate with Effexor and is black boxed: "*A study conducted in Finland followed more than 15,000 patients for 3.4 years. Venlafaxine increased suicide risk by 60% (statistically significant), as compared to no treatment.*" Venlafaxine may lower the seizure threshold – i.e. it increases seizures. Venlafaxine acts as an opioid. Frequent effects (after quitting Effexor) is "flashback" syndrome. Patients stopping venlafaxine commonly experience extreme SSRI discontinuation syndrome.

Trazodone (Desyrel, Oleptro)

An antidepressant of the serotonin antagonist and reuptake inhibitor (SARI) class. It is a phenylpiperazine compound. Trazodone also has antianxiety (anxiolytic) and sleep-inducing (hypnotic) effects. For many patients, the relief from agitation, anxiety, and insomnia can be rapid; for other patients, including those individuals with considerable psychomotor retardation and feelings of low energy, therapeutic doses of trazodone may not be tolerable because of sedation.

Adverse effects: orthostatic hypotension, Mania in patients with bipolar disorder, as well as in patients with previous diagnoses of unipolar depression, Cardiac arrhythmia, Priapism, hepatotoxicity, Blurred vision, Dizziness, Somnolence, Dry mouth, Nausea, Headache, Fatigue, Vomiting, Constipation, Diarrhea, Backache, Confusion, Insomnia, Dream disorder, Disorientation, Incoordination, Nasal congestion, Orthostatic hypotension, Syncope, Tremor, Weight change, Nervous, Hypotension, Edema, Coordination abnormal, Dysgeusia, Memory impairment, Migraine, Paraesthesia, Agitation, Confusional state, Disorientation, Micturition urgency, Dyspnoea, Night sweats, Hypersensitivity reaction, Muscle twitching, Amnesia, Aphasia, Hypoesthesia, Speech disorder, Bladder pain, Urinary incontinence, Gait disturbance, Reflux oesophagitis, Dry eye, Eye pain, Photophobia, Hypoacusis, Tinnitus, Vertigo, Acne, Hyperhidrosis, Photosensitivity reaction, Flushing, Urinary retention, Prolonged QT interval, Torsades de Pointes, Ataxia, Breast enlargement or engorgement, Lactation, Cardiospasm, Stroke, Chills, Cholestasis, Clitorism, Congestive heart failure, Diplopia, Extrapyramidal symptoms, Hallucinations, Haemolytic anaemia, Hirsutism, Hyperbilirubinaemia, Increased amylase, Increased salivation, Leukocytosis, Leukonychia, Jaundice, Liver enzyme alterations, Methemoglobinemia, Paranoid reaction, Stupor, Rash, Seizure, Priapism, Pruritus, Psoriasis, Psychosis, Suicidal ideation, Suicidal behavior, Syndrome of inappropriate antidiuretic hormone secretion, Tardive dyskinesia, Serotonin syndrome, Unexplained death, Urticaria, Vasodilation

Tramadol (Ultram)

An opioid medication used to treat moderate to severe pain. It has two different mechanisms. First, it binds to the μ-opioid receptor. Second, it inhibits the reuptake of serotonin and norepinephrine so it is an SNRI.

Adverse effects: Liver and kidney failure is very common! Dizziness, Nausea, Constipation, Vertigo, Headache, Vomiting, Somnolence, Agitation, Anxiety, Emotional lability, Euphoria, Nervousness, Spasticity, Dyspepsia, Asthenia, Pruritus, Dry mouth, Diarrhea, Fatigue, Sweating, Malaise, Vasodilation, Confusion, Coordination disturbance, Miosis, Sleep disorder, Rash, Hypertonia, Abdominal pain, Weight loss, Visual disturbance, Flatulence, Menopausal symptoms, Urinary frequency, Urinary retention, Cardiovascular regulation anomalies (palpitation, tachycardia, postural hypotension or cardiovascular collapse), Retching, Gastrointestinal irritation, Urticaria, Trembling, Flushing, Bradycardia, Hypertension, Allergic reactions (e.g. dyspnoea), bronchospasm, wheezing, angioneurotic oedema), Anaphylaxis, Changes in appetite, Paraesthesia, Hallucinations, Tremor, Respiratory depression, Epileptiform convulsions, Involuntary muscle contractions, Abnormal coordination, Syncope, Blurred vision, Dyspnoea, Tinnitus, Migraine, Stevens-Johnson syndrome/Toxic epidermal necrolysis, Motorial weakness,

Creatinine increase, Elevated liver enzymes, Hepatitis (liver swelling), Stomatitis, Liver failure, Pulmonary edema, Gastrointestinal bleeding, Pulmonary embolism, Myocardial ischaemia, Speech disorders, Hemoglobin decrease, Proteinuria. Tramadol interacts, potentially fatally, with serotonergics, monoamine oxidase inhibitors, tricyclic antidepressants, selective serotonin reuptake inhibitors, serotonin-norepinephrine reuptake inhibitors, noradrenergic and specific serotonergic antidepressants, serotonin antagonist and reuptake inhibitors, certain analgesics, certain anxiolytics, antibiotics, herbs, amphetamines, phenethylamines, phentermine, lithium, methylene blue as well as numerous other therapeutic agents. A pressor response similar to the so-called "cheese effect" was noted in combinations of amphetamine and tramadol, which appears to cause dysfunction of or toxicity to epinephrine/norepinephrine receptors. Tramadol acts as a μ-opioid receptor agonist, serotonin reuptake inhibitor and releasing agent, norepinephrine reuptake inhibitor, NMDA receptor antagonist receptor antagonist, nicotinic acetylcholine receptor antagonist, TRPV1 receptor agonist, and M1 and M3 muscarinic acetylcholine receptor antagonist.

Tramadol has inhibitory actions on the 5-HT2C receptor. Antagonism of 5-HT2C could be partially responsible for tramadol's reducing effect on depressive and obsessive-compulsive symptoms in patients with pain and co-morbid neurological illnesses. 5-HT2C antagonism may also account for its lowering of the seizure threshold, significantly increasing vulnerability to epileptic seizures, sometimes resulting in spontaneous death. However, the reduction of seizure threshold could be attributed to tramadol's putative inhibition of GABAA receptors at high doses. In addition, tramadol's major active metabolite, O-desmethyltramadol, is a high-affinity ligand of the δ- and κ-opioid receptors, and activity at the former receptor could be involved in tramadol's ability to provoke seizures in some individuals, as δ-opioid receptor agonists are well known to induce seizures.

Celexa (Citalopram)

An antidepressant drug of the selective serotonin reuptake inhibitor (SSRI) class. Nausea is often caused when the 5HT3 receptors actively absorb free serotonin, as this receptor is present within the digestive tract. The 5HT3 receptors stimulate vomiting.

Adverse effects: drowsiness, insomnia, nausea, weight changes, vivid dreams, frequent urination, decreased sex drive, anorgasmia, dry mouth, increased sweating, trembling, diarrhea, excessive yawning, fatigue, bruxism, vomiting, cardiac arrhythmia, blood pressure changes, dilated pupils, anxiety, mood swings, headache, dizziness, convulsions, hallucinations, severe allergic reactions, photosensitivity, dose-dependent QT interval prolongation. Severe discontinuation syndrome with "brain zap" has been very common adverse effects upon trying to titrate down this medicine.

> *"Further clarification issued in March 2012 restricted the maximum dose to 20 mg for subgroups of patients, including those older than 60 years."*

Celebrex (Celecoxib)

An NSAID. It is to treat the pain and inflammation of osteoarthritis, rheumatoid arthritis, ankylosing spondylitis, acute pain in adults, painful menstruation, and juvenile rheumatoid arthritis. It is used off label for migraine.

Adverse effects: myocardial infarction and stroke, New-onset hypertension or exacerbation of hypertension may occur, sodium and fluid retention, serious gastrointestinal ulceration, bleeding, and perforation (may be fatal), Anemia, Moderate to severe liver impairment, allergic reactions in those allergic to other sulfonamide-containing drugs (Aspirin and alike), Heart attack and stroke.

Verapamil (Calan, Verelan, Calan SR, Covera-HS)

An L-type voltage gated calcium channel blocker. It is used in the treatment of hypertension, angina pectoris, cardiac arrhythmia, and most recently, cluster headaches. It is also used for migraine and as a vasodilator.

Adverse effects: headaches, facial flushing, dizziness, lightheadedness, swelling, increased urination, fatigue, nausea, ecchymosis, galactorrhea, constipation, gingival hyperplasia.

Zofran (Ondansetron)

A serotonin 5-HT3 receptor antagonist to prevent nausea and vomiting caused by cancer chemotherapy, radiation therapy, and surgery. It has little effect on vomiting caused by motion sickness, and does not have any effect on dopamine receptors or muscarinic receptors—it is used off-label for migraine.

Adverse effects: Constipation, diarrhea, dizziness, and headache are the most commonly reported side effects, ototoxicity if injected too quickly, QT prolongation, electrolyte imbalances should be corrected before the use of injectable ondansetron.

Zomig (Zolmitriptan)

A selective serotonin receptor agonist of the 1B and 1D subtypes. It is a triptan, used in the acute treatment of migraine attacks with or without aura and cluster headaches. Zolmitriptan may increase blood pressure, it should not be given to patients with uncontrolled hypertension, should not be used within 24 hours of treatment with another 5-HT1 agonist, or an ergotamine-containing or ergot-type medication and should not be administered to patients with hemiplegic or basilar migraine.

Adverse effects: hypesthesia, paresthesia (all types), warm and cold sensations, chest pain, throat and jaw tightness, dry mouth, dyspepsia, dysphagia, nausea, somnolence, vertigo, asthenia, myalgia, myasthenia, sweating.

Buspar (Buspirone)

An anxiolytic psychotropic drug primarily used to treat generalized anxiety disorder (GAD). Buspirone is approved in the United States by the FDA for the treatment of anxiety disorders and the short-term relief of the symptoms of anxiety. It is used off-label for migraines.

Adverse effects: Dizziness/light-headedness, Headache, Somnolence (sleepiness), Premature ejaculation, Nervousness, Insomnia, Sleep disorder, Disturbance in attention, Depression, Confusional state, Anger, Tachycardia, Chest pain, Sinusitis, Pharyngolaryngeal pain, Paraesthesia, Blurred vision, Abnormal coordination, Tremor, Cold sweat, Rash, Nausea, Abdominal pain, Dry mouth, Diarrhea, Constipation, Vomiting, Fatigue, Musculoskeletal pain, Syncope, Hypotension, Hypertension, Redness and itching of the eyes, Altered taste, Conjunctivitis, Flatulence, Anorexia, Increased appetite, Salivation, Rectal bleeding, Urinary frequency, Urinary hesitancy, Menstrual irregularity or spotting, Dysuria, Muscle cramps, Muscle spasms, Muscle rigidity/stiffness, Involuntary movements, Shortness of breath, Chest congestion, Changes in libido, edema, Pruritus, Flushing, Easy bruising, Dry skin, Facial edema, Mild increases in hepatic aminotransferases (AST, ALT), Weight gain, Fever, Roaring sensation in the head, Weight loss, Malaise, Depersonalisation, Noise intolerance, Euphoria, Akathisia, Fearfulness, Loss of interest, Dissociative reaction, Cerebrovascular accident, Myocardial infarction, Cardiomyopathy, Congestive heart failure, Bradycardia, Dysphoria, Hallucinations, Feelings of claustrophobia, Cold intolerance, Stupor, Seizures, Slurred speech, Extrapyramidal symptoms including dyskinesias (acute & delayed), Dystonic reactions, Cogwheel rigidity, Emotional lability, Psychosis, Suicidal ideation, Ataxias, Transient difficulty with recall, Serotonin syndrome, Parkinsonism, Restless leg syndrome, Restlessness, Eye pain, Altered sense of smell, Photophobia, Pressure on eyes, Inner ear abnormality, Tunnel vision, Galactorrhoea, Irritable colon, Burning of the tongue, Arthralgias, Amenorrhoea, Enuresis, Nocturia, Pelvic inflammatory disease, Urinary retention, Hyperventilation, Epistaxis, Delayed ejaculation, Impotence, Acne, Hair loss, Blisters, Thinning of nails, Allergic reactions including urticaria, ecchymosis, Thrombocytopaenia, angioedema, Eosinophilia, Loss of voice, Leucopenia, Alcohol abuse, Bleeding disturbance, Hiccoughs, Thyroid abnormality.

Wellbutrin (bupropion hydrochloride)

An antidepressant and smoking cessation aid. It is a norepinephrine-dopamine reuptake inhibitor (NDRI). An atypical antidepressant. The most important side effect is an increase in risk for epileptic seizures. For this reason the drug was first withdrawn from the market, and then was reintroduces with a reduced recommended dosage. Bupropion is known to affect several different biological targets, and its mechanism of action is only partly understood. Bupropion induces the release of norepinephrine and dopamine in addition to inhibiting their reuptake. It is also known to increase blood pressure and heart rate. Epileptic seizures are the most important adverse effect of Wellbutrin! It is a reuptake inhibitor for the neurotransmitters norepinephrine (noradrenaline) and epinephrine (adrenaline) by blocking the action of the norepinephrine transporter (NET). This in turn leads to increased extracellular concentrations of norepinephrine and epinephrine and therefore can increase in adrenergic neurotransmission (adrenaline). Wellbutrin inhibits the CYP2D6 enzyme thereby reducing the clearance rate. It also lowers the threshold for epileptic seizures—meaning it can cause seizures.

Adverse effects: Headache, Transient insomnia, Abdominal pain, Agitation, Alopecia, Anxiety, Asthenia, Concentration disturbance, Constipation, Depression, Dizziness, Dry mouth, Fever, Nausea, Pruritus, Rash, Sweating, Taste disorders, Tremor, Urticaria, Visual disturbance, Vomiting, Anorexia, Chest pain, Confusion, Flushing, Increased blood pressure, Tachycardia, Tinnitus, Abnormal dreams, Aggression, Anaphylactic shock, Angioedema, Arthralgia, Ataxia, Blood glucose disturbances, Bronchospasm, Delusions, Depersonalization, Dyspnoea, Dystonia, Elevated liver enzymes, Erythema multiforme, Hallucinations, Hepatitis, Hostility, Hypotension, Irritability, Jaundice, Malaise, Memory impairment, Myalgia, Orthostatic hypotension, Palpitations, Paraesthesia, Paranoid ideation, Parkinsonism, Restlessness, Seizures, A condition similar to serum sickness, Stevens Johnson syndrome, Syncope, Twitching, Urinary frequency, Urinary retention, Vasodilation. Wellbutrin is prescribed off label for migraines.

Duloxetine (Cymbalta)

A serotonin-norepinephrine reuptake inhibitor (SNRI) for major depressive disorder, generalized anxiety disorder, fibromyalgia, and neuropathic pain—used off-label for migraine. The results of two clinical trials show that duloxetine treatment resulted in only 1–1.7-point decrease of pain as compared with placebo on an 11-point scale—quite insignificant in terms of pain relief. It makes one wonder if it is worth taking it given its dangers. Cymbalta also increases dopamine (meaning it may make one anxious).

Cymbalta is associated with an increased risk of mydriasis (dilation of the pupil); therefore, its use should be avoided for patients with uncontrolled narrow-angle glaucoma, in which mydriasis can cause sudden worsening. It should be avoided in migraine patients who are sensitive to light (they all are!). CNS acting drugs like duloxetine, should be used with caution when it is taken in combination with or substituted for other centrally acting drugs. In addition, the FDA has reported life-threatening drug interactions when Cymbalta is co-administered with triptans and other drugs acting on serotonin pathways, leading to increased risk for serotonin syndrome.

Adverse effects: Nausea, somnolence, insomnia, dizziness, dry mouth, headache, Sexual dysfunction, difficulty becoming aroused, lack of interest in sex, and anorgasmia, Loss of or decreased response to sexual stimuli and ejaculatory anhedonia.

Ergotamine (Migranal, Cafergot, Migergot)

An ergopeptine and part of the ergot family of alkaloids. It possesses structural similarity to several neurotransmitters, and has biological activity as a vasoconstrictor. It is used medicinally for treatment of acute migraine attacks (sometimes in combination with caffeine). The molecule shares structural similarity with neurotransmitters such as serotonin, dopamine, and epinephrine and can thus bind to several receptors acting as an agonist. The anti-migraine effect is due to constriction of the intracranial extracerebral blood vessels through the 5-HT1B receptor, and by inhibiting trigeminal neurotransmission by 5-HT1D receptors. Ergotamine also has effects on the dopamine and norepinephrine receptors.

Adverse effects: due mainly to its action at the D2 dopamine and 5-HT1A receptors. Ergotamine produces vasoconstriction peripherally as well as damages the peripheral epithelium. In high doses ergotamine is conducive to vascular stasis, thrombosis and gangrene.

Lamictal (Lamotrigine)

An anticonvulsant drug used in the treatment of epilepsy and bipolar disorder. Lamotrigine can induce a type of seizure known as a myoclonic jerk. This is a sodium channel blocking, antiepileptic drug. It inhibits voltage-sensitive sodium channels, leading to voltage gate inactivity of neuronal membranes. Approved for primary use of epileptic seizures, bipolar disorder, depression. Off-label uses include the treatment of peripheral neuropathy, trigeminal neuralgia, cluster headaches, migraines, and reducing neuropathic pain.

Adverse effects: Life-threatening skin reactions (black box), including Stevens–Johnson syndrome, DRESS syndrome and toxic epidermal necrolysis, skin rash--its presence is an indication of a possible serious or even deadly side-effect of the drug. Not all rashes that occur while taking lamotrigine progress to SJS or TEN. Between 5 to 10% of patients will develop a rash, but only one in a thousand patients will develop a serious rash. Rash and other skin reactions are more common in children, so this medication is often reserved for adults. As of December 2010, lamotrigine carries an FDA black box warning for aseptic meningitis. Side-effects such as rash, fever, and fatigue are very serious, as they may indicate incipient Stevens–Johnson syndrome, toxic epidermal necrolysis, DRESS syndrome or aseptic meningitis. Other side-effects include loss of balance or coordination; double vision; crossed eyes; pupil constriction; blurred vision; dizziness and lack of coordination; drowsiness, insomnia; anxiety; vivid dreams or nightmares; dry mouth, mouth ulcers; memory and cognitive problems; mood changes; runny nose; cough; nausea, indigestion, abdominal pain, weight loss; missed or painful menstrual periods; and vaginitis. Lamotrigine has been associated with a decrease in white blood cell count (leukopenia). Lamotrigine does not prolong QT/QTc in TQT studies in healthy subjects. Cases of lamotrigine-induced neuroleptic malignant syndrome have been reported.

In clinical trials women were more likely than men to have side-effects. There is evidence showing interactions between lamotrigine and female hormones, which can be of particular concern for women on estrogen-containing hormonal contraceptives. Ethynyl estradiol, the ingredient of such contraceptives, has been shown to decrease serum levels of lamotrigine. Likewise, women may experience an increase in lamotrigine side-effects upon discontinuation of the pill. This may include the "pill-free" week where lamotrigine serum levels have been shown to increase twofold. Another study showed a significant increase in follicle stimulating hormone (FSH) and luteinizing hormone in women taking lamotrigine with oral contraceptive compared to women taking oral contraceptives alone. However, these increases were not in conjunction with increased progesterone, indicating that oral contraceptives maintained suppression of ovulation. Lamotrigine binds to melanin-containing tissues such as the iris of the eye. The long-term consequences of this are unknown. Some patients have reported experiencing a loss of concentration, even with very small doses. Lamotrigine has been implicated in the apoptotic neurodegeneration of the developing brain. Lamotrigine is known to affect sleep. A study of 109 patients' medical records found that 6.7% of patients experienced an "alerting effect" resulting in intolerable insomnia, for which the treatment had to be discontinued.

Lamotrigine can induce a type of seizure known as a myoclonic jerk, which tends to happen soon after the use of the medication. When used in the treatment of myoclonic epilepsies such as juvenile myoclonic epilepsy, lower doses (and lower plasma levels) are usually needed, as even moderate doses of this drug can induce seizures, including tonic-clonic seizures, which can develop into status epilepticus, a medical emergency. It can also cause myoclonic status epilepticus. In overdose, lamotrigine can cause uncontrolled seizures in most people. Reported results in overdoses involving up to 15 g include increased seizures, coma and death.

Mechanism of action: Lamotrigine is a member of the sodium channel blocking class of antiepileptic drugs. It is a triazine derivate that inhibits voltage-sensitive sodium channels, leading to stabilization of neuronal membranes. It also blocks L-, N-, and P-type calcium channels and has weak 5-hydroxytryptamine-3 (5-HT3) receptor inhibition. These actions are thought to inhibit release of glutamate at cortical projections in the ventral striatum limbic areas. It has been pointed out that its neuroprotective and antiglutamatergic effects are contributors to its mood stabilizing activity. Observations that lamotrigine reduced γ-aminobutyric acid (GABA) A receptor-mediated neurotransmission in rat amygdala suggest that a GABAergic mechanism may also be involved, although this concept is controversial. Lamotrigine inhibites the release of glutamate and aspartate, evoked by the sodium-channel activator veratrine.

Naratriptan (Amerge)

A 5HT (serotonin) agonist triptan.

Adverse effects include: dizziness, drowsiness, tingling of the hands or feet, nausea, dry mouth and unsteadiness, chest pain/pressure, throat pain/pressure, unusually fast/slow/irregular pulse, one-sided muscle weakness, vision problems, cold/bluish hands or feet, stomach pain, bloody diarrhea, mental/mood changes, and fainting.

Symptoms of a serious allergic reaction include: rash, itching, swelling, severe dizziness, trouble breathing. The use of naratriptan with MAOIs and serotonergic drugs may result in the life-threatening serotonin syndrome. Make sure your doctor/pharmacist is aware of all your current medications (including as needed medications) before taking this drug.

Zoloft (Sertraline)

An antidepressant of the selective serotonin reuptake inhibitor (SSRI) class for major depressive disorders.

Adverse effects: Fatigue, Insomnia, Somnolence (sleepiness), Nausea, Dry mouth, Diarrhea, Headache, Ejaculation disorder, Dizziness, Agitation, Anorexia, Constipation, Dyspepsia, Decreased libido, Sweating, Tremor, Vomiting, Impaired concentration, Nervousness, Paroniria, Yawning, Palpitations, Increased sweating, Hot flushes, Weight decrease, Weight increase, Myoclonus, Hypertonia, Bruxism, Hypoesthesia, Menstrual irregularities, Sexual dysfunction, Rash, Vision abnormal, Asthenia, Chest pain, Paranesthesia, Tinnitus, Hypertension, Hyperkinesia, Bronchospasm, Esophagitis, Dysphagia, Hemorrhoids, Periorbital Edema, Purpura, Cold Sweat, Dry skin, Nocturia, Urinary Retention, Polyuria, Vaginal Hemorrhage, Malaise, Chills, Pyrexia, Thirst, Pollakiuria, Micturition disorder, Salivary Hypersecretion, Tongue Disorder, Osteoarthritis, Muscular Weakness, Back Pain, Muscle Twitching, Eructation, Dyspnea, Epistaxis (nose bleed), Edema peripheral, Periorbital edema,

Syncope, Postural dizziness, Tachycardia (high heart rate), Urticaria, Migraine, Abnormal bleeding (esp. in the GI tract), Muscle cramps, Arthralgia, Depressive symptoms, Euphoria, Hallucination, Alopecia, Urinary Retention, Pruritus, Amnesia memory loss., Urinary incontinence, Eye pain, Asymptomatic elevations in serum transaminases, Abnormal semen, Melena, Coffee ground vomiting, Hematochezia, Stomatitis, Tongue ulceration, Tooth Disorder, Glossitis, Mouth Ulceration, Laryngospasm, Hyperventilation, Hypoventilation, Stridor, Dysphonia, Upper Respiratory Tract Infection, Rhinitis, Hiccups, Apathy, Thinking Abnormal, Allergic reaction, Allergy, Anaphylactoid reaction, Face edema, Priapism, Atrial arrhythmia, AV block, Coma, Peripheral Ischemia, Injury, Vasodilation Procedure, Lymphadenopathy, Involuntary muscle contractions, Galactorrhea, Gynecomastia, Hyperprolactinemia, Hypothyroidism, Syndrome of inappropriate secretion of antidiuretic hormone (SIADH), Pancreatitis, Altered platelet function, Hematuria, Leukopenia, Thrombocytopenia, Increased coagulation times, Abnormal clinical laboratory results, Hyponatremia, Conversion Disorder, Drug Dependence, Paranoia, Myocardial Infarction, Bradycardia, Cardiac Disorder, Suicidal Ideation/behavior, Sleep Walking, Premature Ejaculation, Hyperglycemia, Hypoglycemia, Hypercholesterolemia, Vasculitis, Aggressive reaction, Psychosis, Mania, Menorrhagia, Atrophic Vulvovaginitis, Balanoposthitis, Genital Discharge, Angioedema, Photosensitivity skin reaction, Enuresis, Visual field defect, Abnormal liver function, Dermatitis, Dermatitis Bullous, Rash Follicular, Glaucoma, Lacrimal Disorder, Scotoma, Diplopia, Photophobia, Hyphemia, Mydriasis, Hair Texture Abnormal, Neoplasm, Diverticulitis, Choreoathetosis, Dyskinesia, Hyperesthesia, Sensory Disturbance, Gastroenteritis, Otitis Media, Skin Odour Abnormal, QTc prolongation, Anaphylactoid Reaction, Allergic Reaction, Allergy, Neuroleptic malignant syndrome. A potentially fatal reaction that most often occurs using antipsychotic drugs. It is characterized by fever, muscle rigidity, rhabdomyolysis, profuse sweating, tachycardia, tachypnoea, agitation, Stevens-Johnson syndrome a potentially fatal skin reaction, Toxic epidermal necrolysis another potentially fatal skin reaction, Torsades de pointes a potentially fatal change in the heart's rhythm., Cerebrovascular spasm, Serotonin syndrome similar to neuroleptic malignant syndrome but develops more rapidly, Bone fracture, Movement disorders, Diabetes mellitus, Dyspnea, Jaundice yellowing of the skin, mucous membranes and eyes due to an impaired ability of the liver to clear the haem breakdown by product, bilirubin, Hepatitis, Liver failure. This drug is known to cause serotonin syndrome on its own.

Pristiq (Desvenlafaxine)

A serotonin-norepinephrine reuptake inhibitor (SNRI).

Adverse effect: Nausea, Headache, Dizziness, Dry mouth, Hyperhidrosis, Diarrhea, Insomnia, Constipation, Fatigue, Tremor, Blurred vision, Mydriasis, Decreased appetite, Sexual dysfunction, Anxiety, Elevated cholesterol and triglycerides, Proteinuria, Vertigo, Feeling jittery, Asthenia, Nervousness, Hot flush, Irritability, Abnormal dreams, Urinary hesitation, Yawning, Rash, Hypersensitivity,

Syncope, Depersonalization, Hypomania, Withdrawal syndrome, Urinary retention, Epistaxis, Alopecia (hair loss), Orthostatic hypotension, Peripheral coldness, Hyponatremia (low blood sodium), Seizures, Extrapyramidal side effects, Hallucinations,, Angioedema, Photosensitivity reaction, Stevens-Johnson syndrome, Abnormal bleeding (e.g. gastrointestinal bleeds), Narrow-angle glaucoma, Mania, Interstitial lung disease, Eosinophilic pneumonia, Hypertension, Suicidal behavior & thoughts, Serotonin syndrome. It is only approved for use for major depression—not for migraines!

Viibryd (Vilazodone)

A serotonergic antidepressant serotonin reuptake inhibitor and 5-HT1A receptor partial agonist. It has some affinity for other serotonin receptors such as 5-HT1D, 5-HT2A, and 5-HT2C. It also exhibits some inhibitory activity at the norepinephrine and dopamine transporters.

Adverse effects: Nausea, Diarrhea, Headache, Vomiting, Dry mouth, Dizziness, Insomnia, Somnolence, Paraesthesia, Tremor, Abnormal dreams, Libido decreased, Restlessness, Akathisia, Restless legs syndrome, Abnormal orgasms (male persons only), Delayed ejaculations (male persons only), Erectile dysfunction (male persons only), Fatigue, Feeling jittery, Palpitations, Ventricular premature contractions, Arthralgia, Increased appetite, Serotonin syndrome — a possibly fatal side effect signaled by: Nausea, Vomiting, Mental status change (e.g. confusion, hallucinations, agitation, coma, stupor),

Muscle rigidity, Tremor, Myoclonus, Hyperreflexia — overresponsive, overactive reflexes, Hyperthermia — elevated body temperature. Autonomic instability (e.g. tachycardia, dizziness, abnormally excessive sweating, etc.), Mania/hypomania — a potentially dangerously elated/agitated mood. Suicidal ideation, Abnormal bleeding, Seizures, Syndrome of inappropriate antidiuretic hormone secretion (SIADH) — a condition characterized by an abnormally excessive secretion of antidiuretic hormone causing potentially-fatal electrolyte abnormalities. Antidepressants have the potential to induce psychiatric reactions. They are particularly problematic in those with a history of hypomania/mania such as those with bipolar disorder.

Valproate (Depakote)

An anticonvulsant and mood-stabilizing drug for the treatment of epilepsy, bipolar disorder and prevention of migraine headaches. Off-label uses include impulse control disorders, suggested by recent evidence of efficacy in controlling adverse effects of Parkinson's disease medical therapy, as well as treatments of HIV and cancer., A broad spectrum of anticonvulsant, although it is primarily used as a first-line treatment for tonic-clonic seizures, absence seizures and myoclonic seizures, and as a second-line treatment for partial seizures and infantile spasms. It has also been successfully given intravenously to treat status epilepticus. It works by blocking the voltage-dependent sodium channels and the gamma-aminobutyric acid (GABA) reuptake as well. It raises cerebral and cerebellar levels of the inhibitory synaptic neurotransmitter GABA, by inhibiting re-uptake.

Adverse effects: Nausea, Vomiting, Diarrhea, Headache, Low platelet count (dose-related), Tremor (dose-related), Hair loss (usually temporary), Drowsiness, Dizziness, Hyperandrogenism in females, Seeing double, Indigestion, Lazy eye, Infection, Tinnitus, Elevated aminotransferase concentrations (dose-related; indicative of liver injury), Paresthesia, Abdominal pain, Increased appetite, Weight gain, Ataxia, Polycystic ovaries, Memory impairment, Menstrual irregularities, Rash, Back pain, Mood changes, Anxiety, Confusion, Abnormal gait, Hallucinations, Catatonia, Dysarthria, Tardive dyskinesia, Vertigo, High blood levels of ammonia without symptoms, Peripheral edema, Syndrome of inappropriate secretion of antidiuretic hormone, Liver failure, Pancreatitis (these two usually occur in first 6 months and can be fatal), Leukopenia, Neutropenia, Pure red cell aplasia, Agranulocytosis, Extrapyramidal syndrome, Brain problems due to high ammonia levels, Low body temperature, Hypersensitivity reactions including multi-organ, hypersensitivity syndrome, Eosinophilic pleural effusion, Bone fractures.

Section 14

Paradigm Shift

When you no longer know what headache, heartache, or stomachache means without cistern punctures, electrocardiograms and six x-ray plates, you are slipping.

Martin H. Fischer

Medicine is experiencing a major paradigm shift in how health conditions are looked at and how the sick is treated. There is a movement toward two approaches that interlink:

1. Natural dietary modifications
2. Treatments based on genetic testing results

Until recently, it has been sufficient for medical professionals to look for readily observable signs and patterns to identify health conditions and treat their associated symptoms. In the more challenging areas of medicine, causal information has been hard to come by. The sick has appreciated the experts in these fields of medicine for their diagnostic skills and even more for their knowledge of the necessary steps for taking care of the "problem". For a person with a health-related complaint the only possibility for identifying the problem is through describing its symptoms. Not surprisingly the focus of the medical industry has been on symptoms. Treatments and medications are tailored to help relieve the unwanted ones. The commercial interests of the pharmaceutical companies and the financial reward system of physicians do not support simple solutions without chargeable treatments and/or medications. Many medical professionals are not motivated for lifelong learning of continuous scientific advancements in their field without incentives. The good news (for the sick) is that positive changes are afoot. With the age of free information available to the masses, the sick can self-educate and find explanations as well as solutions that their doctors have not kept up with, or have not payed attention to. Grassroots movements for attaining and maintaining health by dietary changes develop and flourish, regardless if the medical community agrees to those changes or even pays attention to them.

We have had a rapid succession of significant research findings about the human body, its metabolic processes, and how when those processes are faulty they become the underlying causes of most diseases, including cancer[115,195,196,202-204,214,877,878]. It is not unreasonable to suspect that metabolic challenges are at the root of most little-understood but well-known common human diseases.

Lack of Trust in Doctors

As I mentioned earlier, many years ago I joined several migraine sufferer groups on Facebook hoping to learn how the members coped. What I found stunned me: members were chatting during their worst migraines asking each other – their fellow migraine sufferers – what medications to take. They were cheering each other on when someone tried a new medicine and posted comments like this: "doctor said yesterday as soon as side effects pass I should increase the dose to 20mg, so here's waiting…", and "You go girl! You're doing great and being so brave!". In some forums, the migraine sufferers call themselves *warriors*.

I have heard many horror stories and some warrant a bit of discussion. The most common complaint about physicians is that they fail to ask basic and relevant questions. To illustrate:

1. A woman was taken to the emergency with a sudden onset of disturbed mental state. Her blood test showed an elevated level of a certain prescription medicine; it showed four times the prescribed dose. The woman had been running as part of her serious exercise routine. Running caused dehydration,

which increased the concentration of this medicine to overdose level! The prescribing physician missed to adjust the dosage to the patient's real-life conditions. This patient was accused of deliberate misuse of her medicine.

2. Another woman, in a disoriented state with migraine, sick stomach, dizziness and general malaise presented herself in the ER. She had severe and constant migraines even though she had a surgically implanted neural stimulator. The stimulator had worked a tad at the beginning but then stopped helping. In the ER waiting room her husband decided to search on the internet for help with migraines and happened to find me. He sent me a PM (private message) on FB on the spot. I knew nothing about his wife's history; I had never talked to her. I just asked one question from the husband; unbelievably, neither the admitting staff nor the ER doctor asked the same simple question: how much water has she drunk today? I just about fainted hearing the answer: the recommended water for the petite wife was 66 oz per day (just over 8 glasses) but she drank 256 oz (32 glasses) of water that day. Wow!!! Water toxicity! Completely missed by the ER doctor by not even asking. Seriously? They just pumped her up with medicines and even more water via the IV! Nightmarish cluelessness! You can read her entire story in more detail here:
https://stantonmigraineprotocol.com/2016/05/16/saved-from-migraine-one-life-at-the-time-story-makes-news/
This migraineur also made the local TV news more than once; you can see her here:

http://www.myeasttex.com/news/local-news/raw-milk-helping-woman-relieve-migraine-pain
The doctor just assumed migraine and started to push medicines without a word. Upon releasing her from the hospital where no change had been achieved in her pain after a week, per my instructions, the husband provisioned the correct amount of water per day and the type and amount of minerals she needed to maintain a proper electrolyte balance. She fully recovered in a few months. A year later her neuronal implant was surgically removed and she is still migraine free.

3. A woman presented in the ER with partial paralysis on one side of her body and severe migraine. She collapsed in the restroom as the paralysis took hold. The ER personnel placed a saline IV into her arm and tried to push a variety of medications into her. Her husband, who accompanied her, did not consent. Instead, he administered one of the steps of the Stanton Migraine Protocol®. After a brief sleep the migraineur recovered and was checked out of the ER. The doctor on ER duty at this hospital did not know that saline IV has salt in it. During a later visit with the same doctor the migraineur found out that this doctor had never heard of hemiplegic migraines either. This incident did not take place in the United States but then this book, the Stanton Migraine Protocol®, and the migraine group on Facebook are international.

The lack of trust in doctors is real and I am not surprised! Many migraineurs go to their appointments to share their medicine-free success, the way they have changed their lifestyles, and that finally all their migraines are gone. The neurologists hearing this, literally kick many migraineurs out of their offices for *non-compliance with the prescribed medication regime*! Doctors punish migraineurs for feeling well! Here is an example message that one of the migraineurs posted in the group:

> *"So, interesting and expected conversation with my doc today. [The doc] asked how my migraines were. I gave [the doc] my very positive update, and explained why. [The doc's] comments: 'there's no evidence on sodium connection, your body regulates its own potassium, milk is bad, eat more carbs'. I also said I want to get off my meds, and [the doc] said 'not yet'. Will be looking for a new doctor I think. I'd also add that [the doc] encouraged me to eat 'natural' sugars, like honey and pure stevia. Clueless!"*

Why was no consideration given to the fact that the migraineur is doing just fine and needs no more medicines? One would expect some curiosity from the doctor to at least ask what is helping and how. I'll leave it to you to speculate on this physician's motivations. Migraineurs are reaching out for anything to get rid of their misery but then learn not to reach out to doctors because they know it is not worth the effort, the money, and the embarrassment.

Migraineurs Have to Hide Quitting Drugs

There are several migraineurs in the migraine group who take a lot of prescribed medications. One of them took this list of medicines:

- Fetzima ER (SNRI),
- Propranolol (beta blocker)
- Protonix (treats GERD or acid reflux),
- Buspar (general anxiety disorder),
- Deplin (folic acid B9),
- Gabapentin (voltage gated calcium channel blocker),
- Zanaflex (muscle relaxant),
- Klonopin (anxiety reducing medicine),
- Ambien (hypnotic sleeping aid),
- Namenda (Alzheimer's disease—she has no Alzheimer's disease),
- Frovatriptan (triptan for migraines),
- Toradol (NSAID like Aleve or similar),
- Benadryl (1st generation antihistamine),
- Phenergan (1st generation antihistamine),
- Perphenazine (antipsychotic for schizophrenia),
- Zofran (anti-nausea),
- Nucynta (opioid narcotic),
- Percocet (combination of Oxycodone (a narcotic) with Tylenol).

This list of medications is not the longest one I've seen but I found 27 pages of major to moderate adverse interactions for this one, some of which could kill the migraineur. It also presents therapeutic duplications—potential overdose. What doctors seem to do is to pile medicines on. If one does not work, another is tried, often without removing the previous one. This creates major health problems for the migraineur, while doctors don't seem to have anything to lose following this practice.

Because support by a doctor is not guaranteed, prior to contacting a doctor, I recommend that all migraineurs check the open payment database:

https://openpaymentsdata.cms.gov/search/physicians

This is available to check on US doctors, starting from the year 2013. I have often found that some doctors who receive payment from pharmaceutical companies when writing prescriptions will try to keep their patients on medications. If a migraineur asks for help to quit, the doctor forces her to quit in a speedy manner that guarantees return to taking those same medicines again. We found doctors who earn millions of dollars from pharmaceutical companies for prescription writing and also for prescribing off-label drugs, so that migraineurs become experimental subjects, supplying clinical data (post clinical trial experience) without knowledge or consent. An example from one of my migraine group members on Citalopram, trying to titrate down with a non-cooperative doctor:

> *"It is like a shooting of tingles with lightening through my head all day. It has been a week and it is not getting better… I can't even think. People probably think I am drunk because I can't speak when this is going on I just stop everything. Help????!!!!... The brain zaps and brain shivers have been happening for over a week now… When it happens it is so intense that I can't remember what I am doing. The brain tremors are fun too, like my brain suddenly just got freezing cold and my body tenses up… My doctor thinks I have been off Escitalopram long enough that I should just tough it out now."*

At this point I checked withdrawal...argh… "discontinuation" syndrome online and this is what I found:

> *"Escitalopram discontinuation, particularly abruptly, may cause certain withdrawal symptoms such as "electric shock" sensations (also known as "brain shivers" or "brain zaps"), dizziness, acute depressions and irritability, as well as heightened senses of akathisia". (Wikipedia)*

And her doctor removed her abruptly to the point that she experienced all of the above. At this point she took a couple of pills she still had and her brain zaps went away. So she wanted to get more of the medication, since it was clear that the abrupt discontinuation caused the problems. Coincidentally I wrote an article about SSRI's being much more addictive than doctor's think and she emailed the article link to her doctor… my blog, *cluelesdoctors.com*, didn't sit well with this doctor at all.

> *"She was PISSED at me that I would send her a link clueless doctor, that insults her education."*
>
> *(http://cluelessdoctors.com/2015/02/23/dependence-ssris-snris-addiction/)*

And what education I wondered? Now, after proper tapering off, helped by another doctor, this migraineur is totally fine. She has been medication and migraine free for over a year.

I understand that doctors do not like to be called clueless and obviously not all doctors are. For whatever reasons, when it comes to migraines, the kind of doctors migraineurs are sent to seem more likely to be completely ignorant about migraines than doctors in fields other than migraines. Migraine doctors (usually neurologists) push drugs on migraineurs without knowing how the medicines work and without asking what the patient is already taking. They ignore the possibility of interactions.

Indeed, migraineurs often find that they do need to hide that they are slowly reducing their medicines, although this can be a dangerous practice. They are forced into lying because of their doctors who increase the dose when the migraineur complains about side effects. Not all doctors are like this but in the history of my migraine group, with several thousand migraineurs, I have only heard from a handful of members whose doctor would consider supporting the reduction in medicines, or accept that their patient has become migraine free without medicines. Only a very few of them are interested in how and why the patient did what she did. It is truly a sad situation when medical professionals, and an entire industry, forces migraineurs on drugs and then call them drug seekers when they get addicted to the very drugs they had been prescribed.

I personally had the "fortunate" experience of having been called a hypochondriac by my neurologist. That ended up being her last week of working for the medical facility I belonged to! I am teaching my migraineurs to stand up for their rights; after all, it is their money that pays for the services the doctors provide. The state of the current medical care of migraineurs is such that, as ugly as it sounds, going to a shoe sales representative for answers to migraine pain is just about as good an option as going to a migraine specialist or neurologist, in approximately 90% of the cases. It is no wonder that I find many of my migraineurs consulting about their migraines with their OBGYN or their chiropractor.

My doctor was very quick in picking up the issues and their implications. No argument about the test, he was on the phone to the department immediately. He said you did really well to pick it up Angela; I agreed. He then asked me about you, although I had told him before. He was very quiet and I wondered how he felt. I could see that he was uncomfortable; he put his arm round me as I left the room. He has never done that before. He has seen me probably 12 times a year on average for 8 years, getting sicker by the year. You have never seen me or even spoken to me and have been helping me for only a short time: you are not an MD. I hope he felt 'I should have been able to pick that up, why couldn't I?' He also asked me if I would send the test results to you, I think knowing that I wasn't going to do their diet [referring to SAD]!! He's not a bad guy! Nice, kind, caring, actually a thinker but obviously clueless.... but the best around here!

--GS

A Member in the Facebook Migraine Group

The Clueless, The Bad, The Ugly, & The Good!

The quote above is from one of my Facebook migraineurs whose response to my questionnaire, made me faint. I was shocked to see how much fruits and vegetables she ate—she was not a vegan or vegetarian but carbohydrates made up over 60% of her diet. Not only is that a problem for migraineurs, it is also a problem for non-migraineurs. As she was not able to fully stabilize on the Stanton Migraine Protocol®, she joined my keto-mild group, in which migraineurs apply the ketogenic nutritional concept but with a few changes to suit their special constraints. Still she was not able to stabilize and after an oral glucose tolerance test, showed diabetes. No doctor would consider her seriously because she was very thin (atypical for diabetics) and her HbA1c was perfect! Of course it was perfect because, on average, her bs was OK as she swung between 50 mg/dL and 14 mg/dL and so her standard evaluation always showed normal. Profiling in medicine based on looks is a dangerous practice!

One of my requirements in the keto-mild group is to check both glucose and β-Hydroxybutyrate (BHB) levels on a regular basis to be sure migraineurs respond to the changes properly, without any danger of reactive hypoglycemia from cutting carbohydrates. This migraineur experienced reactive hypoglycemia plus general hypoglycemia—her blood sugar would drop to 50 with or without eating! She told me about this after a week of experiencing this. I promptly removed her from the ketogenic diet and asked her to head to her doctor's office, hand over her recorded blood sugar readings, and request a check for diabetes—and to calibrate her blood sugar meter in case that was not working well, though she did mention her feeling unwell and shaky, a general sign of true hypoglycemia. The quote above is from her after her visit with her doctor for the first time discussing her blood sugar findings. As you can see, she had gone to the same doctor for 8 years and 12 times a year, so the doctor had more than enough opportunity to check her blood sugar status. However, and here is the catch, she doesn't fit the "profile" of a diabetic: she is not overweight (if anything she would like to gain weight), has low blood pressure, she doesn't appear to have any metabolic syndrome based on standard tests (such as the HbA1c), and because of lack of questions asked and lack of patient health monitoring in general, her extreme condition had gone unnoticed. Although this doctor seems to be a "nice guy", one questions the qualifications of a medical professional who misses a rather simple-to-detect health condition simply by not asking how his patient is doing.

At this point I trust you are properly prepped to read my portrayal of the four types of doctors and nurses that migraineurs often run into when they need help.

The Clueless

Who are the Clueless doctors? Those who literally close all their brain cells after they receive their medical degree, not only refusing to make any effort for updating their knowledge but even forgetting – as time goes by – what they had learned during their education.

I run a website – www.cluelessdoctors.com – to help, prod, and shame doctors, so they recognize the importance of keeping up with scientific advances. A doctor, sarcastically calling himself clueless, responded to one of my postings, an article I had written about the differences between generic and brand name medicines, highlighting the example of Singulair (Montelulast Sodium). I described how some generic manufacturers had changed the active ingredient from Montelukast Sodium to just Montelukast. I made a big deal about this and I had good reasons to do so. I had become a victim of this swap and got very ill.

Here is what the clueless doctor wrote (all spelling errors are his; I left his note in the quote below completely unedited):

> *"I am another 'clueless doctor' Sorry Angela but you're knowledge of basic chemistry is not up to writing this article. All drugs that are swallowed are dissolved before they are absorbed.* ***The molecules you have shown dissociate into ions in the gut.*** *Montelukast is the acid and Montelukast Na is the salt. Therefore the Montelukast ion in solution is the same for both preparations.* ***Given the huge amount of Sodium in your body versus the tiny amount in the tablet; there is no way that the molecule has a special relationship with its own sodium atom. In terms of the methyl group and the hydroxyl group being in a different place, this remember is a 3 dimensional molecule that rotates freely at each attachment.*** *It is not a flat molecule. Both drawings are in reality identical. Yes they are the same. I would take this post down as it is misleading and* ***pandering to hypochondriacs.***

Remember 2% of the world is mad, allergy and madness make close bedfellows."

I highlighted certain parts for emphasizing his cluelessness. His language also places him in the Ugly category. In case you are interested, here is the reason (as in my answer to him) why he is wrong:

"***Montelukast****'s chemical formula is* $C_{35}H_{36}ClNO_3S$ *with a 586.184 molecular weight (active ingredient only).*

Montelukast Sodium *is* $C_{35}H_{35}ClNNaO_3S$ *with a 608.18 molecular weight (active ingredient only).*

Can their ions even closely be the same? Nope!! That molecular weight difference is huge and the chemical formula is very different. Montelukast's active ingredient is only 90% bioequivalent to Montelukast Sodium" (see explanation of the 90% here:

http://www.fda.gov/downloads/drugs/guidancecomplianceregulatoryinformation/guidances/ucm088705.pdf)

Fortunately, most doctors are more flexible in the face of counter indicative reports. Upon learning about my negative experience with this specific generic drug switch, the major healthcare organization I belong to discontinued purchasing generic *Montelukast* and began using a supplier of generic *Montelukast Sodium.*

Just a bit more about this clueless doctor's comment that all drugs dissolve before absorption "in the gut". It must be noted that while the statement that all drugs dissolve is correct (they must dissolve before they are absorbed), *where* a drug dissolves depends on its coating. Many drugs are specifically coated with a material that can resist the acids of the stomach but not all—see the difference between plain Aspirin (dissolves in the stomach) and Buffered Aspirin (dissolves in the intestines). The absorption location makes a big difference.

Doctors are not the only clueless healthcare providers. The following happened to me with a clueless nurse. Some time ago I went to visit an emergency room with a health concern. The nurse assigned to me was also assigned to another woman—about my age. This other patient was missing a lower arm and a foot due to diabetes mellitus that was highly visible by her darkened and thickened skin, looking like the skin of a rhino. She was on an oxygen tank and was shivering as she nodded off time to time, drifting in and out of sleep. She seemed not be able to talk anymore, perhaps was also blind. It seemed to me she was in end-stage diabetes mellitus, perhaps close to diabetic ketoacidosis state. The nurse and I proceeded to discuss the causes of diabetes and other metabolic disorders, and after a while we hit upon the subject of carbohydrates. To my biggest surprise, this RN had no idea that salads, vegetables, fruits, grains, seeds, and nuts are all carbohydrates! She considered carbohydrates to be only simple sugars like candy or table sugar. I tried maintaining my composure and didn't ask her how she had obtained her RN degree without knowing what carbohydrates were. I spent the rest of the time detailing to this RN the basics of macronutrients. I have to remind you this took place in an emergency room of a major hospital.

The Bad

Who are the doctors I call "bad"? They are the ones who not only don't update their knowledge but actively fight anything not in strict compliance with their understanding and practices.

This example is perhaps the most amazing one. It is about one of my migraine group members who, following the Stanton Migraine Protocol® has reduced her level of triglycerides, LDL, and total cholesterol while increasing her HDL to values well within what doctors today consider the normal range in a short time. Prior to this test, her doctor had wanted to put her on statins. I recommended she try the dietary change approach first. She agreed to postpone the statins for a limited time and if her cholesterol was to increase or remain the same she would start the pills. When the results came back, her happiness was obvious and she decided against the statins. Her doctor – having seen the new test results – called her several times and accused her of taking statins in secret. The doctor claimed that it was not possible to achieve such change in cholesterol in such a short time without statins. He also objected to the increased fat in her diet. He repeatedly called her trying to convince her to stop her new diet and to "continue" taking the statins. He is exhibit A for a bad doctor.

The Ugly

Who are the "Ugly" doctors? They are doctors who block any new information from reaching their patients, doctors who stand in the way of their patients' self-help and self-education, and doctors who drag their patients through mud. The story I am about to tell is not unusual. A patient never expects to bump into an ugly doctor but unfortunately many do. This story was posted by one of my migraine group members who is on the ketogenic diet. I am posting her exact comment with her permission.

> *Went to see my GP last week for a referral to a cardiologist (preferably keto-friendly), and ask for the keto-specific tests Angela has recommended. He's been supportive enough with my way of eating, but when we started talking heart monitoring, genetic mutations, new science, keto books, and pork belly for breakfast, his head nearly exploded. He refused to order any test and suggested we may have to part ways. Such a shame he's so uninformed! Searching for another doctor....sigh! Well, we'll see what happens when I meet the (probably like-minded) cardiologist in March. If he spontaneously bursts into flames when I tell him how much butter I eat daily and suggest he read Phinney & Volek, I can't be held responsible. WY*

The ketogenic diet is used as treatment for many health conditions and for some with amazing results[214,544,547,877,879-882]. Migraine is one of them[883,884]. The ketogenic diet is not along the lines of the conventional wisdom about healthy nutrition, neither is it based on the USDA nutritional guidelines. It flies in the face of the "heart health", the "saturated fats are bad", "grains are good", and "carbohydrates are essential for life" dogma of the AHA, the ADA, and the AMA. It is understandable if some doctors are skeptical of, curious about, or against a new nutritional regime. Regardless, it is not a doctor's role to condemn a patient and kick her out on account of her dietary choice. This doctor also refused to order her blood tests she would have needed to ascertain her heart health—she was taking some medicines for a health condition that are known to cause heart problems in ketosis. Refusing to order tests that are essential for patient health is potentially endangering the migraineur's life! What happened to the oath of *Do No Harm*?

The Good

It takes a long time to find a doctor who is "good." What does a "good doctor" mean, particularly for a migraineur? It means a doctor who is willing to accept that he/she may not know everything. One who asks questions from the patient to learn the full story. One who asks relatives – if they happen to be around – about the patient. One who doesn't propose a medicine without examination and checks for interactions and therapeutic duplications.

Everyone understands the pressure placed on doctors by their medical institutions. They press for less time spent with patients and for delivering chargeable care. Health insurance companies want faster diagnoses, fewer tests, and code-able treatments. Pharmaceutical companies press for their medicines to be prescribed. Patients press for more time with their doctors, more tests, and lower costs—and some patients don't feel taken care of if the doctor doesn't prescribe some pills. These are incompatible goals; it is not easy to be a doctor. Doctors are often forced to decide between maintaining their job and treating their patient ethically.

However, physicians do have responsibilities to their patients that are not written anywhere but are assumed by everyone:

- have an open mind
- be respectful of the patient
- know your field of specialty
- keep up with science
- know enough about the patient to prescribe medicines for her with no interactions or therapeutic duplications

For finding a good doctor, I have had to "weed the field" until I could manage to find one who met all of the above criteria. I would like to thank all of the good doctors for their dedication, ethical standards, and for keeping an open mind.

Over the years, I have treated many doctors in the migraine group. They have helped me tremendously with their expert feed-back. Additionally, some members of the group have reported favorably about their doctors who, after seeing the improvement in the health of their patients and their joy of the migraine-free life, helped and supported them in coming off all of their medicines, and encouraged them to keep up with their beneficial dietary changes. Some of these doctors now have the 1st edition of this book in their waiting room for patients to peruse and some have even directly referred their patients to the Stanton Migraine Protocol®. A hospital dietitian I worked with did not only understand the importance of the unique diet migraineurs require but one day she called me from the ER asking me if she could pass on my contact information to a migraineur for whom no medicine was working.

These healthcare providers are open for finding solutions for their patients by noticing and accepting what works, instead of sticking to the dogma. They are at the vanguard of the emerging paradigm shift!

Section 15

End Notes

Medical Disclosure

No part of this book serves as a medical advice. The book discusses findings based on first hand anecdotal evidence, on free exchange of ideas among migraineurs, and my own experience that led me and others to a migraine-free life. Any decision you make in applying the techniques in this book should not replace your medical professional's guidance. I recommend you discuss all changes and steps you take with your doctor.

This book does not promote the taking of any medication (prescription or over-the-counter), herbs, or supplements. If you do use any of these and choose to end using them, I can provide help for a safe discontinuation. I recommend that any medicine(s) you choose to quit, you do so with your doctor's guidance (or with my guidance approved by your healthcare provider).

In my experience, most doctors are not aware how difficult it is to discontinue the medicines they prescribe and they often give a very short timeline for reduction. It frequently happens that such fast reduction causes not only a lot of pain and discomfort but in the case of some medicines the migraineur may end up with brain zaps, seizures, stuttering, heat intolerance, and other damages—including heart attacks or strokes. It is very important for your body's regeneration from the damages and dependence the drugs caused to reduce your medicines very slowly and so if your current doctor cannot provide you with a comfortable solution, please seek a second opinion. While no patient ever needs to have her doctor's approval for discontinuing a medicine, it is necessary to consult with a doctor to ensure that other health conditions are not compromised.

I also recommend that you check out the interactions between your medicines. I use https://www.drugs.com/drug_interactions.html.

If you find major interactions or therapeutic duplications, please head to your doctor immediately for a consultation; your health (and potentially your life) could be in danger. With moderate interactions, you can wait until your next scheduled doctor's visit. At this web site, when you scroll all the way to the bottom, you may see "therapeutic duplications." That refers to your taking more than one medicine for the same condition that works the same way—hence a duplicate. These are also extremely important to clear out, so you have no duplications in your medicine cabinet. Even in the case of duplication, it is important that you don't stop any of them but seek the advice of your physician.

Before you engage in the procedures of this book, you should have a checkup with your doctor to exclude anything that may mimic or cause migraine-pains, such as a brain tumor or a stroke, and discuss the medications prescribed to you. Some medical conditions, such as heart disease, high blood pressure and other circulatory diseases may prevent you from absorbing many of the nutrients found in common food items I recommend—particularly if you take medicines.

Please consult with your doctor prior to any lifestyle and nutritional changes! The author, Angela A. Stanton, Ph.D., Stanton Migraine Protocol®, and the publisher of this book are not responsible for any adverse changes in health conditions that may appear as a result of applying the procedures detailed herein.

Works Cited

1. Noseda R, Burstein R. Migraine pathophysiology: Anatomy of the trigeminovascular pathway and associated neurological symptoms, cortical spreading depression, sensitization, and modulation of pain. *PAIN®* 2013; **154, Supplement 1**: S44-S53.
2. Catterall WA, Dib-Hajj S, Meisler MH, Pietrobon D. Inherited Neuronal Ion Channelopathies: New Windows on Complex Neurological Diseases. *The Journal of Neuroscience* 2008; **28**(46): 11768-77.
3. Schwedt TJ. Multisensory Integration in Migraine. *Curr Opin Neurol* 2013: 248-53.
4. Liu H, Huaiting G, Xiang J, et al. Resting state brain activity in patients with migraine: a magnetoencephalography study. The Journal of headache and Pain. 2015 May 7:16-42.
5. Tessitore A, Russo A, Conte F, et al. Abnormal Connectivity Within Executive Resting-State Network in Migraine With Aura. *Headache* 2015; **55**(6): 794-805.

6. Xue T, Yuan K, Zhao L, et al. Intrinsic Brain Network Abnormalities in Migraines without Aura Revealed in Resting-State fMRI. *PLOS ONE* 2012: e52927.
7. Tso AR, Trujillo A, Guo CC, Goadsby PJ, Seeley WW. The anterior insula shows heightened interictal intrinsic connectivity in migraine without aura. *Neurology* 2015: 1043-50.
8. Guldiken B, Guldiken S, Taskiran B, et al. Migraine in metabolic syndrome. *The neurologist* 2009; **15**(2): 55-8.
9. Casucci G, Villani V, Cologno D, D'Onofrio F. Migraine and metabolism. *Neurological Sciences* 2012; **33**(1): 81-5.
10. Salmasi M, Amini L, Javanmard SH, Saadatnia M. Metabolic syndrome in migraine headache: A case-control study. *Journal of Research in Medical Sciences : The Official Journal of Isfahan University of Medical Sciences* 2014; **19**(1): 13-7.
11. Sachdev A, Marmura MJ. Metabolic Syndrome and Migraine. *Frontiers in Neurology* 2012; **3**: 161.
12. Bhoi SK, Kalita J, Misra UK. Metabolic syndrome and insulin resistance in migraine. *The Journal of Headache and Pain* 2012; **13**(4): 321-6.
13. Shaw SW, Johnson RH, Keogh HJ. Metabolic changes during glucose tolerance tests in migraine attacks. *J Neurol Sci* 1977; **33**(1-2): 51-9.
14. Mohammad SS, Coman D, Calvert S. Glucose transporter 1 deficiency syndrome and hemiplegic migraines as a dominant presenting clinical feature. *Journal of Paediatrics and Child Health* 2014; **50**(12): 1025-6.

15. Sjölund SL, Maria;Olofsson, Jonas, K.;Seubert, Janina; Laukka, Erika J.;. Phantom Smells: Prevalence and Correlates in a Population-Based Sample of Older Adults. *Chemical Senses* 2017; (epub).
16. Mathew PG, Robertson CE. No Laughing Matter: Gelastic Migraine and Other Unusual Headache Syndromes. *Current Pain and Headache Reports* 2016; **20**(5): 32.
17. Stanton AA. Functional Prodrome in Migraines. *Journal of Neurological Disorders* 2016; **4**(1).
18. Seçil Y, Ünde C, Beckmann YY, Bozkaya YT, Özerkan F, Başoğlu M. Blood Pressure Changes in Migraine Patients before, during and after Migraine Attacks. *Pain Practice* 2010; **10**(3): 222-7.
19. Gupta VK. Migraine-associated hypotension and autonomic ganglionitis. *Neurology* 1997; **49**(4): 1186.
20. Lee H-C. Migraine and hypotension. *Neurology* 1997; **49**(3): 900--b.
21. Charles A. Migraine. *New England Journal of Medicine* 2017; **377**(6): 553-61.
22. Laragh JH. Atrial Natriuretic Hormone, the Renin–Aldosterone Axis, and Blood Pressure–Electrolyte Homeostasis. *New England Journal of Medicine* 1985; **313**(21): 1330-40.
23. Barger AC. Regulation of Blood Pressure: Interaction of the Renin-Angiotensin-Aldosterone System, the Autonomic Nervous System, and Sodium Balance. *Angiology* 1978; **29**(4): 326-31.

24. Cohen AS, Burns B, Goadsby PJ. High-flow oxygen for treatment of cluster headache: A randomized trial. *JAMA* 2009; **302**(22): 2451-7.
25. Leroux E, Ducros A. Cluster headache. *Orphanet Journal of Rare Diseases* 2008; **3**(1): 20.
26. Petersen AS, Barloese MC, Jensen RH. Oxygen treatment of cluster headache: A review. *Cephalalgia* 2014; **34**(13): 1079-87.
27. Al Bu Ali WH. Ciprofloxacin-associated posterior reversible encephalopathy. *BMJ Case Reports* 2013; **2013**: bcr2013008636.
28. Sunku B. Cyclic Vomiting Syndrome: A Disorder of All Ages. *Gastroenterology & Hepatology* 2009; **5**(7): 507-15.
29. Hye Ran Y. Recent Concepts on Cyclic Vomiting Syndrome in Children. *J Neurogastroenterol Motil* 2010; **16**(2): 139-47.
30. Weatherall MW. The diagnosis and treatment of chronic migraine. Ther Adv Chronic Dis. 2015 May:115-23.
31. Kurth T. Migraine With Aura and Ischemic Stroke. *Which Additional Factors Matter?* 2007; **38**(9): 2407-8.
32. Loder E. Migraine with aura and increased risk of ischaemic stroke. *BMJ* 2009; **339**.
33. Gudmundsson LS, Scher AI, Aspelund T, et al. Migraine with aura and risk of cardiovascular and all cause mortality in men and women: prospective cohort study. *BMJ* 2010; **341**.
34. Kelman L. The Aura: A Tertiary Care Study of 952 Migraine Patients. *Cephalalgia* 2004; **24**(9): 728-34.

35. Kalra AA, Elliott D. Acute migraine: Current treatment and emerging therapies. *Ther Clin Risk Manag* 2007; **3**(3): 449-59.
36. Iliff JJ, Wang M, Liao Y, et al. A Paravascular Pathway Facilitates CSF Flow Through the Brain Parenchyma and the Clearance of Interstitial Solutes, Including Amyloid β. *Science Translational Medicine* 2012; **4**(147): 147ra11-ra11.
37. Xie L, Kang H, Xu Q, et al. Sleep Drives Metabolite Clearance from the Adult Brain. *Science (New York, NY)* 2013; **342**(6156): 10.1126/science.1241224.
38. Knutson KL, Spiegel K, Penev P, Van Cauter E. The Metabolic Consequences of Sleep Deprivation. *Sleep medicine reviews* 2007; **11**(3): 163-78.
39. Longo DL, Fauci AS, Kasper DL, Hauser SL, Jameson JL, Loscalzo J. Harrison's Manual of Medicine 18th Edition. New York: McGraw Hill Medical; 2013.
40. Scutt D, Manning JT. Ovary and ovulation: Symmetry and ovulation in women. *Human Reproduction* 1996; **11**(11): 2477-80.
41. Thornhill R, Gangestad SW. Facial attractiveness. *Trends in Cognitive Sciences* 1999; **3**(12): 452-60.
42. Peters M, Simmons LW, Rhodes G. Preferences across the Menstrual Cycle for Masculinity and Symmetry in Photographs of Male Faces and Bodies. *PLOS ONE* 2009; **4**(1): e4138.
43. Penton-Voak IS, Perrett DI, Castles DL, et al. Menstrual cycle alters face preference. *Nature* 1999; **399**(6738): 741-2.

44. Siegel GJA, Bernard W.;Albers, R. Wayne;Fisher, Stephen K.;Uhler, Michael D.;. Basic Neurochemistry: Molecular, Cellular and Medical Aspects. 6 ed. Philadeplphia: Lippincott-Raven; 1999.
45. Burbach JPH. What Are Neuropeptides? In: Merighi A, ed. Neuropeptides: Methods and Protocols. Totowa, NJ: Humana Press; 2011: 1-36.
46. Craik FIM, Bialystok E. Cognition through the lifespan: mechanisms of change. *Trends in Cognitive Sciences*; **10**(3): 131-8.
47. Rocca MA, Ceccarelli A, Falini A, et al. Diffusion tensor magnetic resonance imaging at 3.0 tesla shows subtle cerebral grey matter abnormalities in patients with migraine. *Journal of Neurology, Neurosurgery & Psychiatry* 2006; **77**(5): 686-9.
48. Colombo B, Dalla Libera D, Comi G. Brain white matter lesions in migraine: what's the meaning? *Neurol Sci* 2011; **32**.
49. Pusic AD, Mitchell HM, Kunkler PE, Klauer N, Kraig RP. Spreading Depression Transiently Disrupts Myelin via Interferon-gamma Signaling. *Experimental neurology* 2015; **264**: 43-54.
50. Giuliani C, Peri A. Effects of Hyponatremia on the Brain. *Journal of Clinical Medicine* 2014; **3**(4): 1163-77.
51. Stys PK, Zamponi GW, van Minnen J, Geurts JJG. Will the real multiple sclerosis please stand up? *Nature reviews Neuroscience*, 2012. http://europepmc.org/abstract/MED/22714021 https://doi.org/10.1038/nrn3275 (accessed 2012/07//).

52. Ba AM, Guiou M, Pouratian N, et al. Multiwavelength optical intrinsic signal imaging of cortical spreading depression. *J Neurophysiol* 2002; **88**.
53. Barkley GL, Tepley N, Nagel-Leiby S, Moran JE, Simkins RT, Welch KMA. Magnetoencephalographic Studies of Migraine. *Headache: The Journal of Head and Face Pain* 1990; **30**(7): 428-34.
54. Berger M, Speckmann EJ, Pape HC, Gorji A. Spreading depression enhances human neocortical excitability in vitro. *Cephalalgia* 2008; **28**.
55. Charles AC, Baca SM. Cortical spreading depression and migraine. *Nat Rev Neurol* 2013: 637-44.
56. Eikermann-Haerter K, Ayata C. Cortical spreading depression and migraine. *Curr Neurol Neurosci Rep* 2010; **10**.
57. Grafstein B. Mechanism of spreading cortical depression. *J Neurophysiol* 1956; **19**.
58. Hadjikhani N, Sanchez del Rio M, Wu O, et al. Mechanisms of migraine aura revealed by functional MRI in human visual cortex. *Proceedings of the National Academy of Sciences* 2001; **98**(8): 4687-92.
59. Marrannes R, Wauquier A, Reid K, De Prins E. The Prelude to The Migraine Attack. UK: Effects of drugs on cortical spreading depression. Baillière Tindal Oxford; 1986.
60. Schwedt TJ, Dodick DW. Advanced Neuroimaging of Migraine. *Lancet neurology* 2009; **8**(6): 560-8.

61. Smith JM, Bradley DP, James MF, Huang CL. Physiological studies of cortical spreading depression. *Biol Rev Camb Philos Soc* 2006; **81**.
62. Smith JM, James MF, Fraser JA, Huang CL. Translational imaging studies of cortical spreading depression in experimental models for migraine aura. *Expert Rev Neurother* 2008; **8**.
63. Theriot JJ, Toga AW, Prakash N, Ju YS, Brennan KC. Cortical Sensory Plasticity in a Model of Migraine with Aura. *The Journal of Neuroscience* 2012; **32**(44): 15252-61.
64. Anderson TR, Andrew RD. Spreading depression: imaging and blockade in the rat neocortical brain slice. *J Neurophysiol* 2002; **88**.
65. Brennan KC, Beltrán-Parrazal L, López-Valdés HE, Theriot J, Toga AW, Charles AC. Distinct vascular conduction with cortical spreading depression. *J Neurophysiol* 2007; **97**.
66. Chang JC, Shook LL, Biag J, et al. Biphasic direct current shift, haemoglobin desaturation and neurovascular uncoupling in cortical spreading depression. *Brain* 2010; **133**.
67. Chen S-P, Ay I, Lopes de Morais A, et al. VAGUS NERVE STIMULATION INHIBITS CORTICAL SPREADING DEPRESSION. *PAIN* 9000; **Publish Ahead of Print**.
68. Duckrow RB. Regional cerebral blood flow during spreading cortical depression in conscious rats. *J Cereb Blood Flow Metab* 1991; **11**.
69. Eikermann-Haerter K, Yuzawa I, Qin T, et al. Enhanced Subcortical Spreading Depression in Familial Hemiplegic

Migraine Type 1 Mutant Mice. *The Journal of Neuroscience* 2011; **31**(15): 5755-63.

70. Enger R, Tang W, Vindedal GF, et al. Dynamics of Ionic Shifts in Cortical Spreading Depression. *Cerebral Cortex* 2015; **25**(11): 4469-76.
71. Fabricius M, Fuhr S, Bhatia R, et al. Cortical spreading depression and peri-infarct depolarization in acutely injured human cerebral cortex. *Brain* 2006; **129**.
72. Footitt DR, Newberry NR. Cortical spreading depression induces an LTP-like effect in rat neocortex in vitro. *Brain Res* 1998; **781**.
73. Gault LM, Lin CW, LaManna JC, Lust WD. Changes in energy metabolites, cGMP and intracellular pH during cortical spreading depression. *Brain Res* 1994; **641**.
74. Gorji A, Scheller D, Straub H, et al. Spreading depression in human neocortical slices. *Brain Res* 2001; **906**.
75. Haghir H, Kovac S, Speckmann EJ, Zilles K, Gorji A. Patterns of neurotransmitter receptor distributions following cortical spreading depression. *Neuroscience* 2009; **163**.
76. Kleeberg J, Petzold GC, Major S, Dirnagl U, Dreier JP. ET-1 induces cortical spreading depression via activation of the ETA receptor/phospholipase C pathway in vivo. *Am J Physiol Heart Circ Physiol* 2004; **286**.
77. Lambert G, Michalicek J. Cortical Spreading Depression Reduces Dural Blood Flow—A Possible Mechanism for Migraine Pain? *Cephalalgia* 1994; **14**(6): 430-6.

78. Lambert GA, Truong L, Zagami AS. Effect of cortical spreading depression on basal and evoked traffic in the trigeminovascular sensory system. *Cephalalgia* 2011; **31**.
79. Lauritzen, Dreier JP, Fabricius M, Hartings JA, Graf R, Strong AJ. Clinical relevance of cortical spreading depression in neurological disorders: migraine, malignant stroke, subarachnoid and intracranial hemorrhage, and traumatic brain injury. J Cereb Blood Flow Metab. 2011 January 31:17-35.
80. Leo L, Gherardini L, Barone V, et al. Increased susceptibility to cortical spreading depression in the mouse model of familial hemiplegic migraine type 2. *PLoS Genet* 2011; **7**.
81. Passaro D, Rana G, Piscopo M, Viggiano E, De Luca B, Fucci L. Epigenetic chromatin modifications in the cortical spreading depression. *Brain Res* 2010; **1329**.
82. Pietrobon D. Insights into migraine mechanisms and Ca(V)2.1 calcium channel function from mouse models of familial hemiplegic migraine. *The Journal of Physiology* 2010; **588**(Pt 11): 1871-8.
83. Tang YT, Mendez JM, Theriot JJ, et al. Minimum conditions for the induction of cortical spreading depression in brain slices. *Journal of Neurophysiology* 2014; **112**(10): 2572-9.
84. Tottene A, Conti R, Fabbro A, et al. Enhanced excitatory transmission at cortical synapses as the basis for facilitated spreading depression in Ca(v)2.1 knockin migraine mice. *Neuron* 2009; **61**.

85. Tuckwell HC, Hermansen CL. Ion and transmitter movements during spreading cortical depression. *Int J Neurosci* 1981; **12**.
86. van den Maagdenberg AM, Pizzorusso T, Kaja S, et al. High cortical spreading depression susceptibility and migraine-associated symptoms in Cav2.1 S218L mice. *Ann Neurol* 2010; **67**.
87. Goadsby PJ, Ferrari MD, Csanyi A, Olesen J, Mills JG. Tonabersat TON-01-05 Study Group. Randomized, double-blind, placebo-controlled, proof-of-concept study of the cortical spreading depression inhibiting agent tonabersat in migraine prophylaxis. *Cephalalgia* 2009; **29**.
88. Gorelova NA, Koroleva VI, Amemori T, Pavlík V, Burěs J. Ketamine blockade of cortical spreading depression in rats. *Electroencephalogr Clin Neurophysiol* 1987; **66**.
89. Hernándéz-Cáceres J, Macias-González R, Brozek G, Bures J. Systemic ketamine blocks cortical spreading depression but does not delay the onset of terminal anoxic depolarization in rats. *Brain Res* 1987; **437**.
90. Hoffmann U, Dileköz E, Kudo C, Ayata C. Gabapentin suppresses cortical spreading depression susceptibility. *J Cereb Blood Flow Metab* 2010; **30**.
91. Holland PR, Akerman S, Andreou AP, Karsan N, Wemmie JA, Goadsby PJ. Acid-sensing ion channel 1: a novel therapeutic target for migraine with aura. *Ann Neurol* 2012; **72**(4): 559-63.

92. Read SJ, Hirst WD, Upton N, Parsons AA. Cortical spreading depression produces increased cGMP levels in cortex and brain stem that is inhibited by tonabersat (SB-220453) but not sumatriptan. *Brain Res* 2001; **891**.
93. Read SJ, Parsons AA. Sumatriptan modifies cortical free radical release during cortical spreading depression. A novel antimigraine action for sumatriptan? *Brain Res* 2000; **870**.
94. Richter F, Ebersberger A, Schaible HG. Blockade of voltage-gated calcium channels in rat inhibits repetitive cortical spreading depression. *Neurosci Lett* 2002; **334**.
95. Shimazawa M, Hara H, Watano T, Sukamoto T. Effects of Ca2+ channel blockers on cortical hypoperfusion and expression of c-Fos-like immunoreactivity after cortical spreading depression in rats. *Br J Pharmacol* 1995; **115**.
96. Unekawa M, Tomita Y, Toriumi H, Suzuki N. Suppressive effect of chronic peroral topiramate on potassium-induced cortical spreading depression in rats. *Cephalalgia* 2012; **32**.
97. Perret D, Luo ZD. Targeting voltage-gated calcium channels for neuropathic pain management. *Neurotherapeutics : the journal of the American Society for Experimental Neuro-Therapeutics* 2009; **6**(4): 679-92.
98. Letourneau PC. Molecular Bases of Neural Development. 1985.
99. Bentley D, Toroian-Raymond A. Disoriented pathfinding by pioneer neurone growth cones deprived of filopodia by cytochalasin treatment. *Nature* 1986; **323**(6090): 712-5.

100. Boulpaep E, L; Boron, Walter, F;. Foundations of Physiology. In: Boron W, F; Boulpaep, Emile, L;, ed. Medical Physiology. 3 ed. Philadelphia: Elsevier; 2016: 1312.
101. Kalil K, Dent EW. Touch and go: guidance cues signal to the growth cone cytoskeleton. *Current Opinion in Neurobiology* 2005; **15**(5): 521-6.
102. Kimura K, Mizoguchi A, Ide C. Regulation of Growth Cone Extension by SNARE Proteins. *Journal of Histochemistry & Cytochemistry* 2003; **51**(4): 429-33.
103. Lee AC, Suter DM. Quantitative Analysis of Microtubule Dynamics during Adhesion-Mediated Growth Cone Guidance. *Developmental neurobiology* 2008; **68**(12): 1363-77.
104. Legg AT, O'Connor TP. Gradients and Growth Cone Guidance of Grasshopper Neurons. *Journal of Histochemistry & Cytochemistry* 2003; **51**(4): 445-54.
105. Buck KB, Zheng JQ. Growth Cone Turning Induced by Direct Local Modification of Microtubule Dynamics. *The Journal of Neuroscience* 2002; **22**(21): 9358.
106. Paolicelli RC, Bolasco G, Pagani F, et al. Synaptic Pruning by Microglia Is Necessary for Normal Brain Development. *Science* 2011; **333**(6048): 1456.
107. Cowan WM, Fawcett JW, Leary DD, Stanfield BB. Regressive events in neurogenesis. *Science* 1984; **225**(4668): 1258.
108. Webster M. Migraine. Online Dictionary: http://www.merriam-webster.com/medical/migraine?show=0&t=1390806700.

109. Meriam-Webster EBCb. Migraine: http://www.merriam-webster.com/concise/migraine.

110. MedicineNet.com. Definition of a Headache: http://www.medterms.com/script/main/art.asp?articlekey=11396, 2013.

111. Goadsby PJ. Unique Migraine Subtypes, Rare Headache Disorders, and Other Disturbances. *CONTINUUM: Lifelong Learning in Neurology* 2015; **21**(4, Headache): 1032-40.

112. Bers DM, Despa S. Na/K-ATPase – an integral player in the adrenergic fight-or-flight response. *Trends in cardio-vascular medicine* 2009; **19**(4): 111-8.

113. De Fusco M, Marconi R, Silvestri L. Haploinsufficiency of ATP1A2 encoding the Na+/K+ pump 2 subunit associated with familial hemiplegic migraine type 2. *Nat Genet* 2003; **33**.

114. Friedrich T, Tavraz NN, Junghans C. ATP1A2 Mutations in Migraine: Seeing through the Facets of an Ion Pump onto the Neurobiology of Disease. *Frontiers in Physiology* 2016; 7(239).

115. Naviaux RK. Metabolic features of the cell danger response. *Mitochondrion* 2014; **16**: 7-17.

116. Segall L, Mezzetti A, Scanzano R, Gargus JJ, Purisima E, Blostein R. Alterations in the 2 isoform of Na, K-ATPase associated with familial hemiplegic migraine type 2. *Proc Natl Acad Sci USA* 2005; **102**.

117. Shahid SMM, Tabassum;. ELECTROLYTES AND NA+-K+-ATPase: POTENTIAL RISK FACTORS FOR THE DEVELOPMENT OF DIABETIC NEPHROPATHY. *Pakistan Journal of Pharmaceutical Sciences* 2008; **21**(2): 172-9.

118. Vanmolkot KRJ, Kors EE, Hottenga JJ, et al. Novel mutations in the Na+, K+-ATPase pump gene ATP1A2 associated with familial hemiplegic migraine and benign familial infantile convulsions. *Annals of Neurology* 2003; **54**(3): 360-6.

119. Wessman M, Kaunisto MA, Kallela M, Palotie A. The molecular genetics of migraine. *Annals of Medicine* 2004; **36**(6): 462-73.

120. Fazekas F, Koch M, Schmidt R, et al. The Prevalence of Cerebral Damage Varies With Migraine Type: A MRI Study. *Headache: The Journal of Head and Face Pain* 1992; **32**(6): 287-91.

121. Hamedani AG, Rose KM, Peterlin BL, et al. Migraine and white matter hyperintensities: The ARIC MRI study. *Neurology* 2013; **81**(15): 1308-13.

122. Gelfand AA, Reider AC, Goadsby PJ. Cranial autonomic symptoms in pediatric migraine are the rule, not the exception. *Neurology* 2013; **81**(5): 431-6.

123. Willis T. Discourses concerning the soul of brutes (De anima brutorum). . In: O.U.P. O, editor. cited by Spillane JD in The Doctrine of the nerves and Pearce JMS

Historical aspects of migraine; Journal Neurology, Surgery, and Psychiatry 1986; 49:1097-1103. Oxford Oxford O.U.P.; 1672.

124. Fischera M, Marziniak M, Gralow I, Evers S. The Incidence and Prevalence of Cluster Headache: A Meta-Analysis of Population-Based Studies. *Cephalalgia* 2008; **28**(6): 614-8.

125. Faria V, Erpelding N, Lebel A, et al. The migraine brain in transition: girls vs boys. *PAIN* 2015; **156**(11): 2212-21.

126. CLaino C. New Insights Into Triptans and Migraine. Juna 2003 2003. http://journals.lww.com/neurotodayonline/Fulltext/2003/06001/NEW_INSIGHTS_INTO_TRIPTANS_AND_MIGRAINE.10.aspx2).

127. Saper JR. WHat matters is not the differences between triptans, but the differences between patients. *Archives of Neurology* 2001; **58**(9): 1481-2.

128. Wei Y, Ullah G, Schiff SJ. Unification of Neuronal Spikes, Seizures, and Spreading Depression. *The Journal of Neuroscience* 2014: 11733-43.

129. Lauritzen M, Dreier JP, Fabricius M, Hartings JA, Graf R, Strong AJ. Clinical Relevance of Cortical Spreading Depression in Neurological Disorders: Migraine, Malignant Stroke, Subarachnoid and Intracranial Hemorrhage, and Traumatic Brain Injury. *Journal of Cerebral Blood Flow & Metabolism* 2011; **31**(1): 17-35.

130. Kofuji P, Newman EA. POTASSIUM BUFFERING IN THE CENTRAL NERVOUS SYSTEM. *Neuroscience* 2004; **129**(4): 1045-56.

131. Caplan M, J;. Functional Organization of the Cell. In: Boron W, F; Boulpaep, Emile, L;, ed. Medical Physiology. 3 ed. Philadelphia: Elsevier; 2016: 1312.

132. Scharfman HE. The Neurobiology of Epilepsy. *Current neurology and neuroscience reports* 2007; **7**(4): 348-54.

133. Cooper E, C;. Potassium Channels (including KCNQ) and Epilepsy In: BNoebels JA, M;Rogawski, MA;, ed. Jasper's Basic Mechanisms of the Epilepsies. 4 ed. Bethesda, MD: National Center for Biotechnology Information (US); 2012.

134. Stanton AA. Dehydration and Salt Deficiency Trigger Migraines. In: Matter H, editor.; 2014.

135. Silberstei SD. Serotonin (5-HT) and Migraine. *Headache: The Journal of Head and Face Pain* 1994; **34**(7): 408-17.

136. Silberstein S. Preventive Treatment of Migraine. *Cephalalgia* 1997; **17**(2): 67-72.

137. Dobson CF, Tohyama Y, Diksic M, Hamel E. Effects of acute or chronic administration of anti-migraine drugs sumatriptan and zolmitriptan on serotonin synthesis in the rat brain. *Cephalalgia* 2004; **24**(1): 2-11.

138. Bhoi S, Kalita J, Misra U. Metabolic syndrome and insulin resistance in migraine. *The Journal of Headache and Pain* 2012; **13**(4): 321-6.

139. Gozke E, Unal M, Engin H, Gurbuzer N. An Observational Study on the Association between Migraines and Tension Type Headaches in Patients Diagnosed with Metabolic Syndrome. *ISRN Neurology* 2013; **2013**: 4.

140. Sinclair AJ, Matharu M. Migraine, cerebrovascular disease and the metabolic syndrome. *Annals of Indian Academy of Neurology* 2012; **15**(Suppl 1): S72-S7.

141. Castori M. Ehlers-Danlos Syndrome, Hypermobility Type: An Underdiagnosed Hereditary Connective Tissue Disorder with Mucocutaneous, Articular, and Systemic Manifestations. *ISRN Dermatology* 2012; **2012**: 22.

142. Kuo C-Y, Wang C-H. Patulous Eustachian Tube Causing Hypermobile Eardrums. *New England Journal of Medicine* 2014; **371**(25): e37.

143. Campbell NAR, Jane B.;Urry, Lisa A.;Ca in, Michael L.;Minorsky, Peter V.;Wasserman, Steven A.;Jackson, Robert B. . Chapter 44: The Nervous System. Biology. 8th ed: Pearson; 2007.

144. Campbell DA, Tonks EM, Hay KM. An Investigation of the Salt and Water Balance in Migraine. *British Medical Journal* 1951: 1424-9.

145. George AL. Inherited disorders of voltage-gated sodium channels. *Journal of Clinical Investigation* 2005; **115**(8): 1990-9.

146. Kullmann DM, Waxman SG. Neurological channelopathies: new insights into disease mechanisms and ion channel function. *The Journal of Physiology* 2010; **588**(Pt 11): 1823-7.

147. Kim J-B. Channelopathies. *Korean Journal of Pediatrics* 2014; **57**(1): 1-18.

148. Frank CA. How voltage-gated calcium channels gate forms of homeostatic synaptic plasticity. *Frontiers in Cellular Neuroscience* 2014; **8**: 40.

149. CLaino C. New Insights into Triptans and Migraine. *Neurology Today* 2003; **3**(Supplement): 8.

150. Ambrosini A, De Noordhout A, Sándor PS, Schoenen J. Electrophysiological studies in migraine: a comprehensive review of their interest and limitations. *Cephalalgia* 2003; **23**: 13-31.

151. Adeniyi PO. Stress, a Major Determinant of Nutritional and Health Status. *American Journal of Public Health Research* 2015; **3**(1): 15-20.

152. Baigi K, Stewart WF. Chapter 25 - Headache and migraine: a leading cause of absenteeism. In: Marcello L, Margit LB, eds. Handbook of Clinical Neurology: Elsevier; 2015: 447-63.

153. Baidacci F, Lucchesi C, Cafalli M, et al. Migraine features in migraineurs with and without anxiety-depression symptoms: a hospital-based study. Clin Neurol Neurosurg. 2015 March 11:74-8.

154. Baldwin D, Rudge S. The role of serotonin in depression and anxiety. *Int Clin Psychopharm* 1995; **9**: 41-5.

155. Yavuz BG, Aydinlar EI, Dikmen PY, Incesu C. Association between somatic amplification, anxiety, depression, stress and migraine. *The Journal of Headache and Pain* 2013; **14**(1): 53-.

156. Yong N, Hu H, Fan X, et al. Prevalence and risk factors for depression and anxiety among outpatient migraineurs in mainland China. *The Journal of Headache and Pain* 2012; **13**(4): 303-10.

157. Yamada T, Dickins QS, Arensdorf K, Corbett J, Kimura J. Basilar migraine: Polarity-dependent alteration of brainstem auditory evoked potential. *Neurology* 1986; **36**(9): 1256.

158. de Baaij JHF, Hoenderop JGJ, Bindels RJM. Magnesium in Man: Implications for Health and Disease. *Physiological Reviews* 2014; **95**(1): 1-46.

159. Mauskop A, Varughese J. Why all migraine patients should be treated with magnesium. *Journal of Neural Transmission* 2012; **119**(5): 575-9.

160. Lehrer JF, Poole DC, Seaman M, Restivo D, Hartman K. Identification and treatment of metabolic abnormalities in patients with vertigo. *Archives of Internal Medicine* 1986; **146**(8): 1497-500.

161. Nadarajan V, Perry RJ, Johnson J, Werring DJ. Transient ischaemic attacks: mimics and chameleons. *Practical Neurology* 2014; **14**(1): 23-31.

162. Dennis M, Warlow C. Migraine aura without headache: transient ischaemic attack or not? *Journal of Neurology, Neurosurgery, and Psychiatry* 1992; **55**(6): 437-40.
163. Battista RA. Audiometric Findings of Patients with Migraine-Associated Dizziness. *Otology & Neurotology* 2004; **25**(6): 987-92.
164. Tinnitus and Insulin Resistance. https://www.pehni.com/patient_ed/dn_tinnitusinsulin.htm (accessed 5/6/2017 2017).
165. Rocca MA, Ceccarelli A, Falini A, et al. Brain Gray Matter Changes in Migraine Patients With T2-Visible Lesions. *Stroke* 2006; **37**(7): 1765.
166. May A, Ashburner J, Buchel C, et al. Correlation between structural and functional changes in brain in an idiopathic headache syndrome. *Nat Med* 1999; **5**(7): 836-8.
167. Squier W, Mack J, Green A, Aziz T. The pathophysiology of brain swelling associated with subdural hemorrhage: the role of the trigeminovascular system. *Child's Nervous System* 2012; **28**(12): 2005-15.
168. Steffensen AB, Sword J, Croom D, Kirov SA, MacAulay N. Chloride Cotransporters as a Molecular Mechanism underlying Spreading Depolarization-Induced Dendritic Beading. *The Journal of Neuroscience* 2015; **35**(35): 12172-87.
169. Kruit MC, Launer LJ, Ferrari MD, van Buchem MA. Brain stem and cerebellar hyperintense lesions in migraine. *Stroke* 2006; **37**.

170. Wang S-J, Chen P-K, Fuh J-L. Comorbidities of Migraine. *Frontiers in Neurology* 2010; **1**: 16.
171. Etminan M, Takkouche B, Isorna FC, Samii A. Risk of ischaemic stroke in people with migraine: systematic review and meta-analysis of observational studies. *BMJ* 2005; **330**.
172. Tedeschi G, Russo A, Conte F, et al. Increased interictal visual network connectivity in patients with migraine with aura. *Cephalalgia* 2015.
173. Kuburas A, Thompson S, Artemyev NO, Kardon RH, Russo AF. Photophobia and Abnormally Sustained Pupil Responses in a Mouse Model of Bradyopsia. *Investigative Ophthalmology & Visual Science* 2014; **55**(10): 6878-85.
174. Recober A, Kuburas A, Zhang Z, Wemmie JA, Anderson MG, Russo AF. Role of Calcitonin Gene-Related Peptide in Light-Aversive Behavior: Implications for Migraine. *The Journal of neuroscience : the official journal of the Society for Neuroscience* 2009; **29**(27): 8798-804.
175. Vgontzas A, Cui L, Merikangas KR. Are Sleep Difficulties Associated With Migraine Attributable to Anxiety and Depression? *Headache* 2008; **48**(10): 1451-9.
176. Walters AB, Hamer JD, Smitherman TA. Sleep Disturbance and Affective Comorbidity Among Episodic Migraineurs. *Headache: The Journal of Head and Face Pain* 2014; **54**(1): 116-24.

177. Lin Y-K, Lin G-Y, Lee J-T, et al. Associations Between Sleep Quality and Migraine Frequency: A Cross-Sectional Case-Control Study. *Medicine* 2016; **95**(17): e3554.

178. WHO. Headache Disorders: World Health Organization, 2012.

179. Aversi-Ferreira RAGMF, Bretas RV, Maior RS, et al. Morphometric and Statistical Analysis of the Palmaris Longus Muscle in Human and Non-Human Primates. *BioMed Research International* 2014; **2014**: 178906.

180. Shapiro HL. Man--500,000 Years from Now. *Natural History* 1933; **November-December**.

181. Cox HC, Lea RA, Bellis C, et al. A genome-wide analysis of 'Bounty' descendants implicates several novel variants in migraine susceptibility. *Neurogenetics* 2012; **13**(3): 261-6.

182. Tolner EA, Houben T, Terwindt GM, de Vries B, Ferrari MD, van den Maagdenberg AMJM. From migraine genes to mechanisms. *PAIN* 2015; **156**: S64-S74.

183. Gasparini CF, Sutherland HG, Griffiths LR. Studies on the Pathophysiology and Genetic Basis of Migraine. *Current Genomics* 2013; **14**(5): 300-15.

184. Eising E, A Datson N, van den Maagdenberg AMJM, Ferrari MD. Epigenetic mechanisms in migraine: a promising avenue? *BMC Medicine* 2013; **11**(1): 1-6.

185. Anttila V. Genome-wide association study of migraine implicates a common susceptibility variant on 8q22.1. *Nature Genetics* 2010; **42**.

186. Liu A, Menon S, Colson NJ, et al. Analysis of the MTHFR C677T variant with migraine phenotypes. *BMC Research Notes* 2010; **3**: 213-.

187. Montagna P. Migraine genetics. *Expert Rev Neurother* 2008; **8**.

188. van de Ven RobCG, Kaja Simon, Plomp JaapJ, Frants RuneR, van den Maagdenberg ArnMJM, Ferrari MichelD. Genetic Models of Migraine. *Arch Neurol* 2007; **64**.

189. Wessman M, Terwindt GM, Kaunisto MA, Palotie A, Ophoff RA. Migraine: a complex genetic disorder. *Lancet Neurol* 2007; **6**.

190. Scher AI, Terwindt GM, Verschuren WMM, et al. Migraine and MTHFR C677T genotype in a population-based sample. *Annals of Neurology* 2006; **59**(2): 372-5.

191. Lee J-Y, Kim M. Current Issues in Migraine Genetics. *J Clin Neurol* 2005; **1**(1): 8-13.

192. Oterino A, Valle N, Bravo Y, et al. MTHFR T677 Homozygosis Influences the Presence of Aura in Migraineurs. *Cephalalgia* 2004; **24**(6): 491-4.

193. Ulrich V, Gervil M, Kyvik KO, Olesen J, Russell MB. Evidence of a genetic factor in migraine with aura: A population-based Danish twin study. *Annals of Neurology* 1999; **45**.

194. NIH;. Understanding Cancer. In: [Internet] NCSS, editor.: National Institutes of Health (US); 2007.

195. Stefano GB, Kream RM. Cancer: Mitochondrial Origins. *Medical Science Monitor : International Medical*

Journal of Experimental and Clinical Research 2015; **21**: 3736-9.

196. Seyfried TN, Flores RE, Poff AM, D'Agostino DP. Cancer as a metabolic disease: implications for novel therapeutics. *Carcinogenesis* 2014; **35**(3): 515-27.
197. Seyfried T, Shelton L. Cancer as a metabolic disease. *Nutr Metab* 2010; **7**.
198. Coller HA. Is Cancer a Metabolic Disease? *The American Journal of Pathology* 2014; **184**(1): 4-17.
199. Dang CV. Links between metabolism and cancer. *Genes & Development* 2012; **26**(9): 877-90.
200. Martinez-Outschoorn U, Sotgia F, Lisanti MP. Tumor Microenvironment and Metabolic Synergy in Breast Cancers: Critical Importance of Mitochondrial Fuels and Function. *Seminars in Oncology*; **41**(2): 195-216.
201. Martinez-Outschoorn UE, Pestell RG, Howell A, et al. Energy transfer in "parasitic" cancer metabolism: Mitochondria are the powerhouse and Achilles' heel of tumor cells. *Cell Cycle* 2011; **10**(24): 4208-16.
202. Guido C, Whitaker-Menezes D, Lin Z, et al. Mitochondrial Fission Induces Glycolytic Reprogramming in Cancer-Associated Myofibroblasts, Driving Stromal Lactate Production, and Early Tumor Growth. *Oncotarget* 2012; **3**(8): 798-810.
203. Balliet RM, Capparelli C, Guido C, et al. Mitochondrial oxidative stress in cancer-associated fibroblasts drives lactate production, promoting breast cancer tumor growth:

Understanding the aging and cancer connection. *Cell Cycle* 2011; **10**(23): 4065-73.

204. Lee H-C, Wei Y-H. Mitochondrial DNA Instability and Metabolic Shift in Human Cancers. *International Journal of Molecular Sciences* 2009; **10**(2): 674-701.
205. WALLACE DC. Mitochondria and Cancer: Warburg Addressed. *Cold Spring Harbor Symposia on Quantitative Biology* 2005; **70**: 363-74.
206. Sherin JE, Nemeroff CB. Post-traumatic stress disorder: the neurobiological impact of psychological trauma. *Dialogues in Clinical Neuroscience* 2011; **13**(3): 263-78.
207. Shwartz M. Robert Sapolsky discusses physiological effects of stress. Stanford, California: Stanford News, 2007.
208. Science WIo. The Human Gene Database. 2017. http://www.genecards.org/Search/Keyword?queryString=migraine&pageSize=-1&startPage=0 (accessed 1/28/2017 2017).
209. Caspary DM, Ling L, Turner JG, Hughes LF. Inhibitory Neurotransmission, Plasticity and Aging in the Mammalian Central Auditory System. *The Journal of experimental biology* 2008; **211**(Pt 11): 1781-91.
210. Bortolotto ZA, Clarke VRJ, Delany CM, et al. Kainate receptors are involved in synaptic plasticity. *Nature* 1999; **402**(6759): 297-301.
211. Taubes G. Good Calories, Bad Calories: Fats, Carbs, and the Controversial Science of Diet and Health: Anchor; 2008.

212. Taubes G. Why We Get Fat: And What to Do About It. Reprint edition December 27, 2011 ed: Anchor; 2011.

213. Abedini M, Falahi E, Roosta S. Dairy product consumption and the metabolic syndrome. *Diabetes & Metabolic Syndrome: Clinical Research & Reviews* 2015; **9**(1): 34-7.

214. Allen BG, Bhatia SK, Anderson CM, et al. Ketogenic diets as an adjuvant cancer therapy: History and potential mechanism. *Redox Biology* 2014; **2**: 963-70.

215. Bjørnshave A, Hermansen K. Effects of Dairy Protein and Fat on the Metabolic Syndrome and Type 2 Diabetes. *The Review of Diabetic Studies : RDS* 2014; **11**(2): 153-66.

216. Blüher M. Adipokines – removing road blocks to obesity and diabetes therapy. *Molecular Metabolism* 2014; **3**(3): 230-40.

217. Brandhorst S, Choi In Y, Wei M, et al. A Periodic Diet that Mimics Fasting Promotes Multi-System Regeneration, Enhanced Cognitive Performance, and Healthspan. *Cell Metabolism*; **22**(1): 86-99.

218. Conlee RK, Hammer RL, Winder WW, Bracken ML, Nelson AG, Barnett DW. Glycogen repletion and exercise endurance in rats adapted to a high fat diet. *Metabolism* 1990; **39**.

219. Guilherme A, Virbasius JV, Puri V, Czech MP. Adipocyte dysfunctions linking obesity to insulin resistance and type 2 diabetes. *Nat Rev Mol Cell Biol* 2008; **9**(5): 367-77.

220. Kokavec A, Crebbin SJ. Sugar alters the level of serum insulin and plasma glucose and the serum cortisol:DHEAS ratio in female migraine sufferers. *Appetite* 2010; **55**(3): 582-8.
221. Macfarlane DP, Forbes S, Walker BR. Glucocorticoids and fatty acid metabolism in humans: fuelling fat redistribution in the metabolic syndrome. *Journal of Endocrinology* 2008; **197**(2): 189-204.
222. Nseir W, Nassar F, Assy N. Soft drinks consumption and nonalcoholic fatty liver disease. *World Journal of Gastroenterology : WJG* 2010; **16**(21): 2579-88.
223. Ouyang X, Cirillo P, Sautin Y, et al. Fructose Consumption as a Risk Factor for Non-alcoholic Fatty Liver Disease. *Journal of hepatology* 2008; **48**(6): 993-9.
224. Parks EJ. Effect of Dietary Carbohydrate on Triglyceride Metabolism in Humans. *The Journal of Nutrition* 2001; **131**(10): 2772S-4S.
225. Stanhope KL. Sugar consumption, metabolic disease and obesity: The state of the controversy. *Critical Reviews in Clinical Laboratory Sciences* 2015: 1-16.
226. Pogoda JM, Gross NB, Arakaki X, Fonteh AN, Cowan RP, Harrington MG. Severe Headache or Migraine History Is Inversely Correlated With Dietary Sodium Intake: NHANES 1999–2004. *Headache: The Journal of Head and Face Pain* 2016: n/a-n/a.
227. Stanton AA. The Anatomy of a Migraine. 2014. http://www.hormonesmatter.com/anatomy-migraine/ (accessed 9/18 2015).

228. Stanton AA. Migraine Cause and Treatment. *Mental Health in Family Medicine* 2015; **11**(2): 69-72.
229. Karenberg A, Leitz C. Headache in Magical and Medical Papyri of Ancient Egypt. *Cephalalgia* 2001; **21**(9): 911-6.
230. Cordain L, Eaton SB, Sebastian A, et al. Origins and evolution of the Western diet: health implications for the 21st century. *The American Journal of Clinical Nutrition* 2005; **81**(2): 341-54.
231. USDA. National Nutrient Database for Standard Reference Release 26. Washington, DC: http://ndb.nal.usda.gov/ndb/search/list#, 2013, software v.1.3.1.
232. Teicholz N. The Big Fat Surprise: Why Butter, Meat and Cheese Belong in a Healthy Diet. New York: Simon & Schuster; Reprint edition; 2015.
233. Teicholz N. The scientific report guiding the US dietary guidelines: is it scientific? *BMJ : British Medical Journal* 2015; **351**.
234. Taubes G. The Soft Science of Dietary Fat. *Science* 2001; **291**(5513): 2536-45.
235. DiNicolantonio JJ, Lucan SC. The wrong white crystals: not salt but sugar as aetiological in hypertension and cardiometabolic disease. *Open Heart* 2014; **1**(1): e000167.
236. Meneton P, Jeunemaitre X, de Wardener HE, Macgregor GA. Links Between Dietary Salt Intake, Renal Salt Handling, Blood Pressure, and Cardiovascular Diseases. *Physiological Reviews* 2005; **85**(2): 679-715.

237. Blaustein MP, Leenen FHH, Chen L, et al. How NaCl raises blood pressure: a new paradigm for the pathogenesis of salt-dependent hypertension. *American Journal of Physiology - Heart and Circulatory Physiology* 2012; **302**(5): H1031-H49.

238. Hamed SA. Blood pressure changes in patients with migraine: Evidences, controversial views and potential mechanisms of comorbidity. *Journal of Neurology and Neuroscience* 2010; **1**(2:2).

239. Low PA, Sandroni P, Joyner M, Shen W-K. Postural Tachycardia Syndrome (POTS). *Journal of cardiovascular electrophysiology* 2009; **20**(3): 352-8.

240. Pescatore F. Headaches in Children. *Neurology Now* 2013; **9**(4): 8.

241. Pogoda JM, Gross NB, Arakaki X, Fonteh AN, Cowan RP, Harrington MG. Severe Headache or Migraine History Is Inversely Correlated With Dietary Sodium Intake: NHANES 1999-2004: A Response. *Headache: The Journal of Head and Face Pain* 2016; **56**(7): 1216-8.

242. Mente A, O'Donnell M, Rangarajan S, et al. Associations of urinary sodium excretion with cardiovascular events in individuals with and without hypertension: a pooled analysis of data from four studies. *The Lancet* 2016; **388**(10043): 465-75.

243. Moore LL, Singer MR, Bradlee ML. Low Sodium Intakes are Not Associated with Lower Blood Pressure Levels

among Framingham Offspring Study Adults. *The FASEB Journal* 2017; **31**(1 Supplement): 446.6.

244. Intersalt: an international study of electrolyte excretion and blood pressure. Results for 24 hour urinary sodium and potassium excretion. Intersalt Cooperative Research Group. *BMJ : British Medical Journal* 1988; **297**(6644): 319-28.
245. Albert GNT, Hubeck-Graudal; Gesche, Jurgens;. Effects of low sodium diet versus high sodium diet on blood pressure, renin, aldosterone, catecholamines, cholesterol, and triglyceride. *Cochrane Database of Systematic Reviews* 2011; **11**.
246. Alderman MH, Cohen HW. Dietary Sodium Intake and Cardiovascular Mortality: Controversy Resolved? *American Journal of Hypertension* 2012; **25**(7): 727-34.
247. Bucher C, Tapernoux D, Diethelm M, et al. Influence of weather conditions, drugs and comorbidities on serum Na and Cl in 13 000 hospital admissions: Evidence for a subpopulation susceptible for SIADH. *Clinical Biochemistry* 2014; **47**(7–8): 618-24.
248. Chrysant GS, Bakir S, Oparil S. Dietary salt reduction in hypertension—What is the evidence and why is it still controversial? *Progress in Cardiovascular Diseases*; **42**(1): 23-38.
249. DiNicolantonio JJ, Niazi AK, Sadaf R, O' Keefe JH, Lucan SC, Lavie CJ. Dietary Sodium Restriction: Take It

with a Grain of Salt. *The American Journal of Medicine*; **126**(11): 951-5.

250. Dong J, Li Y, Yang Z, Luo J. Low Dietary Sodium Intake Increases the Death Risk in Peritoneal Dialysis. *Clinical Journal of the American Society of Nephrology : CJASN* 2010; **5**(2): 240-7.
251. Jurgens G, Graudal NA. Effects of low sodium diet versus high sodium diet on blood pressure, renin, aldosterone, catecholamines, cholesterols, and triglyceride. 2004.
252. Karppanen H, Karppanen P, Mervaala E. Why and how to implement sodium, potassium, calcium, and magnesium changes in food items and diets? *J Hum Hypertens* 0000; **19**(S3): S10-S9.
253. Konerman MC, Hummel SL. Sodium Restriction in Heart Failure: Benefit or Harm? *Current treatment options in cardiovascular medicine* 2014; **16**(2): 286-.
254. Nichols H. More than salt, sugars may contribute to high blood pressure. 2015.
255. O'Donnell MJ, Mente A, Smyth A, Yusuf S. Salt intake and cardiovascular disease: why are the data inconsistent? *European Heart Journal* 2013; **34**(14): 1034-40.
256. Rodrigues SL, Baldo MP, Machado RC, Forechi L, Molina MdCB, Mill JG. High potassium intake blunts the effect of elevated sodium intake on blood pressure levels. *Journal of the American Society of Hypertension*; **8**(4): 232-8.

257. Haghdoost F. Is There an Inverse Relationship Between Migraine and Dietary Sodium Intake? *Headache: The Journal of Head and Face Pain* 2016; **56**(7): 1212-3.

258. Stanton AA. A Comment on Severe Headache or Migraine History Is Inversely Correlated With Dietary Sodium Intake: NHANES 1999-2004. *Headache: The Journal of Head and Face Pain* 2016; **56**(7): 1214-5.

259. Perlmutter D, Loberg K. Grain Brain: The Surprising Truth About Wheat, Carbs, and Sugar - Your Brain's Silent Killers: Hodder & Stoughton; 2014.

260. Björkhem I, Meaney S. Brain Cholesterol: Long Secret Life Behind a Barrier. *Arteriosclerosis, Thrombosis, and Vascular Biology* 2004; **24**(5): 806-15.

261. Vitali C, Wellington CL, Calabresi L. HDL and cholesterol handling in the brain. *Cardiovascular Research* 2014; **103**(3): 405-13.

262. Björkhem I, Lütjohann D, Diczfalusy U, Ståhle L, Ahlborg G, Wahren J. Cholesterol homeostasis in human brain: turnover of 24S-hydroxycholesterol and evidence for a cerebral origin of most of this oxysterol in the circulation. *Journal of Lipid Research* 1998; **39**(8): 1594-600.

263. Dietschy JM, Turley SD. Cholesterol metabolism in the brain. *Current Opinion in Lipidology* 2001; **12**(2): 105-12.

264. Jurevics H, Morell P. Cholesterol for Synthesis of Myelin Is Made Locally, Not Imported into Brain. *Journal of Neurochemistry* 1995; **64**(2): 895-901.

265. Martín MG, Pfrieger F, Dotti CG. Cholesterol in brain disease: sometimes determinant and frequently implicated. *EMBO reports* 2014; **15**(10): 1036-52.

266. Vance JE. Dysregulation of cholesterol balance in the brain: contribution to neurodegenerative diseases. *Disease Models and Mechanisms* 2012; **5**(6): 746-55.

267. Zhang J, Liu Q. Cholesterol metabolism and homeostasis in the brain. *Protein & Cell* 2015; **6**(4): 254-64.

268. Goluszko P, Nowicki B. Membrane Cholesterol: a Crucial Molecule Affecting Interactions of Microbial Pathogens with Mammalian Cells. *Infection and Immunity* 2005; **73**(12): 7791-6.

269. Jorde R, Grimnes G. Vitamin D and Lipids. *Circulation* 2012; **126**(3): 252.

270. Nordestgaard BG, Zacho J. Lipids, atherosclerosis and CVD risk: Is CRP an innocent bystander? *Nutrition, Metabolism and Cardiovascular Diseases*; **19**(8): 521-4.

271. Muoio DM. Metabolic Inflexibility: When Mitochondrial Indecision Leads to Metabolic Gridlock. *Cell* 2014; **159**(6): 1253-62.

272. Alberts BJ, Alexander; Lewis Julian; Raff, martin; Roberts, Keith; Walter, Peter;. Molecular Biology of the Cell. 4 ed. New York: Garland Science; 2002.

273. Storlien L, Oakes ND, Kelley DE. Metabolic flexibility. *Proceedings of the Nutrition Society* 2007; **63**(2): 363-8.

274. Vos MB, Kaar JL, Welsh JA, et al. Added Sugars and Cardiovascular Disease Risk in Children: A Scientific

Statement From the American Heart Association. *Circulation* 2016.

275. Jayalath VH, Sievenpiper JL, de Souza RJ, et al. Total Fructose Intake and Risk of Hypertension: A Systematic Review and Meta-Analysis of Prospective Cohorts. *Journal of the American College of Nutrition* 2014; **33**(4): 328-39.
276. Ha V, Jayalath V, Cozma A, Mirrahimi A, de Souza R, Sievenpiper J. Fructose-Containing Sugars, Blood Pressure, and Cardiometabolic Risk: A Critical Review. *Current Hypertension Reports* 2013; **15**(4): 281-97.
277. Kim YH, Abris GP, Sung M-K, Lee JE. Consumption of Sugar-Sweetened Beverages and Blood Pressure in the United States: The National Health and Nutrition Examination Survey 2003-2006. *Clinical Nutrition Research* 2012; **1**(1): 85-93.
278. Cohen L, Curhan G, Forman J. Association of Sweetened Beverage Intake with Incident Hypertension. *Journal of General Internal Medicine* 2012; **27**(9): 1127-34.
279. Sharma N, Okere IC, Barrows BR, et al. High-sugar diets increase cardiac dysfunction and mortality in hypertension compared to low-carbohydrate or high-starch diets. *Journal of hypertension* 2008; **26**(7): 1402-10.
280. Johnson RJ, Segal MS, Sautin Y, et al. Potential role of sugar (fructose) in the epidemic of hypertension, obesity and the metabolic syndrome, diabetes, kidney disease, and cardiovascular disease. *Am J Clin Nutr* 2007; **86**.

281. Roysommuti S, Khongnakha T, Jirakulsomchok D, Wyss JM. Excess Dietary Glucose Alters Renal Function Before Increasing Arterial Pressure and Inducing Insulin Resistance. *American Journal of Hypertension* 2002; **15**(9): 773-9.
282. Schaefer EJ, Gleason JA, Dansinger ML. Dietary Fructose and Glucose Differentially Affect Lipid and Glucose Homeostasis. *The Journal of Nutrition* 2009; **139**(6): 1257S-62S.
283. Kearns CE, Schmidt LA, Glantz SA. Sugar industry and coronary heart disease research: A historical analysis of internal industry documents. *JAMA Internal Medicine* 2016.
284. Tomlinson DR, Gardiner NJ. Glucose neurotoxicity. *Nat Rev Neurosci* 2008; **9**(1): 36-45.
285. Cermenati G, Abbiati F, Cermenati S, et al. Diabetes-induced myelin abnormalities are associated with an altered lipid pattern: protective effects of LXR activation. *Journal of Lipid Research* 2012; **53**(2): 300-10.
286. Hans-Christoph D, David WD, Peter JG, Richard BL, Jes O, Stephen DS. Chronic migraine—classification, characteristics and treatment. *Nature Reviews Neurology* 2012.
287. Tikka-Kleemola P, Artto V, Vepsäläinen S. A visual migraine aura locus maps to 9q21-q22. *Neurology* 2010; **74**.
288. Sand T, Zhitniy N, White LR, Stovner LJ. Visual evoked potential latency, amplitude and habituation in migraine:

A longitudinal study. *Clinical Neurophysiology*; **119**(5): 1020-7.

289. de Tommaso M, Ambrosini A, Brighina F, et al. Altered processing of sensory stimuli in patients with migraine. *Nat Rev Neurol* 2014; **10**(3): 144-55.

290. Hodkinson DJ, Veggeberg R, Kucyi A, et al. Cortico–Cortical Connections of Primary Sensory Areas and Associated Symptoms in Migraine. *eneuro* 2016; **3**(6).

291. Borsook D, Maleki N, Becerra L, McEwen B. Understanding Migraine through the Lens of Maladaptive Stress Responses: A Model Disease of Allostatic Load. *Neuron* 2012; **73**(2): 219-34.

292. KPBS. Staying Awake During Brain Surgery. In: Goldberg K, editor.; 2010.

293. Dubin AE, Patapoutian A. Nociceptors: the sensors of the pain pathway. *The Journal of Clinical Investigation* 2010; **120**(11): 3760-72.

294. Faragó P, Tuka B, Tóth E, et al. Interictal brain activity differs in migraine with and without aura: resting state fMRI study. *The Journal of Headache and Pain* 2017; **18**(1): 8.

295. Magon S, May A, Stankewitz A, et al. Morphological Abnormalities of Thalamic Subnuclei in Migraine: A Multicenter MRI Study at 3 Tesla. *The Journal of Neuroscience* 2015; **35**(40): 13800-6.

296. Chen Z, Chen X, Liu M, Dong Z, Ma L, Yu S. Altered functional connectivity of amygdala underlying the neu-

romechanism of migraine pathogenesis. *The Journal of Headache and Pain* 2017; **18**(1): 7.

297. Wikipedia. Electrolyte. http://en.wikipedia.org/wiki/Electrolyte: Wikipedia, 2013.
298. Gunn BG, Cunningham L, Mitchell SG, Swinny JD, Lambert JJ, Belelli D. GABAA receptor-acting neurosteroids: A role in the development and regulation of the stress response. *Frontiers in Neuroendocrinology* 2015; **36**: 28-48.
299. Kono S, Terada T, Ouchi Y, Miyajima H. An altered GABA-A receptor function in spinocerebellar ataxia type 6 and familial hemiplegic migraine type 1 associated with the CACNA1A gene mutation. *BBA Clinical* 2014; **2**: 56-61.
300. Wikipedia. Stress (Biology): http://en.wikipedia.org/wiki/Stress_(biology), 2013.
301. Rada P, Avena NM, Hoebel BG. Daily bingeing on sugar repeatedly releases dopamine in the accumbens shell. *Neuroscience* 2005; **134**(3): 737-44.
302. Avena NM, Rada P, Hoebel BG. Evidence for sugar addiction: Behavioral and neurochemical effects of intermittent, excessive sugar intake. *Neuroscience & Biobehavioral Reviews* 2008; **32**(1): 20-39.
303. Gruber H-J, Bernecker C, Pailer S, et al. Hyperinsulinaemia in migraineurs is associated with nitric oxide stress. *Cephalalgia* 2010; **30**(5): 593-8.

304. Dexter JD, Roberts J, Byer JA. The Five Hour Glucose Tolerance Test and Effect of Low Sucrose Diet in Migraine. *Headache: The Journal of Head and Face Pain* 1978; **18**(2): 91-4.
305. Adair RK. Simple neural networks for the amplification and utilization of small changes in neuron firing rates. *Proceedings of the National Academy of Sciences* 2001; **98**(13): 7253-8.
306. Granli T, Dahl R, Brodin P, Bøckman OC. Nitrate and nitrite concentrations in human saliva: Variations with salivary flow-rate. *Food and Chemical Toxicology* 1989; **27**(10): 675-80.
307. Webb AJ, Patel N, Loukogeorgakis S, et al. Acute blood pressure lowering, vasoprotective, and antiplatelet properties of dietary nitrate via bioconversion to nitrite. *Hypertension* 2008; **51**(3): 784-90.
308. Moncada S, Higgs EA. Nitric Oxide and the Vascular Endothelium. In: Moncada S, Higgs A, eds. The Vascular Endothelium I. Berlin, Heidelberg: Springer Berlin Heidelberg; 2006: 213-54.
309. Tajima Y. Coffee-induced Hypokalaemia. *Clinical Medicine Insights Case Reports* 2010; **3**: 9-13.
310. Zhang Y, Coca A, Casa DJ, Antonio J, Green JM, Bishop PA. Caffeine and diuresis during rest and exercise: A meta-analysis. *Journal of science and medicine in sport / Sports Medicine Australia* 2015; **18**(5): 569-74.

311. Hwang JL, Weiss RE. Steroid-induced diabetes: a clinical and molecular approach to understanding and treatment. *Diabetes/metabolism research and reviews* 2014; **30**(2): 96-102.

312. Costrini NV, Kalkhoff RK. Relative effects of pregnancy, estradiol, and progesterone on plasma insulin and pancreatic islet insulin secretion. *Journal of Clinical Investigation* 1971; **50**(5): 992-9.

313. Batista MR, Smith MS, Snead WL, Connolly CC, Lacy DB, Moore MC. Chronic estradiol and progesterone treatment in conscious dogs: effects on insulin sensitivity and response to hypoglycemia. *American journal of physiology Regulatory, integrative and comparative physiology* 2005; **289**(4): R1064-R73.

314. Gupte AA, Pownall HJ, Hamilton DJ. Estrogen: An Emerging Regulator of Insulin Action and Mitochondrial Function. *Journal of Diabetes Research* 2015; **2015**: 9.

315. Miner JA, Miner JC, Brunt VE, Kaplan PF, Minson CT. A novel relationship between estrogen, insulin resistance, and cardiovagal baroreflex sensitivity in obese PCOS women. *The FASEB Journal* 2013; **27**(1 Supplement): 1118.36.

316. Matsui S, Yasui T, Tani A, et al. Associations of Estrogen and Testosterone With Insulin Resistance in Pre- and Postmenopausal Women With and Without Hormone Therapy. *Int J Endocrinol Metab* 2013; **11**(2): 65-70.

317. Bruns CM, Kemnitz JW. Sex Hormones, Insulin Sensitivity, and Diabetes Mellitus. *ILAR Journal* 2004; **45**(2): 160-9.

318. Wilcox G. Insulin and Insulin Resistance. *Clinical Biochemist Reviews* 2005; **26**(2): 19-39.

319. Ohashi K, Komada H, Uda S, et al. Glucose Homeostatic Law: Insulin Clearance Predicts the Progression of Glucose Intolerance in Humans. *PLoS ONE* 2015; **10**(12): e0143880.

320. Röder PV, Wu B, Liu Y, Han W. Pancreatic regulation of glucose homeostasis. *Experimental & Molecular Medicine* 2016; **48**(3): e219.

321. Burriss RP, Troscianko J, Lovell PG, et al. Changes in Women?s Facial Skin Color over the Ovulatory Cycle are Not Detectable by the Human Visual System. *PLoS ONE* 2015; **10**(7): e0130093.

322. Roney JR, Simmons ZL. Women's estradiol predicts preference for facial cues of men's testosterone. *Hormones and Behavior* 2008; **53**(1): 14-9.

323. Nigel Barber PD. Are Fertile Women More Attractive? http://www.psychologytoday.com/blog/the-human-beast/200907/are-fertile-women-more-attractive: Psychology Today, 2009.

324. Penton-Voak IS, Perrett DI. Female preference for male faces changes cyclically. *Evolution and Human Behavior*; **21**(1): 39-48.

325. Kim JJ, Buzzio OL, Li S, Lu Z. Role of FOXO1A in the regulation of insulin-like growth factor binding protein-1 in human endometrial cells: Interaction with progesterone receptor. *Biology of reproduction* 2005; **73**(4): 833-9.

326. Iwamoto T, Kagawa Y, Naito Y, Kuzuhara S, Kojima M. Steroid-Induced Diabetes Mellitus and Related Risk Factors in Patients with Neurologic Diseases. *Pharmacotherapy: The Journal of Human Pharmacology and Drug Therapy* 2004; **24**(4): 508-14.

327. Di Dalmazi G, Pagotto U, Pasquali R, Vicennati V. Glucocorticoids and Type 2 Diabetes: From Physiology to Pathology. *Journal of Nutrition and Metabolism* 2012; **2012**: 9.

328. Ferris HA, Kahn CR. New mechanisms of glucocorticoid-induced insulin resistance: make no bones about it. *The Journal of Clinical Investigation*; **122**(11): 3854-7.

329. Liu D, Ahmet A, Ward L, et al. A practical guide to the monitoring and management of the complications of systemic corticosteroid therapy. *Allergy, Asthma, and Clinical Immunology : Official Journal of the Canadian Society of Allergy and Clinical Immunology* 2013; **9**(1): 30-.

330. Pagano G, Cavallo-Perin P, Cassader M, Bruno A, Ozzello A, Masciola Dall'omo AM. An in vivo and in vitro study of the mechanism of prednisone-induced insulin resistance in healthy subjects. *J Clin Invest* 1983; **72**.

331. Douaud G, Groves AR, Tamnes CK, et al. A common brain network links development, aging, and vulnerabil-

ity to disease. *Proceedings of the National Academy of Sciences* 2014; **111**(49): 17648-53.

332. Gettler LT, McDade TW, Feranil AB, Kuzawa CW. Longitudinal evidence that fatherhood decreases testosterone in human males. *Proceedings of the National Academy of Sciences* 2011; **108**(39): 16194-9.
333. Hofeldt F. Reactive Hypoglycemia. *Endocrinology and Metabolism Clinics of North America* 1989; **18**(1): 6.
334. Stuart K, Field A, Raju J, Ramachandran S. Postprandial Reactive Hypoglycaemia: Varying Presentation Patterns on Extended Glucose Tolerance Tests and Possible Therapeutic Approaches. *Case Reports in Medicine* 2013; **2013**: 5.
335. Kraft J, R;. Diabetes Epidemic &You. revision 1 ed. North America & International: Trafford; 2011.
336. Ando H, Ushijima K, Shimba S, Fujimura A. Daily Fasting Blood Glucose Rhythm in Male Mice: A Role of the Circadian Clock in the Liver. *Endocrinology* 2016; **157**(2): 463-9.
337. Monnier L, Colette C, Dunseath GJ, Owens DR. The Loss of Postprandial Glycemic Control Precedes Stepwise Deterioration of Fasting With Worsening Diabetes. *Diabetes Care* 2007; **30**(2): 263-9.
338. Stephenson JM, Schernthaner G. Dawn Phenomenon and Somogyi Effect in IDDM. *Diabetes Care* 1989; **12**(4): 245-51.
339. Schmidt MI, Lin QX, Gwynne JT, Jacobs S. Fasting Early Morning Rise in Peripheral Insulin: Evidence of the

Dawn Phenomenon in Nondiabetes. *Diabetes Care* 1984; **7**(1): 32-5.

340. Kendall M. The Blood Glucose, Glucagon, and Insulin Response to Protein. 6/15/2015 2015. https://optimisingnutrition.com/2015/06/15/the-blood-glucose-glucagon-and-insulin-response-to-protein/ (accessed 7/6/2017 2017).

341. Franz MJ. Protein: Metabolism and Effect on Blood Glucose Levels. *The Diabetes Educator* 1997; **23**(6): 643-51.

342. Wolman SL, Fields ALA, Cheema-Dhadli S, Halperin ML. Protein Conversion to Glucose: An Evaluation of the Quantitative Aspects. *Journal of Parenteral and Enteral Nutrition* 1980; **4**(5): 487-9.

343. Gannon MC, Nuttall JA, Damberg G, Gupta V, Nuttall FQ. Effect of Protein Ingestion on the Glucose Appearance Rate in People with Type 2 Diabetes1. *The Journal of Clinical Endocrinology & Metabolism* 2001; **86**(3): 1040-7.

344. The Liver & Blood Sugar. https://dtc.ucsf.edu/types-of-diabetes/type1/understanding-type-1-diabetes/how-the-body-processes-sugar/the-liver-blood-sugar/ (accessed 8/26/2017 2017).

345. Pivovarov R, Albers DJ, Hripcsak G, Sepulveda JL, Elhadad N. Temporal trends of hemoglobin A1c testing. *Journal of the American Medical Informatics Association : JAMIA* 2014; **21**(6): 1038-44.

346. Bersoux S, Cook CB, Wu Q, et al. Hemoglobin A1c Testing Alone Does Not Sufficiently Identify Patients With Prediabetes. *American Journal of Clinical Pathology* 2011; **135**(5): 674-7.
347. Slama G, Klein J-C, Delage A, et al. Correlation Between the Nature and Amount of Carbohydrate in Meal Intake and Insulin Delivery by the Artificial Pancreas in 24 Insulin-dependent Diabetics. *Diabetes* 1981; **30**(2): 101-5.
348. Aizawa T, Yamada M, Katakura M, Funase Y, Yamashita K, Yamauchi K. Hyperbolic correlation between insulin sensitivity and insulin secretion fades away in lean subjects with superb glucose regulation. *Endocrine Journal* 2012; **59**(2): 127-36.
349. Nuttall FQ, Gannon MC. Metabolic response of people with type 2 diabetes to a high protein diet. *Nutrition & Metabolism* 2004; **1**: 6-.
350. Muckelbauer R, Sarganas G, Grüneis A, Müller-Nordhorn J. Association between water consumption and body weight outcomes: a systematic review. *The American Journal of Clinical Nutrition* 2013; **98**(2): 282-99.
351. Popkin BM, Armstrong LE, Bray GM, Caballero B, Frei B, Willett WC. A new proposed guidance system for beverage consumption in the United States. *The American Journal of Clinical Nutrition* 2006; **83**(3): 529-42.
352. El-Sharkawy AM, Sahota O, Maughan RJ, Lobo DN. The pathophysiology of fluid and electrolyte balance in

the older adult surgical patient. *Clinical Nutrition* 2014; **33**(1): 6-13.

353. Armstrong LE. Challenges of linking chronic dehydration and fluid consumption to health outcomes. *Nutrition Reviews* 2012; **70**(suppl 2): S121-S7.
354. Popkin BM, D'Anci KE, Rosenberg IH. Water, Hydration and Health. *Nutrition reviews* 2010; **68**(8): 439-58.
355. Sawka MN, Cheuvront SN, Carter IR. Human water needs. *Nutr Rev* 2005; **63**: S30-S9.
356. Bossingham MJ, Carnell NS, Campbell WW. Water balance, hydration status, and fat-free mass hydration in younger and older adults. *The American journal of clinical nutrition* 2005; **81**(6): 1342-50.
357. Medicine Io. Dietary Reference Intakes for Water, Potassium, Sodium, Chloride, and Sulfate. Washington, DC: The National Academies Press; 2005.
358. Batmanghelidj F. Your Body's Many Cries for Water. You are not sick; You are thirsty. Don't gtreat thirst with medication. 3rd ed. USA: Global Health Solutions, Inc.; 2008.
359. Klein S, Sheard NF, Pi-Sunyer X, et al. Weight Management Through Lifestyle Modification for the Prevention and Management of Type 2 Diabetes: Rationale and Strategies. *A statement of the American Diabetes Association, the North American Association for the Study of Obesity, and the American Society for Clinical Nutrition* 2004; **27**(8): 2067-73.

360. Kitada K, Daub S, Zhang Y, et al. High salt intake reprioritizes osmolyte and energy metabolism for body fluid conservation. *The Journal of Clinical Investigation* 2017; **127**(5): 1944-59.

361. Rakova N, Kitada K, Lerchl K, et al. Increased salt consumption induces body water conservation and decreases fluid intake. *The Journal of Clinical Investigation* 2017; **127**(5): 1932-43.

362. Ruderman N, Chisholm D, Pi-Sunyer X, Schneider S. The metabolically obese, normal-weight individual revisited. *Diabetes* 1998; **47**(5): 699-713.

363. Vitiello MV, Prinz PN, Halter JB. Sodium-Restricted Diet Increases Nighttime Plasma Norepinephrine and Impairs Sleep Patterns in Man*. *The Journal of Clinical Endocrinology & Metabolism* 1983; **56**(3): 553-6.

364. Polyák É, Gombos K, Hajnal B, et al. Effects of artificial sweeteners on body weight, food and drink intake. *Acta Physiologica Hungarica* 2010; **97**(4): 401-7.

365. Suez J, Korem T, Zeevi D, et al. Artificial sweeteners induce glucose intolerance by altering the gut microbiota. *Nature* 2014; **514**(7521): 181-6.

366. Tandel KR. Sugar substitutes: Health controversy over perceived benefits. *Journal of Pharmacology & Pharmacotherapeutics* 2011; **2**(4): 236-43.

367. Pepino MY. METABOLIC EFFECTS OF NON-NUTRITIVE SWEETENERS. *Physiology & behavior* 2015; **152**(0 0): 450-5.

368. Cohen JB, Townsend RR. To Restrict or Not to Restrict? The Enigma of Sodium Intake and Mortality. *American Journal of Kidney Diseases*; **65**(1): 9-11.
369. Perez V, Chang ET. Sodium-to-Potassium Ratio and Blood Pressure, Hypertension, and Related Factors. *Advances in Nutrition* 2014; **5**(6): 712-41.
370. Holbrook JT, Patterson KY, Bodner JE, et al. Sodium and potassium intake and balance in adults consuming self-selected diets. *The American Journal of Clinical Nutrition* 1984; **40**(4): 786-93.
371. Thornton SN. Thirst and hydration: Physiology and consequences of dysfunction. *Physiology & Behavior* 2010; **100**(1): 15-21.
372. Ritz P, Berrut G. The Importance of Good Hydration for Day-to-Day Health. *Nutrition Reviews* 2005; **63**: S6-S13.
373. MD KB. Water, Energy, and the Perils of Dehydration. 2015. http://kellybroganmd.com/article/perils-of-dehydration/#comment-264269 (accessed 7/26/2015 2015).
374. Maughan RJ, Shirreffs SM, Watson P. Exercise, heat, hydration, and the brain. *J Am Coll Nutr* 2007; **26**: 604S-12S.
375. KE DA, Constant F, Rosenberg IH. Hydration and cognitive function in children. *Nutr Rev* 2006; **64**: 457-64.
376. Jequier E, Constant F. Water as an essential nutrient: the physiological basis of hydration. *Eur J Clin Nutr* 2009; **64**(2): 115-23.

377. Haussinger D. The role of cellular hydration in the regulation of cell function. *Biochem J* 1996; **313**: 697-710.

378. Francesconi RP, Hubbard RW, Szlyk PC, Schnakenberg D, Carlson D, Leva N. Urinary and hematologic indexes of hypohydration. *J Appl Physiol* 1987; **62**: 1271-6.

379. Benton D. Dehydration Influences Mood and Cognition: A Plausible Hypothesis? *Nutrients* 2011; **3**(5): 555-73.

380. Fisher L. How Much salt is in a Human Body? July 22, 2009 2009. http://www.sciencefocus.com/qa/how-much-salt-human-body (accessed 8/6/2017 2017).

381. Peroutka SJ. Dopamine and migraine. *Neurology* 1997; **49**(3): 650-6.

382. Cha Y-H, Baloh RW. Migraine Associated Vertigo. *Journal of Clinical Neurology (Seoul, Korea)* 2007; **3**(3): 121-6.

383. Mamontov OV, Babayan L, Amelin AV, Giniatullin R, Kamshilin AA. Autonomous control of cardiovascular reactivity in patients with episodic and chronic forms of migraine. *The Journal of Headache and Pain* 2016; **17**: 52.

384. Tepper D. Migraine and Cardiovascular Disease. *Headache: The Journal of Head and Face Pain* 2014; **54**(7): 1267-8.

385. Watts SW, Morrison SF, Davis RP, Barman SM. Serotonin and Blood Pressure Regulation. *Pharmacological Reviews* 2012; **64**(2): 359-88.

386. Vikenes K, Farstad M, Nordrehaug JE. Serotonin Is Associated with Coronary Artery Disease and Cardiac Events. *Circulation* 1999; **100**(5): 483-9.

387. Friedman D. Headache and hypertension: refuting the myth. *Journal of Neurology, Neurosurgery & Psychiatry* 2002; **72**(4): 431.

388. Becerra L, Bishop J, Barmettler G, et al. Triptans disrupt brain networks and promote stress-induced CSD-like responses in cortical and subcortical areas. *Journal of Neurophysiology* 2016; **115**(1): 208-17.

389. Gupta VK. Triptans to Abort Neurological Symptoms of Prodrome of Migraine: Fact or Fiction? *Headache: The Journal of Head and Face Pain* 2005; **45**(5): 615-6.

390. Stanton AA. Are Statistics Misleading Sodium Reduction Benefits? *Journal of Medical Diagnostic Methods* 2016; **5**(1).

391. O'Brien E. Salt—too much or too little? *The Lancet.*

392. Reidlinger DP, Darzi J, Hall WL, Seed PT, Chowienczyk PJ, Sanders TA. How effective are current dietary guidelines for cardiovascular disease prevention in healthy middle-aged and older men and women? A randomized controlled trial. *The American Journal of Clinical Nutrition* 2015; **101**(5): 922-30.

393. Health NIo. Sodium in Diet: http://www.nlm.nih.gov/medlineplus/ency/article/002415.htm, 2015.

394. Graudal N, Jürgens G. The blood pressure sensitivity to changes in sodium intake is similar in Asians, Blacks and

Whites. An analysis of 92 randomized controlled trials. *Frontiers in Physiology* 2015; **6**.

395. O'Donnell M, Mente A, Yusuf S. Sodium Intake and Cardiovascular Health. *Circulation Research* 2015; **116**(6): 1046-57.
396. O'Donnell M, Mente A, Rangarajan S, et al. Urinary Sodium and Potassium Excretion, Mortality, and Cardiovascular Events. *New England Journal of Medicine* 2014; **371**(7): 612-23.
397. Ha SK. Dietary Salt Intake and Hypertension. *Electrolytes & Blood Pressure : E & BP* 2014; **12**(1): 7-18.
398. Amer M, Woodward M, Appel LJ. Effects of dietary sodium and the DASH diet on the occurrence of headaches: results from randomised multicentre DASH-Sodium clinical trial. *BMJ Open* 2014; **4**(12).
399. He FJ, Li J, MacGregor GA. Effect of longer term modest salt reduction on blood pressure: Cochrane systematic review and meta-analysis of randomised trials. *BMJ* 2013; **346**.
400. Pieske B, Houser SR, Hasenfuss G, Bers DM. Sodium and the heart: a hidden key factor in cardiac regulation. *Cardiovascular Research* 2003; **57**(4): 871-2.
401. Sacks FM. Effects on blood pressure of reduced dietary sodium and the dietary approaches to stop hypertension (DASH) diet. *N Engl J Med* 2001; **334**: 3-10.
402. Gomez-Pinilla F, Tyagi E. Diet and cognition: interplay between cell metabolism and neuronal plasticity. *Cur-*

rent opinion in clinical nutrition and metabolic care 2013; **16**(6): 726-33.

403. Ahmed SH, Guillem K, Vandaele Y. Sugar addiction: pushing the drug-sugar analogy to the limit. *Current Opinion in Clinical Nutrition & Metabolic Care* 2013; **16**(4): 434-9.
404. Bessesen DH. The Role of Carbohydrates in Insulin Resistance. *The Journal of Nutrition* 2001; **131**(10): 2782S-6S.
405. Hudgins LC, Hellerstein MK, Seidman CE, Neese RA, Tremaroli JD, Hirsch J. Relationship between carbohydrate-induced hypertriglyceridemia and fatty acid synthesis in lean and obese subjects. *Journal of Lipid Research* 2000; **41**(4): 595-604.
406. Lustig RH. Fat Chance: Beating the Odds Against Sugar, Processed Food, Obesity, and Disease: Plume; 2013 (reprint edition).
407. Lusting JYwRH. Pure, White, and Deadly: How Sugar is Killing Us and What We can Do To Stop It: Penguin Books, 2013.
408. Mirmiran P, Yuzbashian E, Asghari G, Hosseinpour-Niazi S, Azizi F. Consumption of sugar sweetened beverage is associated with incidence of metabolic syndrome in Tehranian children and adolescents. *Nutrition & Metabolism* 2015; **12**: 25.
409. Robert H. Lustig M.D. MSL. Fat Chance; Beating the Odds Against Sugar, Processed Food, Obesity, and Disease. New York, New York: Penguin; 2012, 2013, 2014.

410. Sanjay Gupta MD, Lustig MD, Robert H. Sugar: https://www.youtube.com/watch?v=HezSlrJ1k7w, 2013.
411. Stanhope KL, Bremer AA, Medici V, et al. Consumption of Fructose and High Fructose Corn Syrup Increase Postprandial Triglycerides, LDL-Cholesterol, and Apolipoprotein-B in Young Men and Women. *The Journal of Clinical Endocrinology and Metabolism* 2011; **96**(10): E1596-E605.
412. Weir MR. Hypervolemia and Blood Pressure. *Powerful Indicators of Increased Mortality Among Hemodialysis Patients* 2010; **56**(3): 341-3.
413. Lee M, Kim MK, Kim S-M, Park H, Park Cg, Park HK. Gender-Based Differences on the Association between Salt-Sensitive Genes and Obesity in Korean Children Aged between 8 and 9 Years. *PLOS ONE* 2015; **10**(3): e0120111.
414. Kawai M. Newly-acquired pre-cultural behavior of the natural troop of Japanese monkeys on Koshima islet. *Primates* 1965; **6**(1): 1-30.
415. Coleman JSF, James D.;Pringle, Carol A.;. Salt-Eating by Black and Turkey Vultures. *The Condor* 1985; **87**: 1.
416. Voigt CC, Capps KA, Dechmann DKN, Michener RH, Kunz TH. Nutrition or Detoxification: Why Bats Visit Mineral Licks of the Amazonian Rainforest. *PLOS ONE* 2008; **3**(4): e2011.
417. Blake JG, Mosquera D, Guerra J, Loiselle BA, Romo D, Swing K. Mineral Licks as Diversity Hotspots in Lowland Forest of Eastern Ecuador. *Diversity* 2011; **3**(2): 217.

418. Samoylovskaya NU, AV;. Use of Salt lick Briquettes «Ivir-salt» on Natural Areas of Preferential Protection in Russia for the Prevention of Parasitic Diseases in Wild Hoofed Animals. *Dairy, Veterinary & Animal Research* 2016; **3**(2).

419. Kern J, Kern S, Blennow K, et al. Calcium supplementation and risk of dementia in women with cerebrovascular disease. *Neurology* 2016.

420. Viera AJW, Noah; . Potassium Disorders: Hypokalemia and Hyperkalemia. *American family Physician* 2015; **92**(6): 8.

421. Whelton PK. Effects of oral potassium on blood pressure. Meta-analysis of randomized controlled clinical trials. *JAMA* 1997; **27**: 1624-32.

422. Haddy FJ, Vanhoutte PM, Feletou M. Role of potassium in regulating blood flow and blood pressure. *American Journal of Physiology - Regulatory, Integrative and Comparative Physiology* 2006; **290**(3): R546.

423. Geleijnse JM. Reduction in blood pressure with a low sodium, high potassium, high magnesium salt in older subjects with mild to moderate hypertension. *Br Med J* 1994; **309**: 436-40.

424. Breschi GL, Cametti M, Mastropietro A, et al. Different Permeability of Potassium Salts across the Blood-Brain Barrier Follows the Hofmeister Series. *PLoS ONE* 2013; **8**(10): e78553.

425. Jiruska P, Csicsvari J, Powell AD, et al. High-Frequency Network Activity, Global Increase in Neuronal Activ-

ity, and Synchrony Expansion Precede Epileptic Seizures <em>In Vitro</em>. *The Journal of Neuroscience* 2010; **30**(16): 5690-701.

426. Nardone R, Brigo F, Trinka E. Acute Symptomatic Seizures Caused by Electrolyte Disturbances. *Journal of Clinical Neurology (Seoul, Korea)* 2016; **12**(1): 21-33.
427. Lederer E. Hyperkalamia. 1/11/2016 2016. http://emedicine.medscape.com/article/240903-overview?pa=mGIbH6TTSRCwwL4FBbTlXL2c6%2BdzV2TqeDeKbcs%2BdfDNiWgf%2B30oIcyyZBW6k6c9dstDE2wTUmjtR6gNOM0yGUj41%2F3Xq%2FwkYYScwkptsbo%3D (accessed 3/7/2017 2017).
428. Dichgans M, Freilinger T, Eckstein G, et al. Mutation in the neuronal voltage-gated sodium channel <em>SCN1A</em> in familial hemiplegic migraine. *The Lancet*; **366**(9483): 371-7.
429. Reichard GA, Haff AC, Skutches CL, Paul P, Holroyde CP, Owen OE. Plasma Acetone Metabolism in the Fasting Human. *Journal of Clinical Investigation* 1979; **63**(4): 619-26.
430. Landau BR, Brunengraber H. The role of acetone in the conversion of fat to carbohydrate. *Trends in Biochemical Sciences* 1987; **12**: 113-4.
431. Kosugi K, Chandramouli V, Kumaran K, Schumann WC, Landau BR. Determinants in the pathways followed by the carbons of acetone in their conversion to glucose. *Journal of Biological Chemistry* 1986; **261**(28): 13179-81.

432. Reichard GA, Skutches CL, Hoeldtke RD, Owen OE. Acetone Metabolism in Humans During Diabetic Ketoacidosis. *Diabetes* 1986; **35**(6): 668-74.

433. Kaleta C, de Figueiredo LF, Werner S, Guthke R, Ristow M, Schuster S. In Silico Evidence for Gluconeogenesis from Fatty Acids in Humans. *PLOS Computational Biology* 2011; 7(7): e1002116.

434. Argilés JM. Has acetone a role in the conversion of fat to carbohydrate in mammals? *Trends in Biochemical Sciences*; **11**(2): 61-3.

435. Richards MP. A brief review of the archaeological evidence for Palaeolithic and Neolithic subsistence. *Eur J Clin Nutr* 2002; **56**(12): 16 p following 1262.

436. Flatt JP. Conversion of carbohydrate to fat in adipose tissue: an energy-yielding and, therefore, self-limiting process. *Journal of Lipid Research* 1970; **11**(2): 131-43.

437. Veldhorst MA, Westerterp-Plantenga MS, Westerterp KR. Gluconeogenesis and energy expenditure after a high-protein, carbohydrate-free diet. *The American Journal of Clinical Nutrition* 2009; **90**(3): 519-26.

438. Pektas MB, Koca HB, Sadi G, Akar F. Dietary Fructose Activates Insulin Signaling and Inflammation in Adipose Tissue: Modulatory Role of Resveratrol. *BioMed Research International* 2016; **2016**: 10.

439. Lustig RH. Fructose: It's "Alcohol Without the Buzz". *Advances in Nutrition: An International Review Journal* 2013; **4**(2): 226-35.

440. Kolderup A, Svihus B. Fructose Metabolism and Relation to Atherosclerosis, Type 2 Diabetes, and Obesity. *Journal of Nutrition and Metabolism* 2015; **2015**: 12.
441. Sun SZ, Empie MW. Fructose metabolism in humans – what isotopic tracer studies tell us. *Nutrition & Metabolism* 2012; **9**(1): 89.
442. Choi HK, Curhan G. Soft drinks, fructose consumption, and the risk of gout in men: prospective cohort study. *BMJ : British Medical Journal* 2008; **336**(7639): 309-12.
443. Angelopoulos TJ, Lowndes J, Zukley L, et al. The Effect of High-Fructose Corn Syrup Consumption on Triglycerides and Uric Acid. *The Journal of Nutrition* 2009; **139**(6): 1242S-5S.
444. Khitan Z, Kim DH. Fructose: A Key Factor in the Development of Metabolic Syndrome and Hypertension. *Journal of Nutrition and Metabolism* 2013; **2013**: 12.
445. Valishkevych BV, Vasylkovska RA, Lozinska LM, Semchyshyn HM. Fructose-Induced Carbonyl/Oxidative Stress in S. cerevisiae: Involvement of TOR. *Biochemistry Research International* 2016; **2016**: 10.
446. Coss-Bu JA, Sunehag AL, Haymond MW. Contribution of galactose and fructose to glucose homeostasis. *Metabolism* 2009; **58**.
447. Gannon MC, Khan MA, Nuttall FQ. Glucose appearance rate after the ingestion of galactose. *Metabolism - Clinical and Experimental*; **50**(1): 93-8.

448. Birt DF, Boylston T, Hendrich S, et al. Resistant Starch: Promise for Improving Human Health. *Advances in Nutrition: An International Review Journal* 2013; **4**(6): 587-601.
449. Paulmann N, Grohmann M, Voigt J-P, et al. Intracellular Serotonin Modulates Insulin Secretion from Pancreatic β-Cells by Protein Serotonylation. *PLoS Biol* 2009; **7**(10): e1000229.
450. Exton JH, Park CR. Control of Gluconeogenesis in Liver: I. GENERAL FEATURES OF GLUCONEOGENESIS IN THE PERFUSED LIVERS OF RATS. *Journal of Biological Chemistry* 1967; **242**(11): 2622-36.
451. Lenoir M, Serre F, Cantin L, Ahmed SH. Intense Sweetness Surpasses Cocaine Reward. *PLoS ONE* 2007; **2**(8): e698.
452. Johnson RK, Appel LJ, Brands M, et al. Dietary Sugars Intake and Cardiovascular Health. *A Scientific Statement From the American Heart Association* 2009; **120**(11): 1011-20.
453. Lustig RH. Fructose: metabolic, hedonic, and societal parallels with ethanol. *J Am Diet Assoc* 2010; **110**.
454. Shapiro A, Mu W, Roncal C, Cheng K-Y, Johnson RJ, Scarpace PJ. Fructose-induced leptin resistance exacerbates weight gain in response to subsequent high-fat feeding. *American Journal of Physiology - Regulatory, Integrative and Comparative Physiology* 2008; **295**(5): R1370.
455. Zhang Y-J, Wang F, Zhou Y, et al. Effects of 20 Selected Fruits on Ethanol Metabolism: Potential Health Benefits

and Harmful Impacts. *International Journal of Environmental Research and Public Health* 2016; **13**(4): 399.

456. Accurso A, Bernstein RK, Dahlqvist A, et al. Dietary carbohydrate restriction in type 2 diabetes mellitus and metabolic syndrome: time for a critical appraisal. *Nutrition & Metabolism* 2008; **5**(1): 9.
457. Lustig RH. Childhood obesity: behavioral aberration or biochemical drive? Reinterpreting the First Law of Thermodynamics. *Nature Clin Pract Endo Metab* 2006; **2**.
458. Nierengarter M. Pediatric nonalcoholic fatty liver disease. In: Walker T, editor. Contemporary Pediiatrics Expert Clinical Advise for Today's Pediatricians. Internet: Modern Medicine Network.
459. Loomba R, Sirlin CB, Schwimmer JB, Lavine JE. Advances in Pediatric Nonalcoholic Fatty Liver Disease. *Hepatology (Baltimore, Md)* 2009; **50**(4): 1282-93.
460. Berardis S, Sokal E. Pediatric non-alcoholic fatty liver disease: an increasing public health issue. *European Journal of Pediatrics* 2014; **173**(2): 131-9.
461. Strawbrige H. Artificial sweeteners: sugar-free, but at what cost? 2012. http://www.health.harvard.edu/blog/artificial-sweeteners-sugar-free-but-at-what-cost-201207165030 (accessed 8/1/2015 2015).
462. Brown RJ, De Banate MA, Rother KI. Artificial Sweeteners: A systematic review of metabolic effects in youth. *International journal of pediatric obesity : IJPO : an offi-*

cial journal of the International Association for the Study of Obesity 2010; **5**(4): 305-12.

463. Yang Q. Gain weight by "going diet?" Artificial sweeteners and the neurobiology of sugar cravings: Neuroscience 2010. *The Yale Journal of Biology and Medicine* 2010; **83**(2): 101-8.
464. Levine R. Monosaccharides in Health and Disease. *Annual Review of Nutrition* 1986; **6**(1): 211-24.
465. Swithers SE. Artificial sweeteners produce the counterintuitive effect of inducing metabolic derangements. *Trends in Endocrinology & Metabolism*; **24**(9): 431-41.
466. Crofts C, Schofield G, Zinn C, Wheldon M, Kraft J. Identifying hyperinsulinaemia in the absence of impaired glucose tolerance: An examination of the Kraft database. *Diabetes Research and Clinical Practice*; **118**: 50-7.
467. Welsh JA, Sharma A, Cunningham SA, Vos MB. Consumption of Added Sugars and Indicators of Cardiovascular Disease Risk Among US Adolescents; Clinical Perspective. *Circulation* 2011; **123**(3): 249-57.
468. Howard BV, Wylie-Rosett J. Sugar and Cardiovascular Disease. *Circulation* 2002; **106**(4): 523.
469. Laron Z. Insulin–a growth hormone. *Archives of Physiology and Biochemistry* 2008; **114**(1): 11-6.
470. Bartke A. Growth hormone and aging: A challenging controversy. *Clinical Interventions in Aging* 2008; **3**(4): 659-65.

471. Ashpole NM, Sanders JE, Hodges EL, Yan H, Sonntag WE. GROWTH HORMONE, INSULIN-LIKE GROWTH FACTOR-1 AND THE AGING BRAIN. *Experimental gerontology* 2015; **68**: 76-81.
472. Taniguchi CM, Emanuelli B, Kahn CR. Critical nodes in signalling pathways: insights into insulin action. *Nat Rev Mol Cell Biol* 2006; **7**(2): 85-96.
473. Saltiel AR, Kahn CR. Insulin signalling and the regulation of glucose and lipid metabolism. *Nature* 2001; **414**(6865): 799-806.
474. Bernstein RK. Dr. Bernstein's Diabetes Solution; The Complete Guide to Achieving Normal Blood Sugars. 4th ed. New York: Little, Brown and Company, Hachette Book group; 2011.
475. Eiselein L, Schwartz HJ, Rutledge JC. The Challenge of Type 1 Diabetes Mellitus. *ILAR Journal* 2004; **45**(3): 231-6.
476. Rigano KS, Gehring JL, Evans Hutzenbiler BD, et al. Life in the fat lane: seasonal regulation of insulin sensitivity, food intake, and adipose biology in brown bears. *Journal of Comparative Physiology B* 2017; **187**(4): 649-76.
477. Pal A, Barber TM, Van de Bunt M, et al. PTEN Mutations as a Cause of Constitutive Insulin Sensitivity and Obesity. *New England Journal of Medicine* 2012; **367**(11): 1002-11.
478. Nelson OJHG, E;Morgenstern, K;Gehring, JL;Rigano, KS;Lee, J;Gong, J;Shaywitz, AJ;Vella, CA;Robbins, CT;

Corbit, KC;. Grizzly bears exhibit augmented insulin sensitivity while obese prior to a reversible insulin resistance during hibernation. *CellPress*; **20**(2): 6.

479. Musselman LP, Fink JL, Narzinski K, et al. A high-sugar diet produces obesity and insulin resistance in wild-type Drosophila. *Disease Models & Mechanisms* 2011; **4**(6): 842-9.
480. Eades MR. A spoonful of sugar. The Blog of Michael R Eades, MD A critical look at nutritional science and anything else that strikes my fancy. Internet; 2005.
481. Rippe JM, Angelopoulos TJ. Sucrose, High-Fructose Corn Syrup, and Fructose, Their Metabolism and Potential Health Effects: What Do We Really Know? *Advances in Nutrition* 2013; **4**(2): 236-45.
482. Martin BC, Warram JH, Krolewski AS, et al. Role of glucose and insulin resistance in development of type 2 diabetes mellitus: results of a 25-year follow-up study. *The Lancet* 1992; **340**(8825): 925-9.
483. Jørgensen ME, Borch-Johnsen K, Stolk R, Bjerregaard P. Fat Distribution and Glucose Intolerance Among Greenland Inuit. *Diabetes Care* 2013; **36**(10): 2988.
484. Yamashita S, Nakamura T, Shimomura I, et al. Insulin resistance and body fat distribution. *Diabetes care* 1996; **19**(3): 287-91.
485. West KM, Ahuja MMS, Bennett PH, et al. The Role of Circulating Glucose and Triglyceride Concentrations and

Their Interactions with Other "Risk Factors" as Determinants of Arterial Disease in Nine Diabetic Population Samples from the WHO Multinational Study. *Diabetes Care* 1983; **6**(4): 361-9.

486. Theophilus PAS, Victoria MJ, Socarras KM, et al. Effectiveness of Stevia Rebaudiana Whole Leaf Extract Against the Various Morphological Forms of Borrelia Burgdorferi in Vitro. *European Journal of Microbiology & Immunology* 2015; **5**(4): 268-80.

487. Prakash I, Markosyan A, Bunders C. Development of Next Generation Stevia Sweetener: Rebaudioside M. *Foods* 2014; **3**(1): 162.

488. Baudier KM, Kaschock-Marenda SD, Patel N, Diangelus KL, O'Donnell S, Marenda DR. Erythritol, a Non-Nutritive Sugar Alcohol Sweetener and the Main Component of Truvia®, Is a Palatable Ingested Insecticide. *PLoS ONE* 2014; **9**(6): e98949.

489. MARENDA DR, O'donnell S. Use of erythritol or compositions comprising same as mammal-safe insecticides. Google Patents; 2015.

490. Jorda A, Zaragosa R, Manuel P. Long-term high-protein diet induces biochemical and ultrastructural changes in rat liver mitochondria. *Arch Biochem Biophys* 1988; **265**.

491. Manninen AH. High-Protein Weight Loss Diets and Purported Adverse Effects: Where is the Evidence? *Journal of the International Society of Sports Nutrition* 2004; **1**(1): 45.

492. Poortmans JR, Dellalieux O. Do regular high-protein diets have potential health risks on kidney function in athletes? *Int J Sports Nutr* 2000; **10**.

493. Street C. High-protein intake – Is it safe? In: Antonio J, Stout JR, eds. Sports Supplements. Philadelphia: Wilkins; 2001.

494. Messina M, Redmond G. Effects of Soy Protein and Soybean Isoflavones on Thyroid Function in Healthy Adults and Hypothyroid Patients: A Review of the Relevant Literature. *Thyroid* 2006; **16**(3): 249-58.

495. Bao J, de Jong V, Atkinson F, Petocz P, Brand-Miller JC. Food insulin index: physiologic basis for predicting insulin demand evoked by composite meals. *The American Journal of Clinical Nutrition* 2009; **90**(4): 986-92.

496. Holt SH, Miller JC, Petocz P. An insulin index of foods: the insulin demand generated by 1000-kJ portions of common foods. *The American Journal of Clinical Nutrition* 1997; **66**(5): 1264-76.

497. Willett WC. Ask the doctor: Coconut oil. March 18, 2016 2011. http://www.health.harvard.edu/staying-healthy/coconut-oil (accessed November 21 2016).

498. Hoenselaar R. Saturated fat and cardiovascular disease: The discrepancy between the scientific literature and dietary advice. *Nutrition* 2012; **28**.

499. Keys A, Anderson JT, Grande F. Serum cholesterol response to changes in the diet. *Metabolism* 1965; **14**(7): 776-87.

500. Keys A, Anderson JT, Grande F. Prediction of serum-cholesterol responses of man to changes in fats in the diet. *Lancet* 1957; **273**.
501. Bünger J, Bünger JF, Krahl J, et al. Combusting vegetable oils in diesel engines: the impact of unsaturated fatty acids on particle emissions and mutagenic effects of the exhaust. *Archives of Toxicology* 2016; **90**(6): 1471-9.
502. Cleaners K. Laundry Fires Due to Spontaneous Combustion. http://www.kelchnercleaners.com/fire-hazards-laundry-spontaneous-combustion/ (accessed 8/27/2017 2017).
503. Swaminathan A, Jicha GA. Nutrition and prevention of Alzheimer's dementia. *Frontiers in Aging Neuroscience* 2014; **6**: 282.
504. Costantini LC, Barr LJ, Vogel JL, Henderson ST. Hypometabolism as a therapeutic target in Alzheimer's disease. *BMC Neuroscience* 2008; **9**(2): S16.
505. Chen Z, Zhong C. Decoding Alzheimer's disease from perturbed cerebral glucose metabolism: Implications for diagnostic and therapeutic strategies. *Progress in Neurobiology* 2013; **108**: 21-43.
506. Doty L. Coconut Oil for Alzheimer's Disease? *Clinical Practice* 2012; **1**(2): 6.
507. Moore RB, Anderson JT, Taylor HL, Keys A, Frantz ID. Effect of dietary fat on the fecal excretion of cholesterol and its degradation products in man. *Journal of Clinical Investigation* 1968; **47**(7): 1517-34.

508. KEYS A, MIENOTTI A, KARVONEN MJ, et al. THE DIET AND 15-YEAR DEATH RATE IN THE SEVEN COUNTRIES STUDY. *American Journal of Epidemiology* 1986; **124**(6): 903-15.

509. Weintraub MS, Zechner R, Brown A, Eisenberg S, Breslow JL. Dietary polyunsaturated fats of the w-6 and w-3 series reduce postprandial lipoprotein levels: chronic and acute effects of fat saturation on postprandial lipoprotein metabolism. *J Clin Invest* 1988; **82**.

510. Ginsberg HN, Kris-Etherton P, Dennis B, et al. Effects of reducing dietary saturated fatty acids on plasma lipids and lipoproteins in healthy subjects- The Delta Study, Protocol 1. *Arterioscler Thromb Vasc Biol* 1998; **18**.

511. Zicha J, Kuneš J. Ontogenetic Aspects of Hypertension Development: Analysis in the Rat. *Physiological Reviews* 1999; **79**(4): 1227-82.

512. Siri-Tarino PW, Sun Q, Hu FB, Krauss RM. Meta-analysis of prospective cohort studies evaluating the association of saturated fat with cardiovascular disease. *The American Journal of Clinical Nutrition* 2010.

513. Hunter JE, Zhang J, Kris-Etherton PM. Cardiovascular risk of dietary stearic acid compared with trans, other saturated and undsaturated fatty acids: a systematic review. *Am J Clin Nutr* 2010; **91**.

514. Cleave TL. DIETARY PREVENTION OF ATHEROSCLEROSIS. *The Lancet*; **294**(7627): 961.

515. Bray G. EFFECT OF CALORIC RESTRICTION ON ENERGY EXPENDITURE IN OBESE PATIENTS. *The Lancet*; **294**(7617): 397-8.

516. Yudkin J, Carey M. THE TREATMENT OF OBESITY BY THE "HIGH-FAT" DIET. *The Lancet*; **276**(7157): 939-41.

517. Kekwick A, Pawan GLS. FATTY FOODS AND OBESITY. *The Lancet*; **275**(7135): 1190.

518. Taubes G. Insulin resistance. Prosperity's plague. *Science* 2009; **325**.

519. Dr. Kendrick M. The Great Cholesterol Con; The trusth about what really causes heart disease and how to avoid it. London, England: John Blake Publishing; 2007.

520. Kendrick M. Doctoring Data: How to sort out medical advice from medical nonsense: Columbus Publishing Ltd; 2015.

521. Grasgruber P, Sebera M, Hrazdira E, Hrebickova S, Cacek J. Food consumption and the actual statistics of cardiovascular diseases: an epidemiological comparison of 42 European countries. *2016* 2016; **60**.

522. Campbell-McBridge N. Cholesterol: Friend or Foe? 2008. http://www.westonaprice.org/know-your-fats/cholesterol-friend-or-foe/.

523. Buchholz AC, Schoeller DA. Is a calorie a calorie? *The American Journal of Clinical Nutrition* 2004; **79**(5): 899S-906S.

524. Rahman K. Studies on free radicals, antioxidants, and co-factors. *Clinical Interventions in Aging* 2007; **2**(2): 219-36.
525. Keys A. Prediction and Possible Prevention of Coronary Disease. *American Journal of Public Health and the Nations Health* 1953; **43**(11): 1399-407.
526. Keys A. Coronary Heart Disease in Young Adults. *American Journal of Public Health and the Nations Health* 1954; **44**(11): 1469-70.
527. Keys A, Grande F. Role of Dietary Fat in Human Nutrition: III. Diet and the Epidemiology of Coronary Heart Disease. *American Journal of Public Health and the Nations Health* 1957; **47**(12): 1520-30.
528. Strom BL, Schinnar R, Karlawish J, Hennessy S, Teal V, Bilker WB. Statin therapy and risk of acute memory impairment. *JAMA Internal Medicine* 2015; **175**(8): 1399-405.
529. Shea TB, Remington R. Nutritional supplementation for Alzheimer's disease? *Current Opinion in Psychiatry* 2015; **28**(2).
530. Engelborghs S, Gilles C, Ivanoiu A, Vandewoude M. Rationale and clinical data supporting nutritional intervention in Alzheimer's disease. *Acta Clinica Belgica* 2014; **69**(1): 17-24.
531. Boateng L, Ansong R, Owusu WB, Steiner-Asiedu M. Coconut oil and palm oil's role in nutrition, health and national development: A review. *Ghana Medical Journal* 2016; **50**(3): 189-96.

532. Kingsbury KJP, S.; Crossley, A.; Morgan, D.M;. The Fatty Acid Composition of Human Depot Fat. *Biochem J* 1960; **78**: 541-50.

533. Volek JS, Noakes T, Phinney SD. Rethinking fat as a fuel for endurance exercise. *European Journal of Sport Science* 2015; **15**(1): 13-20.

534. Forsythe CE, Phinney SD, Feinman RD, et al. Limited Effect of Dietary Saturated Fat on Plasma Saturated Fat in the Context of a Low Carbohydrate Diet. *Lipids* 2010; **45**(10): 947-62.

535. Kershaw EE, Flier JS. Adipose Tissue as an Endocrine Organ. *The Journal of Clinical Endocrinology & Metabolism* 2004; **89**(6): 2548-56.

536. Zhang W, Cline MA, Gilbert ER. Hypothalamus-adipose tissue crosstalk: neuropeptide Y and the regulation of energy metabolism. *Nutrition & Metabolism* 2014; **11**(1): 27.

537. Nakagomi A, Okada S, Yokoyama M, et al. Role of the central nervous system and adipose tissue BDNF/TrkB axes in metabolic regulation. *Npj Aging And Mechanisms Of Disease* 2015; **1**: 15009.

538. Montague CT, Rahilly S. The perils of portliness: causes and consequences of visceral adiposity. *Diabetes* 2000; **49**(6): 883.

539. Siri-Tarino PW, Sun Q, Hu FB, Krauss RM. Saturated fat, carbohydrate, and cardiovascular disease. *The American Journal of Clinical Nutrition* 2010; **91**(3): 502-9.

540. Kris-Etherton PM, Fleming JA. Emerging Nutrition Science on Fatty Acids and Cardiovascular Disease: Nutritionists' Perspectives. *Advances in Nutrition* 2015; **6**(3): 326S-37S.

541. DiNicolantonio JJ. The cardiometabolic consequences of replacing saturated fats with carbohydrates or Ω-6 polyunsaturated fats: Do the dietary guidelines have it wrong? *Open Heart* 2014; **1**(1).

542. Hu FB. Are refined carbohydrates worse than saturated fat? *The American Journal of Clinical Nutrition* 2010; **91**(6): 1541-2.

543. Poplawski MM, Mastaitis JW, Isoda F, Grosjean F, Zheng F, Mobbs CV. Reversal of Diabetic Nephropathy by a Ketogenic Diet. *PLoS ONE* 2011; **6**(4): e18604.

544. Kossoff EH, Hartman AL. Ketogenic Diets: New Advances for Metabolism-Based Therapies. *Current opinion in neurology* 2012; **25**(2): 173-8.

545. Phinney SD. Ketogenic diets and physical performance. *Nutrition & Metabolism* 2004; **1**(1): 1-7.

546. Paoli A. Ketogenic Diet for Obesity: Friend or Foe? *International Journal of Environmental Research and Public Health* 2014; **11**(2): 2092-107.

547. Paoli A, Rubini A, Volek JS, Grimaldi KA. Beyond weight loss: a review of the therapeutic uses of very-low-carbohydrate (ketogenic) diets. *European Journal of Clinical Nutrition* 2013; **67**(8): 789-96.

548. Ectopic Fat and Insulin Resistance: Pathophysiology and Effect of Diet and Lifestyle Interventions. *International Journal of Endocrinology* 2012; **2012**: 18.
549. Kahn BB, Flier JS. Obesity and insulin resistance. *The Journal of Clinical Investigation* 2000; **106**(4): 473-81.
550. Ma Y, Olendzki B, Chiriboga D, et al. Association between Dietary Carbohydrates and Body Weight. *American Journal of Epidemiology* 2005; **161**(4): 359-67.
551. Bray GA, Popkin BM. Dietary Sugar and Body Weight: Have We Reached a Crisis in the Epidemic of Obesity and Diabetes? *Health Be Damned! Pour on the Sugar* 2014; **37**(4): 950-6.
552. Ludwig DS, Majzoub JA, Al-Zahrani A, Dallal GE, Blanco I, Roberts SB. High Glycemic Index Foods, Overeating, and Obesity. *Pediatrics* 1999; **103**(3): e26-e.
553. Brand-Miller JC, Holt SH, Pawlak DB, McMillan J. Glycemic index and obesity. *The American Journal of Clinical Nutrition* 2002; **76**(1): 281S-5S.
554. Moghaddam E, Vogt JA, Wolever TMS. The Effects of Fat and Protein on Glycemic Responses in Nondiabetic Humans Vary with Waist Circumference, Fasting Plasma Insulin, and Dietary Fiber Intake. *The Journal of Nutrition* 2006; **136**(10): 2506-11.
555. Stubbs RJ, Mazlan N, Whybrow S. Carbohydrates, Appetite and Feeding Behavior in Humans. *The Journal of Nutrition* 2001; **131**(10): 2775S-81S.

556. den Biggelaar LJCJ, Eussen SJPM, Sep SJS, et al. Associations of Dietary Glucose, Fructose, and Sucrose with β-Cell Function, Insulin Sensitivity, and Type 2 Diabetes in the Maastricht Study. *Nutrients* 2017; **9**(4): 380.
557. Jeppesen C, Bjerregaard P, Jørgensen ME. Dietary patterns in Greenland and their relationship with type 2 diabetes mellitus and glucose intolerance. *Public Health Nutrition* 2013; **17**(2): 462-70.
558. Pereira MA, Weggemans RM, Jacobs JDR, et al. Within-person variation in serum lipids: implications for clinical trials. *International Journal of Epidemiology* 2004; **33**(3): 534-41.
559. Pfrieger FW, Ungerer N. Cholesterol metabolism in neurons and astrocytes. *Progress in Lipid Research* 2011; **50**(4): 357-71.
560. Stampfer MJ, Krauss RM, Ma J, et al. A prospective study of triglyceride level, low-density lipoprotein particle diameter, and risk of myocardial infarction. *JAMA* 1996; **276**(11): 882-8.
561. Williams VJ, Leritz EC, Shepel J, et al. Interindividual variation in serum cholesterol is associated with regional white matter tissue integrity in older adults. *Hum Brain Mapp* 2013; **34**(8): 1826-41.
562. Warstadt NM, Dennis EL, Jahanshad N, et al. Serum Cholesterol and Variant in Cholesterol-Related Gene CETP Predict White Matter Microstructure. *Neurobiology of aging* 2014; **35**(11): 2504-13.

563. Rinholm JE, Hamilton NB, Kessaris N, Richardson WD, Bergersen LH, Attwell D. Regulation of oligodendrocyte development and myelination by glucose and lactate. *The Journal of neuroscience : the official journal of the Society for Neuroscience* 2011; **31**(2): 538-48.
564. Podbielska M, Banik NL, Kurowska E, Hogan EL. Myelin Recovery in Multiple Sclerosis: The Challenge of Remyelination. *Brain Sciences* 2013; **3**(3): 1282-324.
565. Alizadeh A, Dyck SM, Karimi-Abdolrezaee S. Myelin damage and repair in pathologic CNS: challenges and prospects. *Frontiers in Molecular Neuroscience* 2015; **8**: 35.
566. Mathur D, López-Rodas G, Casanova B, Marti MB. Perturbed Glucose Metabolism: Insights into Multiple Sclerosis Pathogenesis. *Frontiers in Neurology* 2014; **5**: 250.
567. Malone JI. Diabetic Central Neuropathy: CNS Damage Related to Hyperglycemia. *Diabetes* 2016; **65**(2): 355-7.
568. Hyman Dr. M. Eat Fat Get Thin; Why the fat we Eat is the Key to Sustained Weight Loss and Vibrant Health. London, UK: Hodder & Stoughton Ltd.; 2016.
569. School HM. The truth about fats: the good, the bad, and the in-between. 2015. http://www.health.harvard.edu/staying-healthy/the-truth-about-fats-bad-and-good (accessed 8/1/2015 2015).
570. Fernando WMADB, Martins IJ, Goozee KG, Brennan CS, Jayasena V, Martins RN. The role of dietary coconut for the prevention and treatment of Alzheimer's disease:

potential mechanisms of action. *British Journal of Nutrition* 2015; **114**(01): 1-14.

571. Moullé VS, Picard A, Cansell C, Luquet S, Magnan C. Rôle de la détection centrale des lipides dans le contrôle nerveux de la balance énergétique. *Med Sci (Paris)* 2015; **31**(4): 397-403.

572. Fan S. The fat-fueled brain: unnatural or advantageous? Scientific American. 2013 October 1, 2013.

573. Gómez-Pinilla F. Brain foods: the effects of nutrients on brain function. *Nature reviews Neuroscience* 2008; **9**(7): 568-78.

574. MedlinePlus N. Calcium in Diet by Medline Plus: http://www.nlm.nih.gov/medlineplus/ency/article/002412.htm.

575. Doerge DR, Sheehan DM. Goitrogenic and estrogenic activity of soy isoflavones. *Environmental Health Perspectives* 2002; **110**(Suppl 3): 349-53.

576. USDA. 2015-2020 Dietary Guidelines for Americans. In: Promotion CfNPa, editor. Internet: USDA; 2015-2020.

577. Lafiandra D, Riccardi G, Shewry PR. Improving cereal grain carbohydrates for diet and health. *Journal of Cereal Science* 2014; **59**(3): 312-26.

578. Davis W. Wheat Belly Total Health. New York, NY: Rodale; 2014.

579. de Punder K, Pruimboom L. The Dietary Intake of Wheat and other Cereal Grains and Their Role in Inflammation. *Nutrients* 2013; **5**(3): 771-87.

580. Atkinson FS, Foster-Powell K, Brand-Miller JC. International Tables of Glycemic Index and Glycemic Load Values: 2008. *Diabetes Care* 2008; **31**(12): 2281-3.

581. Harvard. Carbohydrates and Blood Sugar. https://www.hsph.harvard.edu/nutritionsource/carbohydrates/carbohydrates-and-blood-sugar/ (accessed 3/7/2017 2017).

582. Diabetes Superfood. February 2, 2015. http://www.diabetes.org/food-and-fitness/food/what-can-i-eat/making-healthy-food-choices/diabetes-superfoods.html?referrer=https://www.google.com/ (accessed 6/11/2017 2017).

583. Andersson A, Tengblad S, Karlström B, et al. Whole-Grain Foods Do Not Affect Insulin Sensitivity or Markers of Lipid Peroxidation and Inflammation in Healthy, Moderately Overweight Subjects. *The Journal of Nutrition* 2007; **137**(6): 1401-7.

584. Moyer MW. Whole-Grain Foods Not Always Healthful. Scientific American. 2013 July 25, 2013.

585. Freed DLJ. Do dietary lectins cause disease? : The evidence is suggestive—and raises interesting possibilities for treatment *BMJ : British Medical Journal* 1999; **318**(7190): 1023-4.

586. Nachbar MS, Oppenheim JD. Lectins in the United States diet: a survey of lectins in commonly consumed foods and a review of the literature. *The American Journal of Clinical Nutrition* 1980; **33**(11): 2338-45.

587. Infantino MM, F; Maccia, D;Manfredi, M;. Anti-gliadin antibodies in non-celiac gluten sensitivity. *Minerva Gastroenterol Dietol* 2017; **63**(Prepub): 5.

588. Murakami T, Nishimura T, Kitabatake N, Tani F. Molecular Analysis of the Polymeric Glutenins with Gliadin-Like Characteristics That Were Produced by Acid Dispersion of Wheat Gluten. *Journal of Food Science* 2016; **81**(3): C553-C62.

589. Hollon J, Leonard Puppa E, Greenwald B, Goldberg E, Guerrerio A, Fasano A. Effect of Gliadin on Permeability of Intestinal Biopsy Explants from Celiac Disease Patients and Patients with Non-Celiac Gluten Sensitivity. *Nutrients* 2015; **7**(3): 1565-76.

590. Martínez ME, Jacobs ET, Baron JA, Marshall JR, Byers T. Dietary Supplements and Cancer Prevention: Balancing Potential Benefits Against Proven Harms. *JNCI Journal of the National Cancer Institute* 2012; **104**(10): 732-9.

591. Harvie M. Nutritional supplements and cancer: potential benefits and proven harms. Am Soc Clin Oncol Educ Book: ASC University; 2014.

592. Kowalska M, Prendecki M, Kozubski W, Lianeri M, Dorszewska J. Molecular factors in migraine. *Oncotarget* 2016; **7**(31): 50708-18.

593. Azimova JE, Sergeev AV, Korobeynikova LA, et al. Effects of MTHFR gene polymorphism on the clinical and electrophysiological characteristics of migraine. *BMC Neurology* 2013; **13**: 103-.

594. Goldie C, Taylor AJ, Nguyen P, McCoy C, Zhao X-Q, Preiss D. Niacin therapy and the risk of new-onset diabetes: a meta-analysis of randomised controlled trials. *Heart* 2016; **102**(3): 198-203.
595. Messina G. Recommended Supplements for Vegans. Novemebr 28, 2010 2010. http://www.theveganrd.com/2010/11/recommended-supplements-for-vegans.html (accessed 5/5/2017 2017).
596. Craig WJ. Nutrition Concerns and Health Effects of Vegetarian Diets. *Nutrition in Clinical Practice* 2010; **25**(6): 613-20.
597. Dwyer J, Loew FM. Nutritional risks of vegan diets to women and children: Are they preventable? *Journal of Agricultural and Environmental Ethics* 1994; **7**(1): 87-109.
598. Ede G. 2015 US Dietary Guidelines Critique. Diagnosis: Diet Nutrition Science meets Common Sense. p. New Dietary Guidelines Hazardous to Your Health?
599. Christie-David DJG, Christian M,; Gunton, Jenny E.;. Effects of vitamins C and D in type 2 diabetes mellitus. *Nutrition and Dietary Supplements* 2015; **2015:7**: 8.
600. Astuya A, Caprile T, Castro M, et al. Vitamin C uptake and recycling among normal and tumor cells from the central nervous system. *Journal of Neuroscience Research* 2005; **79**(1-2): 146-56.
601. Levine M, Conry-Cantilena C, Wang Y, et al. Vitamin C pharmacokinetics in healthy volunteers: evidence for a recommended dietary allowance. *Proceedings of the Na-*

tional Academy of Sciences of the United States of America 1996; **93**(8): 3704-9.

602. Donin AS, Dent JE, Nightingale CM, et al. Fruit, vegetable and vitamin C intakes and plasma vitamin C: cross-sectional associations with insulin resistance and glycaemia in 9–10 year-old children. *Diabetic Medicine* 2016; **33**(3): 307-15.

603. Omar HR, Komarova I, El-Ghonemi M, et al. Licorice abuse: time to send a warning message. *Therapeutic Advances in Endocrinology and Metabolism* 2012; **3**(4): 125-38.

604. Mouritsen OG, Williams L, Bjerregaard R, Duelund L. Seaweeds for umami flavour in the New Nordic Cuisine. *Flavour* 2012; **1**(1): 4.

605. Rodin J. Insulin levels, hunger, and food intake: An example of feedback loops in body weight regulation. *Health Psychology* 1985; **4**(1): 25.

606. Tara S. The Secret Life of Fat: The Science Behind the Body's Greatest Puzzle. US: Blink Publishing; 2016.

607. Lim JS, Mietus-Snyder M, Valente A, Schwarz JM, Lustig RH. The role of fructose in the pathogenesis of NAFLD and the metabolic syndrome. *Nat Rev Gastroenterol Hepatol* 2010; **7**.

608. Lemieux S, Després JP, Moorjani S, et al. Are gender differences in cardiovascular disease risk factors explained by the level of visceral adipose tissue? *Diabetologia* 1994; **37**(8): 757-64.

609. Nestle MN, Malden;. Why Calories Count; From Science to Politics. California, US: University of California Press; 2013.

610. Mozaffarian RS, Lee RM, Kennedy MA, Ludwig DS, Mozaffarian D, Gortmaker SL. Identifying whole grain foods: a comparison of different approaches for selecting more healthful whole grain products. *Public health nutrition* 2013; **16**(12): 2255-64.

611. Unwin T. Hedonic price indexes and the qualities of wines. *Journal of Wine Research* 1999; **10**(2): 95-104.

612. NHS. Blueberries: antioxidant powerhouse? 8/26/2015 2015. http://www.nhs.uk/Livewell/superfoods/Pages/are-blueberries-a-superfood.aspx2017).

613. Know L. Life - The Epic Story of Our Mitochondria: How the Original Probiotic Dictates Your Health, Illness, Ageing, and Even Life Itself FriesenPress; 2014.

614. Post TH. Diet Coke vs. Coca-Cola Zero: What's The Difference? Taste; 2016.

615. Nettleton JA, Lutsey PL, Wang Y, Lima JA, Michos ED, Jacobs DR. Diet Soda Intake and Risk of Incident Metabolic Syndrome and Type 2 Diabetes in the Multi-Ethnic Study of Atherosclerosis (MESA). *Diabetes Care* 2009; **32**(4): 688-94.

616. Anton SD, Martin CK, Han H, et al. Effects of stevia, aspartame, and sucrose on food intake, satiety, and postprandial glucose and insulin levels. *Appetite* 2010; **55**(1): 37-43.

617. News; B. Youngest toddler with type 2 diabetes raises concern, 2015.
618. Fernstrom JD, Munger SD, Sclafani A, de Araujo IE, Roberts A, Molinary S. Mechanisms for Sweetness. *The Journal of Nutrition* 2012; **142**(6): 1134S-41S.
619. Hellfritsch C, Brockhoff A, Stähler F, Meyerhof W, Hofmann T. Human Psychometric and Taste Receptor Responses to Steviol Glycosides. *Journal of Agricultural and Food Chemistry* 2012; **60**(27): 6782-93.
620. Blázquez E, Velázquez E, Hurtado-Carneiro V, Ruiz-Albusac JM. Insulin in the Brain: Its Pathophysiological Implications for States Related with Central Insulin Resistance, Type 2 Diabetes and Alzheimer's Disease. *Frontiers in Endocrinology* 2014; **5**: 161.
621. Havrankova J, Schmechel D, Roth J, Brownstein M. Identification of insulin in rat brain. *Proceedings of the National Academy of Sciences of the United States of America* 1978; **75**(11): 5737-41.
622. Szabo O, Szabo A. Evidence for an insulin-sensitive receptor in the central nervous system. *American Journal of Physiology -- Legacy Content* 1972; **223**(6): 1349-53.
623. Abdul-Ghani MA, DeFronzo RA. Pathogenesis of Insulin Resistance in Skeletal Muscle. *Journal of Biomedicine and Biotechnology* 2010; **2010**.
624. Savage DB, Petersen KF, Shulman GI. Mechanisms of Insulin Resistance in Humans and Possible Links With Inflammation. *Hypertension* 2005; **45**(5): 828-33.

625. Heinrich G, Ghadieh HE, Ghanem SS, et al. Loss of Hepatic CEACAM1: A Unifying Mechanism Linking Insulin Resistance to Obesity and Non-Alcoholic Fatty Liver Disease. *Frontiers in Endocrinology* 2017; **8**(8).

626. Zheng S, Xu H, Zhou H, et al. Associations of lipid profiles with insulin resistance and β cell function in adults with normal glucose tolerance and different categories of impaired glucose regulation. *PLOS ONE* 2017; **12**(2): e0172221.

627. Kuhlmann J, Neumann-Haefelin C, Belz U, et al. Intramyocellular Lipid and Insulin Resistance. *<span class=”subtitle”>A Longitudinal In Vivo ¹H-Spectroscopic Study in Zucker Diabetic Fatty Rats </span>* 2003; **52**(1): 138-44.

628. Sears B, Perry M. The role of fatty acids in insulin resistance. *Lipids in Health and Disease* 2015; **14**(1): 121.

629. Kowalski GM, Moore SM, Hamley S, Selathurai A, Bruce CR. The Effect of Ingested Glucose Dose on the Suppression of Endogenous Glucose Production in Humans. *Diabetes* 2017.

630. Kanauchi M. A New Index of Insulin Sensitivity Obtained From the Oral Glucose Tolerance Test Applicable to Advanced Type 2 Diabetes. *Diabetes Care* 2002; **25**(10): 1891-2.

631. Gutch M, Kumar S, Razi SM, Gupta KK, Gupta A. Assessment of insulin sensitivity/resistance. *Indian Journal of Endocrinology and Metabolism* 2015; **19**(1): 160-4.

632. Matsuda M, DeFronzo RA. Insulin sensitivity indices obtained from oral glucose tolerance testing: comparison with the euglycemic insulin clamp. *Diabetes Care* 1999; **22**(9): 1462-70.

633. Soonthornpun S, Setasuban W, Thamprasit A, Chayanunnukul W, Rattarasarn C, Geater A. Novel Insulin Sensitivity Index Derived from Oral Glucose Tolerance Test. *The Journal of Clinical Endocrinology & Metabolism* 2003; **88**(3): 1019-23.

634. Odegaard JI, Chawla A. Pleiotropic actions of insulin resistance and inflammation in metabolic homeostasis. *Science* 2013; **339**.

635. Draznin B. Molecular Mechanisms of Insulin Resistance: Serine Phosphorylation of Insulin Receptor Substrate-1 and Increased Expression of p85α. *The Two Sides of a Coin* 2006; **55**(8): 2392-7.

636. Watanabe H, Rose MT, Aso H. Role of peripheral serotonin in glucose and lipid metabolism. *Current Opinion in Lipidology* 2011; **22**(3): 186-91.

637. Ohara-Imaizumi M, Kim H, Yoshida M, et al. Serotonin regulates glucose-stimulated insulin secretion from pancreatic β cells during pregnancy. *Proceedings of the National Academy of Sciences* 2013; **110**(48): 19420-5.

638. Cataldo LR, Mizgier ML, Bravo Sagua R, et al. Prolonged Activation of the Htr2b Serotonin Receptor Impairs Glucose Stimulated Insulin Secretion and Mitochon-

drial Function in MIN6 Cells. *PLOS ONE* 2017; **12**(1): e0170213.

639. Robinson R. Serotonin's Role in the Pancreas Revealed at Last. *PLoS Biol* 2009; **7**(10): e1000227.
640. Isaac R, Boura-Halfon S, Gurevitch D, Shainskaya A, Levkovitz Y, Zick Y. Selective Serotonin Reuptake Inhibitors (SSRIs) Inhibit Insulin Secretion and Action in Pancreatic β Cells. *Journal of Biological Chemistry* 2013; **288**(8): 5682-93.
641. Tötterman K, Groop L, Groop P-H, Kala R, Tolppanen E-M, Fyhrquist F. Effect of beta-blocking drugs on beta-cell function and insulin sensitivity in hypertensive non-diabetic patients. *European Journal of Clinical Pharmacology* 1984; **26**(1): 13-7.
642. Blackburn DF, Wilson TW. Antihypertensive medications and blood sugar: Theories and implications. *The Canadian journal of cardiology* 2006; **22**(3): 229-33.
643. Moores S. Experts warn of detox diet dangers. 5/18/2007 2007. http://www.nbcnews.com/id/18595886/ns/health-diet_and_nutrition/t/experts-warn-detox-diet-dangers/#.WUHd-evysuU (accessed 6/14/2017 2017).
644. Whitehouse CR, Boullata J, McCauley LA. The Potential Toxicity of Artificial Sweeteners. *AAOHN Journal* 2008; **56**(6): 251-61.
645. Esmaillzadeh A, Azadbakht L. Different kinds of vegetable oils in relation to individual cardiovascular risk factors

among Iranian women. *British Journal of Nutrition* 2011; **105**(6): 919-27.

646. Mozaffarian D, Clarke R. Quantitative effects on cardiovascular risk factors and coronary heart disease risk of replacing partially hydrogenated vegetable oils with other fats and oils. *Eur J Clin Nutr* 0000; **63**(S2): S22-S33.
647. Halvorsen BL, Blomhoff R. Determination of lipid oxidation products in vegetable oils and marine omega-3 supplements. *Food & Nutrition Research* 2011; **55**: 10.3402/fnr.v55i0.5792.
648. Choe E, Min DB. Mechanisms and Factors for Edible Oil Oxidation. *Comprehensive Reviews in Food Science and Food Safety* 2006; **5**(4): 169-86.
649. Noakes TD, Windt J. Evidence that supports the prescription of low-carbohydrate high-fat diets: a narrative review. *British Journal of Sports Medicine* 2017; **51**(2): 133-9.
650. Wheless JW. History of the ketogenic diet. *Epilepsia* 2008; **49**: 3-5.
651. Kim DY, Hao J, Liu R, Turner G, Shi F-D, Rho JM. Inflammation-Mediated Memory Dysfunction and Effects of a Ketogenic Diet in a Murine Model of Multiple Sclerosis. *PLOS ONE* 2012; **7**(5): e35476.
652. Rho J, Stafstrom C. The Ketogenic Diet as a Treatment Paradigm for Diverse Neurological Disorders. *Frontiers in Pharmacology* 2012; **3**(59).

653. Reger MA, Henderson ST, Hale C, et al. Effects of Beta-hydroxybutyrate on cognition in memory-impaired adults. *Neurobiology of Aging*; **25**(3): 311-4.
654. Costantini LC, Barr LJ, Vogel JL, Henderson ST. Hypometabolism as a therapeutic target in Alzheimer's disease. *BMC Neuroscience* 2008; **9**(Suppl 2): S16-S.
655. Tay J, Zajac IT, Thompson CH, et al. A randomised-controlled trial of the effects of very low-carbohydrate and high-carbohydrate diets on cognitive performance in patients with type 2 diabetes. *British Journal of Nutrition* 2016; **116**(10): 1745-53.
656. Tay J, Luscombe-Marsh ND, Thompson CH, et al. Comparison of low- and high-carbohydrate diets for type 2 diabetes management: a randomized trial. *The American Journal of Clinical Nutrition* 2015; **102**(4): 780-90.
657. Bougneres PF, Lemmel C, Ferré P, Bier DM. Ketone body transport in the human neonate and infant. *Journal of Clinical Investigation* 1986; **77**(1): 42-8.
658. Dametti S, Faravelli I, Ruggieri M, Ramirez A, Nizzardo M, Corti S. Experimental Advances Towards Neural Regeneration from Induced Stem Cells to Direct In Vivo Reprogramming. *Molecular Neurobiology* 2016; **53**(4): 2124-31.
659. El-Mallakh RS, Gao Y, Jeannie Roberts R. Tardive dysphoria: The role of long term antidepressant use in-inducing chronic depression. *Medical Hypotheses*; **76**(6): 769-73.

660. Verdoux H, Cougnard A, Thiébaut A, Tournier M. Impact of Duration of Antidepressant Treatment on the Risk of Occurrence of a New Sequence of Antidepressant Treatment. *Pharmacopsychiatry* 2011; **44**(03): 96-101.

661. Mula M. Topiramate and cognitive impairment: evidence and clinical implications. *Therapeutic Advances in Drug Safety* 2012; **3**(6): 279-89.

662. Mula M, Trimble MR. Antiepileptic Drug-Induced Cognitive Adverse Effects. *CNS Drugs* 2009; **23**(2): 121-37.

663. Sachs H, Wolf A, Russell JG, Christman DR. Effect of reserpine on regional cerebral glucose metabolism jjss in control and migraine subjects. *Archives of Neurology* 1986; **43**(11): 1117-23.

664. Shaw SWJ, Johnson RH, Keogh HJ. Metabolic changes during glucose tolerance tests in migraine attacks. *Journal of the Neurological Sciences*; **33**(1): 51-9.

665. Clinch CR. Evaluation of Acute Headaches in Adults. *American Family Physician* 2001; **63**(4): 8.

666. Mayo. Cluster Headaches. https://www.gstatic.com/healthricherkp/pdf/cluster_headaches.pdf (accessed 2/3/2017 2017).

667. Adler AR, Charnin JA, Quraishi SA. Serotonin Syndrome: The Potential for a Severe Reaction Between Common Perioperative Medications and Selective Serotonin Reuptake Inhibitors. *A&A Case Reports* 2015; **5**(9): 156-9.

668. Haberzettl R, Fink H, Bert B. The murine serotonin syndrome – Evaluation of responses to 5-HT-enhancing

drugs in NMRI mice. *Behavioural Brain Research* 2015; **277**: 204-10.

669. Dale E, Bang-Andersen B, Sánchez C. Emerging mechanisms and treatments for depression beyond SSRIs and SNRIs. *Biochemical Pharmacology* 2015; **95**(2): 81-97.
670. Hertz L, Rothman DL, Li B, Peng L. Response: Commentary: Chronic SSRI Stimulation of Astrocytic 5-HT(2B) Receptors Change Multiple Gene Expressions/Editings and Metabolism of Glutamate, Glucose and Glycogen: A Potential Paradigm Shift. *Frontiers in Behavioral Neuroscience* 2015; **9**: 308.
671. De Long NE, Barry EJ, Pinelli C, et al. Antenatal exposure to the selective serotonin reuptake inhibitor fluoxetine leads to postnatal metabolic and endocrine changes associated with type 2 diabetes in Wistar rats. *Toxicology and Applied Pharmacology* 2015; **285**(1): 32-40.
672. Thériault O, Poulin H, Beaulieu J-M, Chahine M. Differential modulation of Nav1.7 and Nav1.8 channels by antidepressant drugs. *European Journal of Pharmacology* 2015; **764**: 395-403.
673. Homberg JR, Schubert D, Gaspar P. New perspectives on the neurodevelopmental effects of SSRIs. *Trends Pharmacol Sci* 2010; **31**: 60-5.
674. Safarinejad MR. Reversal of SSRI-induced female sexual dysfunction by adjunctive bupropion in menstruating women: a double-blind, placebo-controlled and randomized study. *Journal of Psychopharmacology* 2010; **25**(3): 370-8.

675. Evans RW. The FDA Alert on Serotonin Syndrome With Combined Use of SSRIs or SNRIs and Triptans: An Analysis of the 29 Case Reports. *Medscape General Medicine* 2007; **9**(3): 48-.

676. Dams R, Benijts THP, Lambert WE, et al. A Fatal Case of Serotonin Syndrome after Combined Moclobemide-Citalopram Intoxication. *Journal of Analytical Toxicology* 2001; **25**(2): 147-51.

677. Ferguson JM. SSRI Antidepressant Medications: Adverse Effects and Tolerability. *Primary Care Companion to The Journal of Clinical Psychiatry* 2001; **3**(1): 22-7.

678. Sample I. Nobel winner declares boycott of top science journals. The Guardian. 2013 9 December 2013.

679. Seife C. Research misconduct identified by the us food and drug administration: Out of sight, out of mind, out of the peer-reviewed literature. *JAMA Internal Medicine* 2015; **175**(4): 567-77.

680. Lee CJ, Sugimoto CR, Zhang G, Cronin B. Bias in peer review. *Journal of the American Society for Information Science and Technology* 2013; **64**(1): 2-17.

681. Jefferson T, Alderson P, Wager E, Davidoff F. Effects of editorial peer review: A systematic review. *JAMA* 2002; **287**(21): 2784-6.

682. Sackett DL, Rosenberg WMC, Gray JAM, Haynes RB, Richardson WS. Evidence based medicine: what it is and what it isn't. *BMJ* 1996; **312**(7023): 71-2.

683. Ceh E, S.;. Adverse Event Reporting and Treatment after the Study. *Journal of Clinical Research Best Practices* 2010; **6**(9).

684. Reardon S. US government cracks down on clinical-trials reporting, 2014.

685. Jones N. Half of US clinical trials go unpublished, 2013.

686. Suissa S. The Number Needed to Treat: 25 Years of Trials and Tribulations in Clinical Research. *Rambam Maimonides Medical Journal* 2015; **6**(3): e0033.

687. Ranganathan P, Pramesh CS, Aggarwal R. Common pitfalls in statistical analysis: Absolute risk reduction, relative risk reduction, and number needed to treat. *Perspectives in Clinical Research* 2016; **7**(1): 51-3.

688. Thompson A, Temple NJ. The case for statins: has it really been made? *Journal of the Royal Society of Medicine* 2004; **97**(10): 461-4.

689. Riveros C, Dechartres A, Perrodeau E, Haneef R, Boutron I, Ravaud P. Timing and Completeness of Trial Results Posted at ClinicalTrials.gov and Published in Journals. *PLOS Medicine* 2013; **10**(12): e1001566.

690. Hopewell S, Loudon K, Clarke MJ, Oxman AD, Dickersin K. Publication bias in clinical trials due to statistical significance or direction of trial results. *Cochrane Database of Systematic Reviews* 2009; (1).

691. Marco CA, Larkin GL. Research Ethics: Ethical Issues of Data Reporting and the Quest for Authenticity. *Academic Emergency Medicine* 2000; **7**(6): 691-4.

692. DiNicolantonio JJ, Lucan SC. The wrong white crystals: not salt but sugar as aetiological in hypertension and cardiometabolic disease. *Open Heart* 2014; **1**(1).

693. Graudal N, Jürgens G, Baslund B, Alderman MH. Compared With Usual Sodium Intake, Low- and Excessive-Sodium Diets Are Associated With Increased Mortality: A Meta-Analysis. *American Journal of Hypertension* 2014.

694. Liamis G, Liberopoulos E, Barkas F, Elisaf M. Diabetes mellitus and electrolyte disorders. *World Journal of Clinical Cases : WJCC* 2014; **2**(10): 488-96.

695. Parati G. Blood pressure variability: its measurement and significance in hypertension. *Journal of Hypertension* 2005; **23**: S19-S25.

696. Espeland MA, Kumanyika S, Wilson AC, et al. Statistical Issues in Analyzing 24-Hour Dietary Recall and 24-Hour Urine Collection Data for Sodium and Potassium Intakes. *American Journal of Epidemiology* 2001; **153**(10): 996-1006.

697. Lantelme P, Milon H, Gharib C, Gayet C, Fortrat J-O. White Coat Effect and Reactivity to Stress: Cardiovascular and Autonomic Nervous System Responses. *Hypertension* 1998; **31**(4): 1021-9.

698. Frese EM, Fick A, Sadowsky HS. Blood Pressure Measurement Guidelines for Physical Therapists. *Cardiopulmonary Physical Therapy Journal* 2011; **22**(2): 5-12.

699. Fisher NDL. Stress raising your blood pressure? Take a deep breath. 2016. http://www.health.harvard.edu/

blog/stress-raising-your-blood-pressure-take-a-deep-breath-201602159168 (accessed 2/4/2017 2017).

700. Jennings JR, Heim AF. From Brain to Behavior: Hypertension's Modulation of Cognition and Affect. *International Journal of Hypertension* 2012; **2012**: 12.

701. Agarwal R, Bunaye Z, Bekele DM. Prognostic Significance of Between-Arm Blood Pressure Differences. *Hypertension* 2008; **51**(3): 657-62.

702. Eguchi K, Yacoub M, Jhalani J, Gerin W, Schwartz JE, Pickering TG. Consistency of blood pressure differences between the left and right arms. *Archives of Internal Medicine* 2007; **167**(4): 388-93.

703. Handler J. The Importance of Accurate Blood Pressure Measurement. *The Permanente Journal* 2009; **13**(3): 51-4.

704. Pickering TG, Hall JE, Appel LJ, et al. Recommendations for Blood Pressure Measurement in Humans and Experimental Animals. *Part 1: Blood Pressure Measurement in Humans: A Statement for Professionals From the Subcommittee of Professional and Public Education of the American Heart Association Council on High Blood Pressure Research* 2005; **111**(5): 697-716.

705. Vloet LCM, Smits R, Jansen RWMM. The Effect of Meals at Different Mealtimes on Blood Pressure and Symptoms in Geriatric Patients With Postprandial Hypotension. *The Journals of Gerontology: Series A* 2003; **58**(11): M1031-M5.

706. Jakulj F, Zernicke K, Bacon SL, et al. A High-Fat Meal Increases Cardiovascular Reactivity to Psychological Stress in Healthy Young Adults. *The Journal of Nutrition* 2007; **137**(4): 935-9.
707. He F, MacGregor G. Salt and sugar: their effects on blood pressure. *Pflügers Archiv - European Journal of Physiology* 2015; **467**(3): 577-86.
708. Laura P, Rosa Maria B, Angelo G, Chiara B, Lorenzo G, Dieter R. Sleep Loss and Hypertension: A Systematic Review. *Current Pharmaceutical Design* 2013; **19**(13): 2409-19.
709. Graudal NA, Galløe AM, Garred P. Effects of sodium restriction on blood pressure, renin, aldosterone, catecholamines, cholesterols, and triglyceride: A meta-analysis. *JAMA* 1998; **279**(17): 1383-91.
710. Stolarz-Skrzypek K, Staessen JA. Reducing Salt Intake for Prevention of Cardiovascular Disease—Times Are Changing. *Advances in Chronic Kidney Disease*; **22**(2): 108-15.
711. Frisoli TM, Schmieder RE, Grodzicki T, Messerli FH. Salt and Hypertension: Is Salt Dietary Reduction Worth the Effort? *The American Journal of Medicine*; **125**(5): 433-9.
712. Alderman MH. Salt, Blood Pressure, and Human Health. *Hypertension* 2000; **36**(5): 890-3.
713. FH MSB. Dietary salt reduction; further lowering of target lowers blood pressure but may increase risk. *Evidence Based Medicine* 2014; **19**(1): 22.

714. Goldman JJS, Tiffany L. The Limitations of Evidence-Based Medicine—Applying Population-Based Recommendations to Individual Patients. *AMA Journal of Ethics* 2011; **13**(1): 4.

715. Greenhalgh T, Howick J, Maskrey N. Evidence based medicine: a movement in crisis? *The BMJ* 2014; **348**: g3725.

716. van der Meer AJ, Veldt BJ, Feld JJ, et al. The number needed to treat to prevent mortality and cirrhosis-related complications among patients with cirrhosis and HCV genotype 1 infection. *Journal of Viral Hepatitis* 2014; **21**(8): 568-77.

717. Sanmuganathan P, Ghahramani P, Jackson P, Wallis E, Ramsay L. Aspirin for primary prevention of coronary heart disease: safety and absolute benefit related to coronary risk derived from meta-analysis of randomised trials. *Heart* 2001; **85**(3): 265-71.

718. Dorsey E, Ritzer G. THe mcdonaldization of medicine. *JAMA Neurology* 2015: 1-2.

719. Burstein R, Noseda R, Borsook D. Migraine: Multiple Processes, Complex Pathophysiology. *The Journal of Neuroscience* 2015; **35**(17): 6619-29.

720. Afridi SK, Giffin NJ, Kaube H, et al. A positron emission tomographic study in spontaneous migraine. *Archives of Neurology* 2005; **62**(8): 1270-5.

721. Signs and Symptoms of Sensory Processing Disorder. https://www.brainbalancecenters.com/blog/2012/04/

signs-and-symptoms-of-sensory-processing-disorder/ (accessed 4/4/2017 2017).

722. Mawson AR. Toward a Theory of Childhood Learning Disorders, Hyperactivity, and Aggression. *ISRN Psychiatry* 2012; **2012**: 19.

723. Cermak SA, Curtin C, Bandini LG. Food selectivity and sensory sensitivity in children with autism spectrum disorders. *Journal of the American Dietetic Association* 2010; **110**(2): 238-46.

724. Fuller GN, Guiloff RJ. Migrainous olfactory hallucinations. *Journal of Neurology, Neurosurgery, and Psychiatry* 1987; **50**(12): 1688-90.

725. Klinov V, Syrow L. The Case Of Migraine With Visual And Olfactory Hallucination Related To Food Allergy (P5.205). *Neurology* 2014; **82**(10 Supplement).

726. Coleman ER, Grosberg BM, Robbins MS. Olfactory hallucinations in primary headache disorders: Case series and literature review. *Cephalalgia* 2011; **31**(14): 1477-89.

727. Migraine is an extraordinarily prevalent neurological disease, affecting 38 million men, women and children in the U.S. and 1 billion worldwide. http://migraineresearchfoundation.org/about-migraine/migraine-facts/ (accessed 4/4/2017.

728. Headache Disorders. April 2016 2016. http://www.who.int/mediacentre/factsheets/fs277/en/ (accessed 4/4/2017 2017).

729. Ehlers-Danlos Syndrome. April 4, 2017 2015. https://ghr.nlm.nih.gov/condition/ehlers-danlos-syndrome#statistics (accessed 4/5/2017 2017).

730. Kenny TT, Colin;. Raynaud's Phenomenon. 4/1/2016 2016. https://patient.info/health/raynauds-phenomenon-leaflet (accessed 4/5/2017 2017).

731. Richards JR. Why are cats so flexible? http://www.ccmr.cornell.edu/faqs/why-are-cats-so-flexible/ (accessed 4/5/2017 2017).

732. Jindal R, Choong A, Arul D, Dhanjil S, Chataway J, Cheshire NJW. Vascular Manifestations of Type IV Ehlers–Danlos Syndrome. *EJVES Extra* 2005; **9**(6): 135-8.

733. Enko D, Meinitzer A, Mangge H, et al. Concomitant Prevalence of Low Serum Diamine Oxidase Activity and Carbohydrate Malabsorption. *Canadian Journal of Gastroenterology and Hepatology* 2016; **2016**: 4.

734. Korterink J, Devanarayana NM, Rajindrajith S, Vlieger A, Benninga MA. Childhood functional abdominal pain: mechanisms and management. *Nat Rev Gastroenterol Hepatol* 2015; **12**(3): 159-71.

735. Guldiken B, Guldiken S, Taskiran B, et al. Migraine in metabolic syndrome. *Neurologist* 2009; **15**.

736. Bhoi SK, Kalita J, Misra UK. Metabolic syndrome and insulin resistance in migraine. *J Headache Pain* 2012; **13**.

737. Sefidbakht S, Johnson-Down L, Young TK, Egeland GM. High protein and cholesterol intakes associated with emergence of glucose intolerance in a low-risk Ca-

nadian Inuit population. *Public Health Nutrition* 2016; **19**(10): 1804-11.

738. Kuhnlein HV, Receveur O, Soueida R, Egeland GM. Arctic Indigenous Peoples Experience the Nutrition Transition with Changing Dietary Patterns and Obesity. *The Journal of Nutrition* 2004; **134**(6): 1447-53.

739. Latulippe ME, Skoog SM. Fructose Malabsorption and Intolerance: Effects of Fructose with and without Simultaneous Glucose Ingestion. *Critical Reviews in Food Science and Nutrition* 2011; **51**(7): 583-92.

740. MalaCards - Human Disease Database. http://www.malacards.org/ (accessed 8/28/2017 2017).

741. Gracey MB, Valerie;. Sugar-induced diarrhoea in children. *Archives of Disease in Childhood; BMJ* 1973; **48**(5): 6.

742. Berni Canani R, Pezzella V, Amoroso A, Cozzolino T, Di Scala C, Passariello A. Diagnosing and Treating Intolerance to Carbohydrates in Children. *Nutrients* 2016; **8**(3): 157.

743. Kyaw MH, Mayberry JF. Fructose Malabsorption: True Condition or a Variance From Normality. *Journal of Clinical Gastroenterology* 2011; **45**(1): 16-21.

744. Liu R, Geng P, Ma M, et al. MTHFR C677T polymorphism and migraine risk: A meta-analysis. *Journal of the Neurological Sciences*; **336**(1): 68-73.

745. Alluri RV, Mohan V, Komandur S, Chawda K, Chaudhuri JR, Hasan Q. MTHFR C677T gene mutation as a

risk factor for arterial stroke: a hospital based study. *European Journal of Neurology* 2005; **12**(1): 40-4.

746. Essmeister R, Kress H-G, Zierz S, Griffith L, Lea R, Wieser T. MTHFR and ACE Polymorphisms Do Not Increase Susceptibility to Migraine Neither Alone Nor in Combination. *Headache: The Journal of Head and Face Pain* 2016; **56**(8): 1267-73.
747. Mitchell ES, Conus N, Kaput J. B vitamin polymorphisms and behavior: Evidence of associations with neurodevelopment, depression, schizophrenia, bipolar disorder and cognitive decline. *Neuroscience & Biobehavioral Reviews* 2014; **47**: 307-20.
748. Di Lorenzo C, Grieco GS, Santorelli FM. Migraine headache: a review of the molecular genetics of a common disorder. *The Journal of Headache and Pain* 2012; **13**(7): 571-80.
749. de Vries B, Frants RR, Ferrari MD, van den Maagdenberg AMJM. Molecular genetics of migraine. *Human Genetics* 2009; **126**(1): 115.
750. Suzuki M, Van Paesschen W, Stalmans I, et al. Defective membrane expression of the Na+-HCO3-cotransporter NBCe1 is associated with familial migraine. *Proc Natl Acad Sci USA* 2010; **107**.
751. FDA. Topamax Highlights of Prescribing Information. 2012 2012. http://www.accessdata.fda.gov/drugsatfda_docs/label/2012/020844s041lbl.pdf (accessed 1/1/2017 2017).

752. Faloon W. Mainstream Doctors Still Confused About Homocysteine. Life Extension Magazine. 2006 June 2006.
753. Zhang D, Wen X, Wu W, Guo Y, Cui W. Elevated Homocysteine Level and Folate Deficiency Associated with Increased Overall Risk of Carcinogenesis: Meta-Analysis of 83 Case-Control Studies Involving 35,758 Individuals. *PLoS ONE* 2015; **10**(5): e0123423.
754. Huh HJ, Chi HS, Shim EH, Jang S, Park CJ. nutrition interactions in coronary artery disease: Correlation between the MTHFR C677T polymorphism and folate and homocysteine status in a Korean population. *Thrombosis Research*; **117**(5): 501-6.
755. Alizadeh S, Djafarian K, Moradi S, Shab-Bidar S. C667T and A1298C polymorphisms of methylenetetrahydrofolate reductase gene and susceptibility to myocardial infarction: A systematic review and meta-analysis. *International Journal of Cardiology*; **217**: 99-108.
756. Khandanpour N, Willis G, Meyer FJ, et al. Peripheral arterial disease and methylenetetrahydrofolate reductase (MTHFR) C677T mutations: A case-control study and meta-analysis. *Journal of Vascular Surgery*; **49**(3): 711-8.
757. Liew S-C, Gupta ED. Methylenetetrahydrofolate reductase (MTHFR) C677T polymorphism: Epidemiology, metabolism and the associated diseases. *European Journal of Medical Genetics* 2015; **58**(1): 1-10.
758. Grabowski M, Banecki B, Kadziński L, et al. The model homologue of the partially defective human 5,10-methy-

lenetetrahydrofolate reductase, considered as a risk factor for stroke due to increased homocysteine level, can be protected and reactivated by heat shock proteins. *Metabolic Brain Disease* 2016; **31**(5): 1041-5.

759. Dodick DW. Chronic Daily Headache. *New England Journal of Medicine* 2006; **354**(2): 158-65.
760. Mayo Clinic DD, M.D. Complex migraine: https://www.youtube.com/watch?v=9PHb8gcEw1M, 2011.
761. Bigal ME, Serrano D, Reed M, Lipton RB. Chronic migraine in the population: Burden, diagnosis, and satisfaction with treatment. *Neurology* 2008; **71**(8): 559-66.
762. Eroglu C, Allen NJ, Susman MW, et al. Gabapentin Receptor alpha 2 delta-1 Is a Neuronal Thrombospondin Receptor Responsible for Excitatory CNS Synaptogenesis.
763. Headache Classification C, Olesen J, Bousser MG, et al. New appendix criteria open for a broader concept of chronic migraine. *Cephalalgia* 2006; **26**(6): 742-6.
764. Mathew NT, Frishberg BM, Gawel M, et al. Botulinum Toxin Type A (BOTOX®) for the Prophylactic Treatment of Chronic Daily Headache: A Randomized, Double-Blind, Placebo-Controlled Trial. *Headache: The Journal of Head and Face Pain* 2005; **45**(4): 293-307.
765. Goadsby PJ. Pathophysiology of migraine. *Annals of Indian Academy of Neurology* 2012; **15**(Suppl 1): S15-S22.
766. Nouchine Hadjikhani MSdR, Ona Wu, Denis Schwartz, Dick Bakker, Bruce Fischl. Mechanisms of migraine

aura revealed by functional MRI in human visual cortex. *PNAS* 2001; **98**(8): 4687–92.

767. James MF, Smith JM, Boniface SJ, Huang CL-H, Leslie RA. Cortical spreading depression and migraine: new insights from imaging? *TRENDS In Neuroscience* 2001: 226-71.
768. Thie A, Fuhlendorf A, Spitzer K, Kunze K. Transcranial Doppler Evaluation of Common and Classic Migraine. Part II. Ultrasonic Features During Attacks. *Headache: The Journal of Head and Face Pain* 1990; **30**(4): 209-15.
769. Holtzheimer PE, Kelley ME, Gross RE, et al. Subcallosal Cingulate Deep Brain Stimulation for Treatment-Resistant Unipolar and Bipolar Depression. Arch Gen Psychiatry. 2012 January 2:150-8.
770. Leone M. Hypothalamic deep brain stimulation in the treatment of chronic cluster headache. Ther Adv Neurol Disord. 2010 May 3:187-95.
771. Lozano AM, Giacobbe P, Hamani C, et al. A multicenter pilot study of subcallosal cingulate area deep brain stimulation for treatment-resistant depression. *J Neurosurg* 2012: 315-22.
772. Mayberg HS, Lozano AM, Voon V, et al. Deep brain stimulation for treatment-resistant depression. Neuron. 2005 March 3:651-60.
773. Taghva AS, Malone DA, Rezai AR. Deep brain stimulation for treatment-resistant depression. *World Neurosurg* 2013: 826-31.

774. Schwedt TJ. Neurostimulation for Primary Headache Disorders. Curr Neurol Neurosci Rep. 2013 March 4:101-7.

775. Akerman S, Holland PR, Goadsby PJ. Mechanically-induced cortical spreading depression associated regional cerebral blood flow changes are blocked by Na+ ion channel blockade. *Brain Res* 2008; **1229**.

776. Guiou M, Sheth S, Nemoto M, et al. Cortical spreading depression produces long-term disruption of activity-related changes in cerebral blood volume and neurovascular coupling. *J Biomed Opt* 2005; **10**.

777. Olesen J, Friberg L, Olsen TS, et al. Timing and topography of cerebral blood flow, aura, and headache during migraine attacks. *Ann Neurol* 1990; **28**.

778. Coppola G, Di Renzo A, Tinelli E, et al. EHMTI-0177. Evidence for plastic brain morphometric changes during the migraine cycle. *The Journal of Headache and Pain* 2014; **15**(Suppl 1): E10-E.

779. Avci AY, Lakadamyali H, Arikan S, Benli US, Kilinc M. High sensitivity C-reactive protein and cerebral white matter hyperintensities on magnetic resonance imaging in migraine patients. *The Journal of Headache and Pain* 2015; **16**: 9.

780. Bashir A, Lipton RB, Ashina S, Ashina M. Migraine and structural changes in the brain: A systematic review and meta-analysis. *Neurology* 2013; **81**(14): 1260-8.

781. Weller CM, Leen WG, Neville BGR, et al. A novel SLC2A1 mutation linking hemiplegic migraine with alternating hemiplegia of childhood. *Cephalalgia* 2014; **35**(1): 10-5.

782. Freilinger T, Koch J, Dichgans M. A novel mutation in SLC1A3 associated with pure hemiplegic migraine. *J Headache Pain* 2010; **11**.
783. Morth JP, Poulsen H, Toustrup-Jensen MS, et al. The structure of the Na+, K+-ATPase and mapping of isoform differences and disease-related mutations. *Philosophical Transactions of the Royal Society B: Biological Sciences* 2009; **364**(1514): 217-27.
784. Dichgans M, Freilinger T, Eckstein G. Mutation in the neuronal voltage-gated sodium channel SCN1A in familial hemiplegic migraine. *Lancet* 2005; **366**.
785. De Marchis ML, Barbanti P, Palmirotta R, et al. Look beyond Catechol-O-Methyltransferase genotype for cathecolamines derangement in migraine: the BioBIM rs4818 and rs4680 polymorphisms study. *The Journal of Headache and Pain* 2015; **16**: 37.
786. Schurks M, Rist PM, Kurth T. MTHFR 677C > T and ACE D/I polymorphisms in migraine: a systematic review and meta-analysis. *Headache* 2010; **50**.
787. Roecklein KA, Scher AI, Smith A, et al. Haplotype analysis of the folate-related genes MTHFR, MTRR, and MTR and migraine with aura. *Cephalalgia : an international journal of headache* 2013; **33**(7): 469-82.
788. Tana C, Tafuri E, Tana M, et al. New insights into the cardiovascular risk of migraine and the role of white matter hyperintensities: is gold all that glitters? *The Journal of Headache and Pain* 2013; **14**(1): 9.

789. Pizza V, Bisogno A, Lamaida E, et al. Migraine and Coronary Artery Disease: An Open Study on the Genetic Polymorphism of the 5, 10 Methylenetetrahydrofolate (MTHFR) and Angiotensin I-Converting Enzyme (ACE) Genes. *Central Nervous System Agents in Medicinal Chemistry* 2010; **10**(2): 91-6.

790. Tronvik E, Stovner LJ, Bovim G, et al. Angiotensin-converting enzyme gene insertion/deletion polymorphism in migraine patients. *BMC Neurology* 2008; **8**: 4-.

791. Strassman A, Raymond S, Burstein R. Sensitization of meningeal sensory neurons and the origin of headaches. *Nature* 1996; **384**: 560 - 4.

792. Goadsby PJ, Akerman S. The trigeminovascular system does not require a peripheral sensory input to be activated–migraine is a central disorder. Focus on 'Effect of cortical spreading depression on basal and evoked traffic in the trigeminovascular sensory system'. *Cephalalgia* 2012; **32**.

793. Whiting AC, Marmura MJ, Hegarty SE, Keith SW. Olfactory Acuity in Chronic Migraine: A Cross-Sectional Study. *Headache: The Journal of Head and Face Pain* 2015; **55**(1): 71-5.

794. Gracey M, Burke V. Sugar-induced diarrhoea in children. *Archives of Disease in Childhood* 1973; **48**(5): 331-6.

795. Bernecker C, Ragginer C, Fauler G, et al. Oxidative stress is associated with migraine and migraine-related metabolic risk in females. *Eur J Neurol* 2011; **18**.

796. Frazer S, Otomo K, Dayer A. Early-life serotonin dysregulation affects the migration and positioning of cortical interneuron subtypes. *Transl Psychiatry* 2015; **5**: e644.
797. Afarideh M, Behdadnia A, Noshad S, et al. ASSOCIATION OF PERIPHERAL 5-HYDROXYINDOLE-3-ACETIC ACID, A SEROTONIN DERIVATIVE, WITH METABOLIC SYNDROME AND LOW-GRADE INFLAMMATION. *Endocrine Practice* 2015; **21**(7): 711-8.
798. Crane JD, Palanivel R, Mottillo EP, et al. Inhibiting peripheral serotonin synthesis reduces obesity and metabolic dysfunction by promoting brown adipose tissue thermogenesis. *Nat Med* 2015; **21**(2): 166-72.
799. Ouchi Y, Yoshikawa E, Futatsubashi M, Yagi S, Ueki T, Nakamura K. Altered Brain Serotonin Transporter and Associated Glucose Metabolism in Alzheimer Disease. *Journal of Nuclear Medicine* 2009; **50**(8): 1260-6.
800. Smith GS, Kramer E, Hermann C, et al. Serotonin Modulation of Cerebral Glucose Metabolism in Depressed Older Adults. *Biological psychiatry* 2009; **66**(3): 259-66.
801. Duarte AI, Moreira PI, Oliveira CR. Insulin in Central Nervous System: More than Just a Peripheral Hormone. *Journal of Aging Research* 2012; **2012**: 21.
802. Gray SM, Meijer RI, Barrett EJ. Insulin Regulates Brain Function, but How Does It Get There? *Diabetes* 2014; **63**(12): 3992-7.

803. Bohár ZP, Árpád; Vécsei, László;. Tryptophan catabolites and migraine *Current Pharmaceutical Design* 2015; **22**(E-pu ahead of print).

804. Donovan MH, Tecott LH. Serotonin and the regulation of mammalian energy balance. *Frontiers in Neuroscience* 2013; **7**: 36.

805. Kleinridders A, Ferris HA, Cai W, Kahn CR. Insulin Action in Brain Regulates Systemic Metabolism and Brain Function. *Diabetes* 2014; **63**(7): 2232.

806. Andersen H, Friis UG, Hansen PBL, Svenningsen P, Henriksen JE, Jensen BL. Diabetic nephropathy is associated with increased urine excretion of proteases plasmin, prostasin and urokinase and activation of amiloride-sensitive current in collecting duct cells. *Nephrology Dialysis Transplantation* 2015; **30**(5): 781-9.

807. Gerich JE. Role of the kidney in normal glucose homeostasis and in the hyperglycaemia of diabetes mellitus: therapeutic implications. *Diabetic Medicine* 2010; **27**(2): 136-42.

808. Poole CJML, S L;. Inhibition of vasopressin secretion during migraine. *Journal of Neurology, Neurosurgery, and Psychiatry* 1988; **51**: 4.

809. Gasior M, Rogawski MA, Hartman AL. Neuroprotective and disease-modifying effects of the ketogenic diet. *Behavioural pharmacology* 2006; **17**(5-6): 431-9.

810. Hartman AL. Neuroprotection in Metabolism-Based Therapy. *Epilepsy Research* 2012; **100**(3): 286-94.
811. Li H-f, Zou Y, Ding G. Therapeutic Success of the Ketogenic Diet as a Treatment Option for Epilepsy: a Meta-analysis. *Iranian Journal of Pediatrics* 2013; **23**(6): 613-20.
812. Allaman I, Fiumelli H, Magistretti PJ, Martin J-L. Fluoxetine regulates the expression of neurotrophic/growth factors and glucose metabolism in astrocytes. *Psychopharmacology* 2011; **216**(1): 75-84.
813. Goldberg S, Smith GS, Barnes A, et al. Serotonin modulation of cerebral glucose metabolism in normal aging. *Neurobiology of Aging* 2004; **25**(2): 167-74.
814. Smith GS, Ma Y, Dhawan V, et al. Serotonin modulation of cerebral glucose metabolism measured with positron emission tomography (PET) in human subjects. *Synapse* 2002; **45**(2): 105-12.
815. Oler JA, Fox AS, Shelton SE, et al. Serotonin Transporter Availability in the Amygdala and Bed Nucleus of the Stria Terminalis Predicts Anxious Temperament and Brain Glucose Metabolic Activity. *The Journal of neuroscience : the official journal of the Society for Neuroscience* 2009; **29**(32): 9961-6.
816. Arab L, Sadeghi R, Walker DG, Lue LF, Sabbagh MN. Consequences of Aberrant Insulin Regulation in the Brain: Can Treating Diabetes be Effective for Alzheimer's Disease. *Current Neuropharmacology* 2011; **9**(4): 693-705.

817. de la Monte SM. Brain Insulin Resistance and Deficiency as Therapeutic Targets in Alzheimer's Disease. *Current Alzheimer Research* 2012; **9**(1): 35-66.

818. Chen J, Diesburg-Stanwood A, Bodor G, Rasouli N. Led Astray by Hemoglobin A1c. *Journal of Investigative Medicine High Impact Case Reports* 2016; **4**(1): 2324709616628549.

819. Mosconi L. Brain glucose metabolism in the early and specific diagnosis of Alzheimer's disease. *European Journal of Nuclear Medicine and Molecular Imaging* 2005; **32**(4): 486-510.

820. Simpson IA, Chundu KR, Davies-Hill T, Honer WG, Davies P. Decreased concentrations of GLUT1 and GLUT3 glucose transporters in the brains of patients with Alzheimer's disease. *Annals of Neurology* 1994; **35**(5): 546-51.

821. Kennedy AM, Frackowiak RSJ, Newman SK, et al. Deficits in cerebral glucose metabolism demonstrated by positron emission tomography in individuals at risk of familial Alzheimer's disease. *Neuroscience Letters* 1995; **186**(1): 17-20.

822. Yokoyama JS, Bonham LW, Sturm VE, et al. The 5-HTTLPR variant in the serotonin transporter gene modifies degeneration of brain regions important for emotion in behavioral variant frontotemporal dementia. *Neuroimage Clin* 2015; **9**: 283-90.

823. Is Sugar Making My Neuropathy Worse? http://www.neuropathytreatmentgroup.com/is-sugar-making-my-neuropathy-worse/ (accessed 2/7/2017 2017).

824. Materazzi S, Fusi C, Benemei S, et al. TRPA1 and TRPV4 mediate paclitaxel-induced peripheral neuropathy in mice via a glutathione-sensitive mechanism. *Pflugers Arch* 2012; **463**: 561 - 9.

825. Uauy R, Dangour AD. Nutrition in Brain Development and Aging: Role of Essential Fatty Acids. *Nutrition Reviews* 2006; **64**(suppl 2): S24-S33.

826. Llewelyn JG, Tomlinson DR, Thomas PK. Peripheral neuropathy. Nature Publishing Group; 2005. p. 1951-91.

827. Oyibo SO, Prasad YD, Jackson NJ, Jude EB, Boulton AJ. The relationship between blood glucose excursions and painful diabetic peripheral neuropathy: a pilot study. *Diabet Med* 2002; **19**: 870-3.

828. Tottene A, Urbani A, Pietrobon D. Role of different voltage-gated Ca2+ channels in cortical spreading depression: specific requirement of P/Q-type Ca2+ channels. *Channels (Austin)* 2011; **5**.

829. Lauritzen M, Dreier JP, Fabricius M, Hartings JA, Graf R, Strong AJ. Clinical relevance of cortical spreading depression in neurological disorders: migraine, malignant stroke, subarachnoid and intracranial hemorrhage, and traumatic brain injury. *J Cereb Blood Flow Metab* 2011; **31**.

830. Levy D. Endogenous mechanisms underlying the activation and sensitization of meningeal nociceptors: the role

of immuno-vascular interactions and cortical spreading depression. *Curr Pain Headache Rep* 2012; **16**.

831. Jahnen-Dechent W, Ketteler M. Magnesium basics. *Clinical Kidney Journal* 2012; **5**(Suppl_1): i3-i14.
832. Saris NE. Magnesium. An update on physiological, clinical and analytical aspects. *Clin Chim Acta* 2000; **29**: 1-26.
833. van der Hel WS, van den Bergh WM, Nicolay K, Tulleken KA, Dijkhuizen RM. Suppression of cortical spreading depressions after magnesium treatment in the rat. *Neuroreport* 1998; **9**.
834. Mauskop A, Altura BM. Role of magnesium in the pathogenesis and treatment of migraines. *Clin Neurosci* 1998; **5**.
835. Zandt B-J, Stigen T, ten Haken B, Netoff T, van Putten MJAM. Single neuron dynamics during experimentally induced anoxic depolarization. *Journal of Neurophysiology* 2013; **110**(7): 1469-75.
836. physics.illinois.edu. Physics 212 James Scholar Assignment #2. https://courses.physics.illinois.edu/phys212/JamesScholars/02/index.html.
837. Covey E. CHAPTER 4 STRUCTURE AND CELL BIOLOGY OF THE NEURON. In: Washington Uo, editor. Washington; 1980.
838. AUSTINCC. Membrane Potentials. http://www.austincc.edu/lesalbin/Membrane%20Potentials.htm (accessed 2/8/2017 2017).

839. Mokri B. Spontaneous Low Pressure, Low CSF Volume Headaches: Spontaneous CSF Leaks. *Headache: The Journal of Head and Face Pain* 2013; **53**(7): 1034-53.

840. Yun DJ, Choi HN, Oh G-S. A Case of Postural Orthostatic Tachycardia Syndrome Associated with Migraine and Fibromyalgia. *The Korean Journal of Pain* 2013; **26**(3): 303-6.

841. Vaillend C, Mason SE, Cuttle MF, Alger BE. Mechanisms of Neuronal Hyperexcitability Caused by Partial Inhibition of Na⁺-K⁺-ATPases in the Rat CA1 Hippocampal Region. *Journal of Neurophysiology* 2002; **88**(6): 2963-78.

842. Cho C-H. New mechanism for glutamate hypothesis in epilepsy. *Frontiers in Cellular Neuroscience* 2013; **7**: 127.

843. Mistovich J. Blood pressure assessment in the hypovolemic shock patient. 2009. https://www.ems1.com/ems-products/Ambulance-Disposable-Supplies/articles/479223-Blood-pressure-assessment-in-the-hypovolemic-shock-patient/ (accessed 3/4/2017 2017).

844. TheFranklinInstitute;. BLOOD VESSELS. https://www.fi.edu/heart/blood-vessels (accessed 2/9/2017 2017).

845. Harrison-Bernard LM. The renal renin-angiotensin system. *Advances in Physiology Education* 2009; **33**(4): 270-4.

846. Tronvik E, Stovner LJ, Hagen K, Holmen J, Zwart J-A. High pulse pressure protects against headache: Prospective and cross-sectional data (HUNT study). *Neurology* 2008; **70**(16): 1329-36.

847. Feng G-H, Li H-P, Li Q-L, Fu Y, Huang R-B. Red blood cell distribution width and ischaemic stroke. *Stroke and Vascular Neurology* 2017.

848. Badar VA, Hiware SK, Shrivastava MP, Thawani VR, Hardas MM. Comparison of nebivolol and atenolol on blood pressure, blood sugar, and lipid profile in patients of essential hypertension. *Indian Journal of Pharmacology* 2011; **43**(4): 437-40.

849. Roysommuti S, Suwanich A, Jirakulsomchok D, Wyss JM. Perinatal taurine depletion increases susceptibility to adult sugar-induced hypertension in rats. *Advances in experimental medicine and biology* 2009; **643**: 123-33.

850. Varma V, Boros L, Nolen G, et al. Metabolic fate of fructose in human adipocytes: a targeted 13C tracer fate association study. *Metabolomics* 2015; **11**(3): 529-44.

851. Ma Y, Chiriboga DE, Olendzki BC, et al. Association between Carbohydrate Intake and Serum Lipids. *Journal of the American College of Nutrition* 2006; **25**(2): 155-63.

852. Besir FH, Koçer A, Dikici S, Yazgan S, Ozdem S. The evaluation of atherosclerosis in migraine patients. Pain Pract; 2012.

853. Hamed SA, Hamed EA, Ezz Eldin AM, Mahmoud NM. Vascular risk factors, endothelial function, and carotid thickness in patients with migraine: relationship to atherosclerosis. *J Stroke Cerebrovasc Dis* 2010; **19**.

854. Schwaiger J, Kiechl S, Stockner H, et al. Burden of atherosclerosis and risk of venous thromboembolism in patients with migraine. *Neurology* 2008; **71**.

855. Rose KM, Wong TY, Carson AP, Couper DJ, Klein R, Sharrett AR. Migraine and retinal microvascular abnormalities: the atherosclerosis risk in communities study. *Neurology* 2007; **68**.

856. Miron VE, Zehntner SP, Kuhlmann T, et al. Statin Therapy Inhibits Remyelination in the Central Nervous System. *The American Journal of Pathology* 2009; **174**(5): 1880-90.

857. Love S. Demyelinating diseases. *Journal of Clinical Pathology* 2006; **59**(11): 1151-9.

858. Statins a Possible Treatment for Prevention of Migraine. October 17, 2016 2016. http://www.headaches.org/2016/10/17/statins-possible-treatment-prevention-migraine/ (accessed 3/2/2017 2017).

859. Buettner C, Nir R-R, Bertisch SM, et al. Simvastatin and Vitamin D for Migraine Prevention: A Randomized Controlled Trial. *Annals of neurology* 2015; **78**(6): 970-81.

860. Lesaffre E, Boon P, Pledger GW. The Value of the Number-Needed-to-Treat Method in Antiepileptic Drug Trials. *Epilepsia* 2000; **41**(4): 440-6.

861. Gray SL, Lai KV, Larson EB. Drug-Induced Cognition Disorders in the Elderly. *Drug Safety* 1999; **21**(2): 101-22.

862. Kanner AM, Palac S. Depression in Epilepsy: A Common but Often Unrecognized Comorbid Malady. *Epilepsy & Behavior*; **1**(1): 37-51.

863. Puustinen J, Nurminen J, Löppönen M, et al. Use of CNS medications and cognitive decline in the aged: a longitudinal population-based study. *BMC Geriatrics* 2011; **11**(1): 70.

864. Sommer BR, Mitchell EL, Wroolie TE. Topiramate: Effects on cognition in patients with epilepsy, migraine headache and obesity. *Therapeutic Advances in Neurological Disorders* 2013; **6**(4): 211-27.

865. Pacher P, Kecskemeti V. Cardiovascular Side Effects of New Antidepressants and Antipsychotics: New Drugs, old Concerns? *Current pharmaceutical design* 2004; **10**(20): 2463-75.

866. Sharma AT, Lemeneh; Aminzay, Aman;Tarabar, Asim;. Beta-Blocker Toxicity. 2016. http://emedicine.medscape.com/article/813342-overview?pa=s8KU38uDdjE5NPKOpcXu%2FbJogD4T7q3V8JSYlnU2dABKmmVGcyYcNXGNdz96IOYL4zIzYhbg9jPgPsdfGl3K3TyZ53MRiVvLb0nlgNqJi1E%3D (accessed 2/23/2017 2017).

867. Aburawi SM, Al-Tubuly RA, Alghzewi EA, Gorash ZM. Effects of calcium channel blockers on antidepressant action of Alprazolam and Imipramine. *The Libyan Journal of Medicine* 2007; **2**(4): 169-75.

868. Lavoie PB, G;Elie, R;. Tricyclic antidepressants inhibit voltage-dependent calcium channels and Na(+)-Ca2+ exchange in rat brain cortex synaptosomes. *Canadian Journal of Physiology and Pharmacology* 1990; **68**(11): 5.

869. Zahradník I, Minarovič I, Zahradníková A. Inhibition of the Cardiac L-Type Calcium Channel Current by Antidepressant Drugs. *Journal of Pharmacology and Experimental Therapeutics* 2008; **324**(3): 977-84.
870. Sproule BA, Naranjo CA, Bremner KE, Hassan PC. Selective Serotonin Reuptake Inhibitors and CNS Drug Interactions. *Clinical Pharmacokinetics* 1997; **33**(6): 454-71.
871. Alexander W. The Uphill Path to Successful Clinical Trials: Keeping Patients Enrolled. *Pharmacy and Therapeutics* 2013; **38**(4): 225-7.
872. Harris R. Results Of Many Clinical Trials Not Being Reported. march 11, 2015 2015. http://www.npr.org/sections/health-shots/2015/03/11/392355433/results-of-many-clinical-trials-not-being-reported (accessed 9/18 2015).
873. Steinbrook R, Redberg RF. REporting research misconduct in the medical literature. *JAMA Internal Medicine* 2015; **175**(4): 492-3.
874. Shank RP, Gardocki JF, Streeter AJ, Maryanoff BE. An Overview of the Preclinical Aspects of Topiramate: Pharmacology, Pharmacokinetics, and Mechanism of Action. *Epilepsia* 2000; **41**.
875. Mula M, Cavanna AE, Monaco F. Psychopharmacology of topiramate: from epilepsy to bipolar disorder. *Neuropsychiatric Disease and Treatment* 2006; **2**(4): 475-88.
876. Wang DW, Mistry AM, Kahlig KM, Kearney JA, Xiang J, George AL. Propranolol Blocks Cardiac and Neuronal

Voltage-Gated Sodium Channels. *Frontiers in Pharmacology* 2010; **1**: 144.

877. Meidenbauer JJ, Mukherjee P, Seyfried TN. The glucose ketone index calculator: a simple tool to monitor therapeutic efficacy for metabolic management of brain cancer. *Nutrition & Metabolism* 2015; **12**: 12.
878. Kleppe R, Martinez A, Doskeland SO, Haavik J. The 14-3-3 proteins in regulation of cellular metabolism. *Semin Cell Dev Biol* 2011; **22**(7): 713-9.
879. Erickson N, Boscheri A, Linke B, Huebner J. Systematic review: isocaloric ketogenic dietary regimes for cancer patients. *Medical Oncology* 2017; **34**(5): 72.
880. Tan-Shalaby JL, Carrick J, Edinger K, et al. Modified Atkins diet in advanced malignancies - final results of a safety and feasibility trial within the Veterans Affairs Pittsburgh Healthcare System. *Nutrition & Metabolism* 2016; **13**: 52.
881. Poff A, Ari C, Seyfried T, D'Agostino D. The ketogenic diet and hyperbaric oxygen therapy prolong survival in mice with systemic metastatic cancer. *PLoS ONE* 2013; **8**.
882. Stafstrom CE, Rho JM. The Ketogenic Diet as a Treatment Paradigm for Diverse Neurological Disorders. *Frontiers in Pharmacology* 2012; **3**: 59.
883. Di Lorenzo C, Coppola G, Bracaglia M, et al. Cortical functional correlates of responsiveness to short-lasting preventive intervention with ketogenic diet in migraine:

a multimodal evoked potentials study. *The Journal of Headache and Pain* 2016; **17**: 58.

884. Di Lorenzo C, Coppola G, Sirianni G, Pierelli F. Short term improvement of migraine headaches during ketogenic diet: a prospective observational study in a dietician clinical setting. *The Journal of Headache and Pain* 2013; **14**(Suppl 1): P219-P.

Made in the
USA
Columbia, SC

81867930R00361